# Embodying the Soul

THE MIDDLE AGES SERIES

Ruth Mazo Karras, *Series Editor*
Edward Peters, *Founding Editor*

A complete list of books in the series is available from the publisher.

# EMBODYING THE SOUL

Medicine and Religion in Carolingian Europe

Meg Leja

PENN

UNIVERSITY OF PENNSYLVANIA PRESS

PHILADELPHIA

Published by
University of Pennsylvania Press
Philadelphia, Pennsylvania 19104-4112
www.upenn.edu/pennpress

Printed in the United States of America on acid-free paper
10 9 8 7 6 5 4 3 2 1

Hardcover ISBN 9780812253894
Ebook ISBN 9780812298505

Library of Congress Cataloging-in-Publication Data

Names: Leja, Meg, author.
Title: Embodying the soul : medicine and religion in Carolingian Europe / Meg Leja.
Other titles: Middle Ages series.
Description: 1st edition. | Philadelphia : University of Pennsylvania Press, [2022] | Series: The Middle Ages series | Includes bibliographical references and index.
Identifiers: LCCN 2021042968 | ISBN 9780812253894 (hardcover)
Subjects: LCSH: Medicine, Medieval—Europe, Western. | Medicine, Medieval—Europe, Western—Sources. | Carolingians—Health and hygiene. | Carolingians—Religion. | Medicine—Religious aspects—Christianity—History—To 1500. | Human body—Religious aspects—Christianity—History—To 1500. | Mind and body—Religious aspects—Christianity—History—To 1500.
Classification: LCC R141 .L44 2022 | DDC 610.94—dc23
LC record available at https://lccn.loc.gov/2021042968

*For my parents, Allison and Mark Leja*

CONTENTS

# NOTE ON MANUSCRIPT TRANSCRIPTIONS AND TRANSLATIONS

Due to space limitations, Latin is provided only for transcriptions from manuscripts, not from published editions. I have maintained the spelling exactly as it appears in the manuscripts, with the exception of expanding abbreviations and regularizing *u/v*. All punctuation in these transcriptions is my own. All translations are my own unless otherwise indicated. Sometimes my translations replace the Latin masculine with feminine subjects/pronouns. References to the Bible follow the Vulgate. Names follow standardized English spelling (with the exception of Asclepius/Aesculapius/Scolapius, where I have maintained the variant spellings found in the sources even though these variants *usually* refer to the same figure).

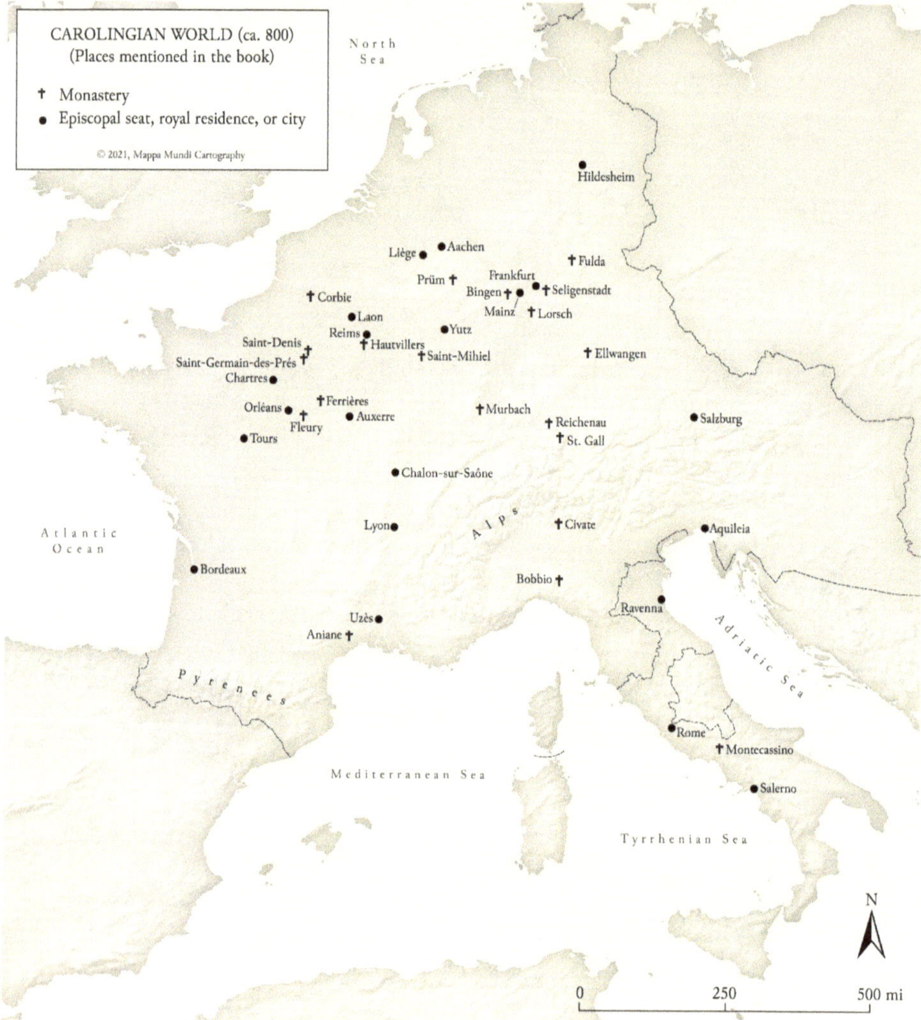


Figure 1. The boundaries of the Carolingian Empire, with sites of relevance indicated. Erik Goosmann, Mappa Mundi Cartography.

# INTRODUCTION

Hair removal was serious business in the Carolingian period. Indeed, the very act of seizing the title "king of the Franks" from the long-established Merovingian dynasty was symbolically associated with a haircut.[1] In 751, the last Merovingian king was deposed, shaved and tonsured, and consigned to a monastery—the "long-haired" royals, whose tresses had been imbued with a mysterious potency, were relegated to the past.[2] The new Carolingian dynasty would favor a closely cropped hairstyle with a longer mustache, as sported by the illustrious Charlemagne.[3]

Yet it was not only head grooming to which the Carolingian elite devoted their attention. Within medical writings that survive from the ninth century, we find a sustained interest in procedures that promise to eradicate unwanted hair on the torso of the body. The most famous compendium of medical cures produced by a Carolingian hand includes several recipes for "driving away hair."[4] Similarly, one of the brightest young scholars at the court of Charlemagne's son, Louis the Pious, devoted over a page of his personal handbook to depilatory lotions (*psilotra*).[5] And a lengthy set of instructions on hair removal continued to be copied centuries after Carolingian rule with a note at the end praising the efficacy of the formula and its use by several ninth-century notables at the court of Charlemagne's grandson, Charles the Bald.[6] The reader is promised that the bishop of Laon used this depilatory unguent frequently and that it was endorsed by learned Greeks.[7] Concocted from lime and arsenic, the unguent was to be spread all over the body with gentle strokes after one had sweated in a warm bath; it was then rinsed off with an infusion of flax seeds, mallow plants, and wheat husks boiled in water. The procedure was guaranteed to denude the body of hair like a feather stripped of its barbs. The hairless body served as an external sign of internal health, for the recipe proclaimed that the unguent "not only expunges hair but also represses a noxious attack of humors," drying them out and preventing spring and summer fevers.[8] Charles the Bald may not have attained the hairlessness of which his epithet boasts, but it would seem as though the ninth-century Frankish elite were not well disposed toward the hairy.[9]

* * *

This is not a book about hair. But just as an attention to hair crossed the political, medical, and religious spheres of Carolingian society, so does this book examine how ideas surrounding physical health, spiritual well-being, and the imperial mission of the Carolingian elite became intersecting concerns. Historians have recognized the myriad ways in which this dynasty cultivated the advancement of education and have revealed the vital links between this "renaissance" of learning and reforms carried out within secular, ecclesiastical, and monastic domains to emend and eradicate faults—whether in words, Christian doctrine, moral behavior, or the administration of justice.[10] At base, this entangled political and religious fixation on correction was oriented toward the improvement of the individual and the goal of securing salvation for everyone.[11] Medicine, however, has never been considered central to the Carolingian *correctio*, despite the period's belief that the integrity of the individual was the building block of a righteous Christian empire and that this integrity rested, in turn, on the stable union of body and soul.

How two such contrary entities—the mortal body and the immortal soul—could remain fastened together and form the nexus of personhood was a great Christian mystery. As a truth concealed from human knowledge, this problem could be probed from various angles but never fully resolved, or so I suggest in the coming pages. Although Carolingian intellectuals tackled the thorny nature of the soul directly starting around the turn of the ninth century, they never composed writings that explicitly outlined a theory of the body. Indeed, the greatest scholar of Charlemagne's reign, Alcuin of Tours, declared the character of the body to be self-evident and not in need of further elaboration.[12]

That said, a new genre of source material exists from the late eighth century onward, which offers an exceptional avenue through which to approach early medieval understandings of the material human form. These are manuscripts with medical material, copied in Carolingian scriptoria.[13] While there survive only twenty-five or so manuscripts and fragments with Latin medical texts from across Europe between the sixth and eighth centuries, at least four times that number (and probably many more) are extant from the ninth-century Carolingian Empire alone.[14] Of course, a variety of factors affecting the survival of pre-Carolingian manuscripts makes numerical comparisons difficult, but there is little doubt that, alongside many other genres, medical writing witnessed a dramatic upsurge in the ninth century (numbers decreased in the tenth century and did not peak again until the twelfth).[15]

Medicine was not simply a genre that enjoyed an efflorescence over the reigns of Charlemagne and his heirs. It was an art—a sacred art, as one text claimed—that itself was reconfigured over this period, becoming not simply a method of physical rehabilitation but also a tool of spiritual transformation. Medical knowledge, and its activation in self-care and charitable healing, had the potential to influence the ineffable bonds uniting spirit and matter. By focusing on preventative regimens, in particular, we are able to see that early medieval care of the body was never simply about renunciation or denigration of the physical. Rather, relations between body and soul existed on a spectrum: at one end was a vision of two sparring foes, yoked together but ever in conflict; at the other end was a model of partnership, centered upon the ideal of harmonious unity. Writings from the middle decades of the ninth century outlining a pious mode of life evince a marked shift toward the latter, favoring language that defined the body as fragile, rather than aggressive, and vulnerable, rather than wicked. Accordingly, it is possible to trace a theological move to redeem the body that occurred simultaneously with a new attention to ancient medical texts and their value.

In the year 800, Charlemagne received the title of emperor from Pope Leo III.[16] Although a pivotal moment in European history, this event did not mark a stark shift in Carolingian priorities. New modes of governing and key reforming efforts had already been introduced, and responses to the imperial title for the most part built on this momentum. It was over these years prior to and immediately following 800 that Alcuin composed the first Latin treatise on the nature of the soul since the sixth century, that the royal monastery of Lorsch put together a compendium of remedies prefaced by a unique Christian defense of the medical art, and that Bishop Paulinus of Aquileia launched a new genre of spiritual manuals directed at the lay elite. Due to a long-standing assumption that these works consist merely of assembled snippets of ancient and patristic writings (whether theological, medical, or moral), they have not typically been treated as products of original thought.[17] Consequently, though recent scholarship has advanced innovative perspectives, these three genres have historically suffered scholarly neglect. Here, I argue for an approach that both draws attention to their originality and charts the intersecting themes, ideas, and priorities among the three literary modes. Though these genres are rarely found alongside one another in extant manuscripts from the Carolingian age, they were all fixated on the importance of *salus* (a Latin term meaning both health and salvation) and contributed to a common, emergent discourse about the importance of personal regulation.

Self-governance, ninth-century authors emphasized, could only be achieved by gaining wisdom about the body's relationship to the material cosmos and the soul's relationship to God.[18] A "more perfect union" between the soul and body was the enterprise of every Christian, not only those in the purified space of the monastery—indeed, as these three genres make clear, the moral lessons of the monastery were by no means so rarefied as to be useless to the lives of lay men and women. One of those lessons centered upon the value of classical medicine for a God-fearing individual, one who had been taught to accept the penitential usefulness of suffering. Works like the *Lorscher Arzneibuch*, a medical compendium assembled at a royal monastery, contended that human medicine was a mirror of divine mercy and should be employed in all cases of illness and injury, no matter whether the cause of such anguish was physical or spiritual.[19]

Medical learning was not subsumed unconsciously within the fold of Carolingian educational programs, which themselves evinced a deep ambivalence toward the classical tradition.[20] To ask how the writings of Hippocrates and Galen ought to be treated was not an entirely new question, but for us to assume that all such questions were fully resolved by the patristics is to ignore the ever-evolving nature of Christian doctrine and theological "kinks" that continued to trouble early medieval societies. The Latin Fathers of Late Antiquity were far less likely than their contemporaries in the East to adamantly condone or condemn a medical corpus that most inherently saw as "Greek" within the Roman world. As Carolingian intellectuals confronted this inherited doctrinal ambiguity, debate ensued regarding the legitimacy of ancient humoral teachings.

The material legacy of the period reveals that debate's results; that a consensus ultimately cohered around the belief that medicine could be refashioned as righteous is evident in the codices that have come down to us. As a subject with pagan origins that *could* arouse suspicions about magical activities and *could* evoke a challenge to God's authority over life and death, medicine was nevertheless incorporated within the sphere of Christian bodily techniques.[21] The process of that incorporation was a significant intellectual project, one of central concern to this book. My aim is to show how medicine formed one aspect of an enduring synthesis that took shape as Carolingian scholars, in propagating their own vision of a Christian empire, implicitly acted as gatekeepers of classical and early Christian texts and ideas. During the last decades of the eighth century and first half of the ninth century, Carolingian deliberations about orthodoxy precipitated the fashioning of ancient medicine as a Christian art. It is in this context of fervent religious inquiry that *Embodying the Soul* explores the possibilities and limitations of human intervention in the body's health, intervention that accrued significance because of the body's "spiritual weight."[22]

* * *

The care of the self was not an agenda important only in the formation of empire. As the realm began to break apart in the fraternal civil war that ensued after Louis the Pious's death in 840, reflections on the bonds uniting Christian society continued to stimulate fresh discussions. In 844, Louis's three sons and the bishops of their respective kingdoms gathered at Yutz in northeastern Francia to resolve how the divided empire of the Franks was to be ruled. As they set forth a vision of idealized political order, the assembled clergy appealed to the structure of the human individual as a means to explain the coordination of various roles within Christian society. Instead of speaking about the "two persons" by which the Church was governed, in language that harkened back to Pope Gelasius, the bishops at Yutz implied that the relationship between royal power and episcopal authority mirrored the bond between the body and soul.[23] Their aim was to stress that the empty seats of certain bishoprics urgently needed to be filled if the realm was to be properly governed, for "the soul is more precious than the body."[24]

By including this explanation, they alluded to the type of relation that ought to exist between body and soul. Their choice of metaphor was grounded not simply in the understanding that the soul was superior to the body; rather, it depended upon the belief that the body and soul were *both* necessary partners in the pursuit of salvation. The body (royal power) ought to be guided by the soul (episcopal authority), with its divine reason, but it was a spirit of cooperation, not antagonism, that characterized the union of these two entities. Just as the common good of the empire depended upon kings and bishops striving for justice and righteousness in a mutually reinforcing way, so did body and soul need to struggle together, not against one another.

This was a vision of the body politic that hinged on theological "work" in which Carolingian intellectuals had already been immersed for decades. If, around 800, Alcuin addressed questions that had been circulating at Charlemagne's court concerning the nature of the soul, this was far from the last word on the subject. Letters and treatises on the soul produced over the next several decades plumbed deeper into the matter of the soul's attachment to its body, with debate cresting around 850. The emerging consensus served to underscore, above all, not the utter disparity between spirit and matter but the mysterious affinity between the two. Concurrent with this line of doctrinal argument was the emphasis within spiritual guidebooks on the partnership that existed between body and soul. In this way, when the Council of Yutz called up an image of political harmony, it was one that evoked a string of recent writings on the governance of the self.

At the heart of these writings that grappled with the cohesion of a discrete person composed of dissimilar parts was a persistent Carolingian uneasiness regarding the nature of personal responsibility. We can trace the roots of this angst to developments in the "Celtic Mediterranean" that were already beginning to coalesce around the year 700—the spread of a tariffed system of penance from Ireland, new depictions of purgatory as a geographical space, a conviction that each soul was marked by its own unique acts, and a conversation about which deeds performed on earth could affect the fate of souls in the afterlife.[25] Such emergent beliefs vested the average person with a heavy responsibility for ensuring that the soul was constantly decontaminated of its sin. However, this focus on human agency simultaneously projected an optimism that society could establish rhythms to purge sin wherever it was to be found, in life or after death.

Carolingian kings were strongly attuned to these ideas as they sought to secure their royal authority amid a rapidly expanding kingdom. Questions raised throughout the reforming movement concentrated not so much on the generation of sin in a cosmological sense as on the processes by which effective "cleanup" could occur. The elite worked to create a series of interlocking safeguards, which functioned alongside the hope that improved education would diminish the production of sin. The realm was fortified against the disorder of iniquity at various levels: first, that of the individual, then the supervision of the local priest, the community leadership of bishops and counts, the prayers supplied by monastic powerhouses, the oversight expected of the king, and, finally, the intercession offered by relics and saintly patrons.[26] Unto themselves, these tools were not necessarily innovative, nor should we call this a system because its function varied by geography and local whim.[27] Yet, in their scope, the councils and legislation that mandated these structures sharpened a new notion of Christian subjecthood—one that emphasized, above all, how techniques of self-governance could strengthen the webs of mutual responsibility uniting the empire.[28]

In the past decade, scholarship on the Carolingians has taken what we might call a penitential turn, as historians have delved into the practices of penance and the ways that they undergirded political and pastoral authority. Monographs by Courtney Booker, Abigail Firey, and Mayke de Jong have revealed the dynamics by which officeholders in the Carolingian Empire (whether kings, bishops, abbots, or counts) secured their authority through the promise that they would "render an account" on the Day of Judgment not only for their own souls but also for the souls of all others in their care.[29] This research draws on a now firmly rooted trend of treating religious rhetoric seriously and not as a means of masking political goals. At the same time, it has transformed our understanding of Carolingian power in demonstrating how monastic concerns regarding purity and iniquity became embedded in developing legal and governmental structures.[30]

The centrality of the care of the soul to ideologies of power has driven scholars to expose the mechanics by which sin (especially the sins of kings) could be detected, examined, exposed, and repaired. Yet, if the nature of "care" has been interrogated, the other term of this equation—soul—has remained quietly overlooked. That the soul and its salvation were the chief enterprise of Carolingian reform is well established, but the attention that Carolingians devoted to illuminating the makeup of the soul itself has been little explored. Nor have historians considered how Carolingian society dealt with the question of extending such modes of care to the physical realm of existence. If the soul was an invisible, immaterial entity lodged within the body, it could never be accessed and inspected directly; to the extent that it was indirectly legible, the body was a crucial conduit to it. And yet, the bodies of average Christians (as opposed to saints and their relics) have remained on the fringes of our delineation of this early medieval society, even as we recognize the brisk religious and political transformations pushed by Carolingian initiatives.[31]

This book suggests that a new awareness of the material insides of the body complemented and extended an intensifying interest in the moral state of the soul, thereby making care for the body a crucial component of spiritual progress. Some of the earliest forays into the history of the body were studies that drew attention to the interplay between Christian ascetic movements and new modes of inhabiting a troublesome flesh. Peter Brown's *The Body and Society* and Caroline Walker Bynum's *Holy Feast and Holy Fast* exposed the creativity and dynamism with which late antique and late medieval men and women manipulated their bodies so as to challenge the weakness of human nature. But if studies of the body have continued apace in both these periods, the early Middle Ages has remained the neglected middle child. Typecast either as the crude barbarian warrior or the neurotically disciplined monk, the early medieval individual has not been seen to participate in the type of boundary-crossing bodily cultures that have given the premodern world a special place in this field.[32] Studies by Janet Nelson, Celia Chazelle, and Stuart Airlie, and most especially Lynda Coon's recent *Dark Age Bodies*, have indicated that we should rethink these stereotypes.[33] Following in their footsteps, I propose that the early decades of the ninth century constituted a period of cautious experimentation when it came to developing "somatic styles" for the tending and nurture of the body.[34] Materials from imperial Rome and other early medieval societies were marshaled as fodder for the imagination, but judiciously, so as to guard against falsehood and deviance.

* * *

In the last three decades, scholarship on medieval medicine has blossomed, and from this new premodern angle, diverse avenues of inquiry have expanded the types of questions pursued within the history of medicine. From an emphasis on classical authorities, we have come to appreciate the complex and multifaceted work of medieval translators. From an elite, male-centered story of intellectual growth, we have come to see the ways in which female, domestic expertise shaped the evolution of medical practice. And from an assumption regarding the hegemonic authority of the physician, we have come to realize the essential roles played by the patient and the local populace in establishing the structure of a healing contract and the contours of a medical marketplace.[35]

Although these studies have effectively challenged a belief in the unchanging nature of medical science before the Renaissance, many of them have continued to employ the specter of the Dark Ages as a backdrop.[36] To argue that medical learning was a crucial intellectual endeavor in the early Middle Ages has proven difficult in the face of a resilient narrative that paints this period as the nadir of Western medicine.[37] This attitude persists, despite exceptional articles by Peregrine Horden, Faith Wallis, and Florence Eliza Glaze, among others.[38] Stereotypes regarding the backwardness of early medieval medical learning are easy to slip into, in large part because of how Galen and his synthetic philosophical system shaped the contours of medical knowledge in much of the last two millennia.[39] But here, the early medieval West is the exception, since only one or two works out of the immense Greek Galenic corpus were translated into Latin.[40] Just as Galen had brought order to a disparate (even contradictory) set of Hippocratic ideas, so did his writings implicitly carry with them an ordering structure. The ebbs and flows of translations and commentaries on his various texts impelled many developments within Mediterranean medicine, perhaps the most important of which was the reconstruction of his ideas into a system called Galenism in the Islamic world beginning in the eighth century.[41]

If ninth-century Baghdad is recognized as a hotbed of medical learning (alongside many other fields of philosophical and scientific inquiry), this world is not seen to bear any relationship to the contemporary court of Aachen on the other side of the Mediterranean.[42] Despite gifts of elephants, spices, and silks from the Abbasid caliph to Charlemagne, historians seem reluctant to speculate on the movement of medical texts from the Arabs to the Franks.[43] Nevertheless, these two dynasties seized power at approximately the same moment (the Abbasids in 750, the Carolingians in 751), and both patronized a significant scholarly revival.[44] The Abbasids had access to the heritage of Greek Alexandria and multilingual physician-translators from Syria.[45] The Carolingians had more limited medical resources but must have scoured Merovingian libraries and imported texts from English monasteries and archives in Italy.[46] The product of the Carolingian revival is witnessed in the hundreds of manuscripts that survive from the ninth and tenth centuries, written in distinctive Caroline minuscule script and exhibiting a diversity of medical writings (from Hippocratic works through to early medieval recipes). The achievement of the Abbasids was the preservation and revitalization of an immense corpus of Greek medical writings that otherwise would have been lost to posterity. Despite differences in the long-term impact of these two enterprises, there appears to be a more fundamental similarity in how both regimes cultivated a vigorous medical tradition as they consolidated their political and spiritual legitimacy.

Early medieval attitudes to medicine were enveloped within a pan-Mediterranean jostling over Greek intellectual goods, as different kingdoms tried to assert their religious-historical supremacy. In a reevaluation of grand narratives of science, Maria Mavroudi has demonstrated that just as the great Arabic translation movement presented itself as a "rescue mission" in the face of Christian failure, so can we locate Byzantine works that appear to respond to these Abbasid initiatives in order to reassert Greek superiority.[47] Likewise, contemporaneous with the Muslim sanction of classical medicine, we find evidence of the direct endorsement of that same antique tradition by Charlemagne and advisors close to the court. Ancient medical learning thus ought to be recognized as one of the resources of the past to which the Carolingian elite turned in order to further their status as God's new chosen people.[48]

And here the designation "court" needs to be understood in its broadest sense, as encompassing not only those scholars around the king but also key monasteries and bishoprics that were closely allied with the royal family.[49] Monasteries were not (despite their claims) institutions segregated from the secular world, and their libraries and scriptoria frequently functioned as "laboratories for research," in the words of Helmut Reimitz.[50] This period in the history of medicine is often designated using the disparaging nineteenth-century term *Mönchsmedizin* (monastic medicine)—a word that harbors the implication that monasteries could never be true sponsors of rational healing given their ingrained ambivalence toward the body.[51] Such a framing imposes a counterproductive dichotomy between medicine and religion. Instead, we should recognize how extensively the Carolingian religious environment both informed medical scholarship *and* gave it new dynamism and purpose. The status of medical literature was heightened, not diminished, by the many ways it intersected with theological concerns and imperial ambitions.

The standard narrative of medicine's regeneration in the West—beginning in the late eleventh century when the first translations of Arabic literature into Latin were produced—often seems to assume that the translations themselves catalyzed a dormant interest in medical learning. But it is equally likely that a growing fascination with medicine spurred on the work of the translators.[52] Constantine the African, whose translations were fundamental in reshaping the medical literature available in western Europe, has typically been cast as a symbol of Salernitan culture rather than traditions at the monastery of Montecassino where he undertook most of his scholarship.[53] To be sure, the diverse mixing of peoples and languages found in Salerno and southern Italy proved fertile ground for medicine. Yet, the work of Florence Eliza Glaze and Monica Green has demonstrated the speed with which Constantine's new translations were diffused from Montecassino across

Europe, in part via Benedictine monastic networks.[54] Perhaps we should ask, then, why was there such an eager audience for Constantine's writings in the first place?

Recognizing the foundation laid by the Carolingian reforms—reforms that, at base, sought to standardize monastic life across the empire through adherence to one common rule—allows for Constantine's work to be viewed as an extension of developments already underway by the early ninth century. Alongside processes by which all monasteries adopted the sixth-century Rule of Benedict of Nursia, increased their production of manuscripts (and began using new Caroline minuscule script), and opened schools to educate young monks, secular clergy, and sometimes lay children too, there occurred a more wide-ranging questioning of what a Christian education should encompass.[55] Therapeutic knowledge and the texts of classical and late antique medical authorities were one subject that came under scrutiny. And although there was not universal agreement, the trajectory of Carolingian scholarship was to make medicine "intellectually respectable," as John Contreni observed many decades ago.[56]

But medicine was not simply intellectual knowledge. Indeed, what made it special was in part how well it fit into Carolingian models that stressed the need to link thought with action. To read royal decrees, hagiography, and other didactic literature from the reigns of Charlemagne and his heirs is to be constantly reminded of the partnership between word and deed.[57] The *vita* of Saint Leoba (ca. 835), for example, emphasizes that Leoba's holiness was due not simply to her devotion to studying the Bible and liberal arts from a young age but to the fact that her conduct was always a reflection of what she had learned.[58] The spiritual handbook written by the laywoman Dhuoda in the 840s similarly defines the very genre of handbook (*liber manualis*) as a call to link reading with deeds, "for 'hand' means action carried out."[59] In this vein of thought, medicine epitomized the twinned pursuit of a contemplative art (for knowledge of healing reflected God's wisdom) *and* of an applied practice, which translated thought into charitable care. Faith Wallis and Brigitte Englisch have argued that early medieval scholars reimagined the essence of ancient sciences, shifting their focus from philosophical speculation to problem-oriented techniques.[60] From this perspective, ninth-century compendia can be seen as the culmination of a trend, already evident in Late Antiquity, to focus on the practical elements of medical learning.[61] Similarly, they highlight an embrace of pre-Carolingian schemas that included medicine within the liberal arts (rather than validating those that excluded it), a move that firmly defined it as part of the divine "house of wisdom," in Alcuin's terminology.[62] It was the ninth century that saw the true fulfillment of an inherited belief that medicine naturally paired with theology to treat the afflictions of body and soul, respectively.[63]

* * *

This book devotes more space to the work of anonymous scribes and editors than it does to writings that fall within the standard medical canon. We encounter numerous treatises ascribed to Hippocrates and Galen, and a few to Aristotle, but almost none of these are found within the modern corpora attributed to those classical authors.[64] As Faith Wallis has articulated, there was little textual stability when it came to early medieval medical manuscripts, where "reverence for ancient authority coincide[d] with extraordinary indifference to textual authenticity."[65] Those unnamed individuals who put together ninth-century medical compendia freely mixed and matched titles and authors, added and deleted words and passages, and rearranged the formats of the different texts according to particular motives or sensibilities. Scholars like Klaus-Dietrich Fischer, Arsenio Ferraces Rodríguez, Gerhard Baader, Gundolf Keil, M. E. Vázquez Buján, Innocenzo Mazzini, and Monica Green have already produced invaluable studies of the relationships among the different textual witnesses, yet much work remains to be done on the extant manuscripts.[66]

Although healing-oriented texts crop up in all kinds of Carolingian collections, this does not undermine the fact that medicine was understood to be a discrete genre. I use the term medical manuscripts throughout the book because this terminology best encapsulates the Carolingians' own organizational impulses. Library catalogues produced by Carolingian monasteries often labeled codices as "medical books" (*libri medicinales*) or stated simply that an institution possessed "a volume on the art of medicine" or "excerpts from medical books."[67] These labels fittingly correspond to numerous manuscripts extant from the period, which contain a variety of shorter and longer texts, adapted, shortened, and interpolated quite freely.[68] Brief herbal recipes, prognostic guidelines for the ill, and calendrical dietary recommendations were frequently included in miscellanies and written into the margins and spaces that remained in nonmedical codices.[69] But most texts authored by prominent medical authorities survive in compilations that consist entirely of similar material (or concern the liberal arts in general);

they are not scattered across liturgical, theological, legal, or hagiographic collections.[70]

Texts were typically assigned to one of a small number of authorities, with Hippocrates being the most common. Correspondingly, the names of ancient and late antique authors were also used to designate entries in library catalogues; at Lorsch, for example, a scribe recorded "in one codex, three books of medical responses by the methodist Caelius Aurelianus of Sicca."[71] This method of categorization set pagan medical authorities alongside the Fathers and other theologians whose names proliferated across the pages of these catalogues.[72] Yet, authorship was only one variable used in organizing medical knowledge.[73] Entries might highlight instead the type of therapy: a cataloguer in Reichenau described one codex as "information on the preparation of poultices, antidotes, and plasters, and a medical diet."[74] Similar labels of this type focused on prognostication, the making of oils, diet, the virtues of herbs, anatomy (or the position of members), and miscellaneous cures and remedies. Cataloguers' decisions to record these codices according to author or treatment point, respectively, to an emphasis on medicine-as-text and medicine-as-tool.

That none of the medical manuscripts extant from the ninth century are identical or derive in their entirety from the same exemplar reveals not only the creative license of Carolingian scribes but also the large volume of material that must have been in circulation.[75] Whether medical texts suffered a higher rate of destruction because they were being carried around for use in therapeutic settings must remain an open-ended question.[76] We do possess one folded manuscript that may well have been owned by an itinerant physician.[77] However, many other extant codices were clearly intended for display or consultation in the library, given their large size. Though the surviving manuscripts are unique in their format, they generally include a similar array of contents.[78] In broad strokes, the shorter texts tend toward a more philosophical subject matter, while the longer present applied knowledge.[79]

The bulk of a ninth-century medical codex typically consisted of *materia medica* texts (with descriptions of different plants, animals, and minerals and their medicinal properties) and recipe collections (lists of bodily conditions, often from head to toe, with various remedies for each condition). Alongside these were shorter treatises on subjects such as medical training, anatomy, the causes of disease, acute and chronic illnesses, phlebotomy, urines, pulses, diet, prognosis, and gynecology. Some of these shorter treatises originally derived from a longer work, which is representative of what happened to many classical and late antique texts: they were broken down into smaller units, condensed, reformulated, and expanded with additional material; at some point, new textual groupings formed.[80] There was no standard core of medical writings in the early Middle Ages, although the reading recommendations of Cassiodorus (d. ca. 585), the Ostrogothic statesman-turned-monk, may have served as a guide for later monastic collections.[81] The difficulty, as scholars have long noted, is that we cannot be certain of the identity of the texts Cassiodorus names.[82] Thus, perhaps the most important point to be drawn from his recommendations is the authority he endowed to the names Dioscorides, Hippocrates, and Galen—all of whom continued to figure as prominent "authors" in Carolingian manuscripts.[83]

Foucault contends that scientific texts in the Middle Ages were especially in need of an "author function" to validate them, but it is, ironically, the lack of authorial identity that has led to their modern dismissal.[84] We have moved well beyond the idea that early medical texts were mere scribal exercises, thanks to Linda Voigts and John Riddle, but an inability to pin down their origins, in conjunction with the messiness of their Latin, has endowed them with an aura of suspicion.[85] What is certain is that the first witness to the majority of texts is a ninth-century manuscript. But there remain a variety of possibilities about how and when any particular medical text that circulated in the ninth century came into existence. In most cases, Carolingian medical codices stand at the end of several long processes—they reflect the continuous recycling of home remedies, as first collected (in Latin) by Roman estate owners like Pliny the Elder (d. 79 C.E.) and then adapted over the centuries; they testify to the venerable authority accrued by ancient herbals, like that written by Dioscorides (ca. 70 C.E.) and that falsely attributed to Apuleius of Madaura (ca. 300 C.E.); and they participate (albeit, many times removed) in the drive already evident in the late Roman period to condense, summarize, and interpret the massive corpus of Galen.[86] Oribasius, physician to the Emperor Julian (r. 361–363), composed some of the most popular abridgments of Galen (with one that nevertheless filled seventy books!), and two of his shorter synopses, alongside pseudo-Pliny and pseudo-Apuleius, are some of the few medical texts to survive from Merovingian Gaul, Visigothic Spain, and early medieval Italy.[87]

A figure such as Marcellus Empiricus, who was able to access many of these works to compose his own book of remedies around 400 C.E. in Bordeaux, generally exemplifies the situation faced by the anonymous Carolingian scribe.[88] Marcellus prefaced his cures with a series of pseudonymous letters attributed to well-known medical authorities, a conceit that was especially popular with late antique and early medieval writers. Indeed, in addition to works by Dioscorides, Oribasius, and Soranus of Ephesus (ca. 100), and those drawn from the Hippocratic Corpus, pseudonymous letters seem to have been some of the chief texts chosen for translation from Greek into Latin by those bilingual scholars undertaking such activities in Italy and North Africa as the western empire was fragmenting.[89]

An entrenched tradition among historians of medicine has been to assume a Ravenna school of medicine in the sixth century, where numerous Greek medical works were translated and thereby put into circulation in the early medieval West.[90] Certainly, as the seat of Byzantine power in Italy, Ravenna was an ideal location for bilingual scholarship. At the same time, as Nicholas Everett observes, "Many of these attributions . . . rely on historical assumptions about Italy's role in preserving classical traditions," assumptions that sustain a circular argument concerning the origins of these translations.[91] That Italy seems to have been a region in which lay people continued to practice medicine after the end of the western Roman Empire has also buttressed a tendency to assign all innovative intellectual activity to Italy, even beyond the clear phases of medical scholarship in eleventh-century Salerno or in sixth-century Ravenna.

Such suppositions can easily drift toward a narrative that scientific innovation *must* have taken place in Italy because it could not have occurred in an environment dominated by ecclesiastical (rather than lay) practitioners. Thus, even studies attuned to the nuances of early medieval thought sometimes fall back on the argument that Carolingian scribes increased the volume of medical literature but added little new to its character.[92] While there are good reasons to conclude that a large number of texts whose first witnesses are Carolingian copies had earlier origins in Italy, Africa, or the Byzantine east, there are also reliable indications of new compositions: a dietary treatise from the Merovingian period, a veterinary manual for hawks by Louis the German's archchaplain, verses about gardening (modeled on a late antique herbal poem) by Charles the Bald's tutor.[93] These, and the examples discussed in the following chapters, signal a need to question any sweeping assumption that medical texts did not originate in early medieval Francia.[94]

Regardless, the sheer variety among the extant codices forces us to confront what historians working on exegesis, historiography, moral literature, and many other genres have persuasively argued—in excerpting, rearranging, editing, organizing, and "clarifying," scribes and compilers were authors.[95] Manuscripts were carefully planned undertakings, intellectual endeavors that offer a window onto authorial intentions and convictions. Though Carolingian scribes remain for the most part anonymous, that is no reason to discount the effects that they had in shaping discourse.[96] They were agents who worked as members of scriptoria, monasteries, regional communities, court schools, and scholarly lineages—and their editorial decisions reflect those networks.[97] Even the copying that they undertook should be considered productive and not simply reproductive. This is an argument already expertly put forth by scholars working on historical narratives, who have treated the variations among manuscript witnesses as clues to contemporary values and ongoing debates.[98] It is an argument that applies equally to the medical, moral, and theological treatises examined throughout this book, all of which evince a ninth-century fascination with assembling and arranging discrete morsels of knowledge.

It is likewise an argument that extends beyond text to encompass the images found in early medieval medical codices. Art historians have long directed attention to the illuminations and line drawings of plants and animals in herbals and *materia medica* collections. But investigations have traditionally been limited to questions of continuity with classical models, and little interest has been shown to the other visual elements in these manuscripts. Recent work, however, has been more inclined to grant creative license to the early medieval artist in the development of medical, natural philosophical, and astronomical images, linking figures like Scolapius (on the cover of this book) to styles at the Carolingian court and recognizing intersections between scientific diagrams and Christian iconography.[99] Consideration, then, of artistic motifs within ninth-century medical manuscripts again leads us into the orbit of contemporary conversations about theology and piety.

* * *

This book proposes a variety of ways in which medical manuscripts share emphases and preoccupations with other literary productions clearly originating in the Carolingian age. My premise—that at least some medical texts may have had ninth-century origins and that, regardless, their organization reflects ninth-century concerns—is foundational to my argument that therapeutics must be seen as a significant aspect of the Carolingian *correctio*. In analyzing a diverse array of evidence (including medical manuscripts, theological and pastoral treatises, monastic rules, court poetry, capitularies, hagiographies, biographies, and exegetical works), I look beyond Galen for frameworks of thought that structured the care of the body. It was ultimately a Carolingian penitential culture, not a natural philosophy grounded in classical authorities, that provided rational coherence to a diverse set of texts and ideas.

*Embodying the Soul* insists on an understanding of medical scholarship anchored in the question of the body-soul relationship and the project of moral education that was at the core of the Carolingian reforms. One could assume, consequently, that most of the extant medical corpus should be read as focused primarily on monks and male bodies, but here I believe the didactic approach of the Carolingian period teaches us to be cautious. Children often received a similar type of education, whether male or female, lay or monastic; moral literature addressed to laymen was owned and consumed by female readers; and the same spiritual advice frequently passed among texts intended for kings, lay nobles, and regular and secular clergy without being adapted.[100] From this perspective, the care of the self transcended many of the binaries that, in other ways, were fundamental to ninth-century conceptions of duty and responsibility, including the divide between clergy and laity as well as that between men and women.[101] Indeed, the book begins with a soul that was not gendered, at least not in any of the theological elucidations produced by male Carolingian ecclesiastics. Gender distinctions certainly do surface in many of the issues considered here—for example, the question of who had the right to assume the title "doctor"—but medical theories of the body did not necessarily follow a consistent male/female binary.[102] Thus, *Embodying the Soul* employs a deliberate openness in discussions of the care of the body, to accommodate the way in which most medical texts offer advice in general terms and do not identify this advice as applying to only one gender.[103] Even as there were multiple and competing discourses that *did* attempt to underscore differences between the lay/religious and the female/male body, I argue that grappling with embodiment was a universal Carolingian problem that shared certain common denominators.[104]

We do well to heed Caroline Bynum's reminder that there was not a singular medieval body.[105] Nevertheless, to assume that an early medieval society distinguished by its concern for consensus pursued no synthesis on the secrets beneath the skin is to fall into the stereotype of Dark Ages chaos.

Though the last synthetic narrative about early medieval medicine was published by Loren MacKinney in 1937, I do not offer here a comprehensive overview of medical texts and theories or of human health and disease in the early Middle Ages.[106] Instead, this is an effort to bring together theology and medicine—which Nancy Caciola calls two "universalizing discourses"—in order to chart the imaginary scope of embodiment in the ninth century.[107]

*Embodying the Soul* is divided into three parts. The first examines the nature of the bond between body and soul. The second demonstrates how attempts to redefine the practice of medicine as a Christian endeavor went hand in hand with the gradual move toward viewing the body in a more positive light. The third connects the medical impulses of the Carolingian age to the reflective, penitential culture that was integral to the religious reforms of the era. The book thus begins where a ninth-century author would have begun—with the care of the soul. This means that material covered in Chapters 1 and 2 may seem somewhat tangential to a more typical history of medicine. It is, however, crucial to understanding the arguments in Part III and, I believe, essential to approaching medicine from a premodern viewpoint. That said, readers interested primarily in a snapshot of early medieval healing and its practitioners may wish to start with Chapters 4 and 5.

Chapter 1 argues that the soul-body union was a topic that came under renewed scrutiny in the ninth century and that investigations into the ontology of the soul were driven primarily by pastoral concerns rather than broader philosophical systems. The focus is a series of treatises composed by Carolingian intellectuals on the soul's nature. These have never been studied together as evidence of early medieval religious thought, and yet a close analysis demonstrates that the authors were not simply regurgitating patristic doctrines but were responding to new concerns and seeking to create a consensus regarding the fundamental components of individual identity. Their assertions coalesced around points that emphasized the binary nature of identity but also the strength of the ties binding the soul to the body and the rational order that existed within each person. Furthermore, these works persistently resisted a wholly incorporeal definition of the soul in order to make more accessible and tangible the interface between the material and spiritual components of the self.

Chapter 2 explores the moral implications of a binary notion of identity, concentrating on four manuals written for the Carolingian lay nobility that constituted a new genre of spiritual advice on regulating habits, behavior, and thoughts in daily life. Drawing attention to the stark contrast over a forty-year period in how the forces of good and evil were mapped onto the components of personhood, I chart a shift from depicting the body as the enemy of the soul to framing the soul-body relationship as more of a partnership. Likewise, I show how the lay manuals were intended to stimulate a kind of mindfulness about the inner state of the self and what it meant for a soul to show good governance to its own proper body throughout its earthly existence.

Chapter 3 brings the previous chapters' discussions of the soul-body relationship into conversations about health and, in doing so, contemplates how metaphors, terms, and images constantly crossed the boundaries of the physical and the spiritual. Using hagiography, epistles, penitential handbooks, anatomical treatises, and visions of the afterlife, it reveals the imagined contours of the inside of the body, an invisible space that was in some ways knowable as a material entity but was also subject to invisible, opposing forces. In its analysis of internal ambiguity, this chapter points to the simultaneous operation of two discourses: in one, physical health and religious purity ran together; in the other, the meaning of illness was inherently obscure and could not function as a cipher for hidden sinfulness.

Chapter 4 argues that the survival of significant numbers of medical manuscripts from the ninth century reflects new attitudes toward the care of the body that emerged in concert with the Carolingian reforms. In contending that these extant manuscripts bear witness to an open-ended deliberation about the validity of medical learning, it aligns with recent scholarly claims that debate did not cease with the advent of the Middle Ages but was, in fact, part of early medieval ecclesiastical culture. I direct particular attention to the *Lorscher Arzneibuch* (ca. 800), a medical codex that has typically been deemed exceptional for its time. I show, however, that the strategies for legitimizing medicine employed by the Lorsch author can be compared to arguments subtly deployed by other contemporaneous compilers, all of whom were contributing to a gradual process of Christianizing medical therapies for the body.

Chapter 5 probes the nebulous frontiers between the physician (*medicus*) and the magician, on the one hand, and the physician and the saint, on the other. Not only was pagan magic a growing concern in the Carolingian world, but a boom in the relic trade and the emergence of new rituals for anointing the sick also intensified competition among diverse healers in the Frankish medical marketplace. I demonstrate how the production of ninth-century medical manuscripts responded to threats against the physician's reputation by presenting the *medicus* as a sanctified and learned figure. In doing so, these writings reframed the care of the body as a worthy endeavor and a skill to be entrusted only to someone with the highest qualifications. The physician, I argue, came to occupy a position closer to a saintly healer and received a set of duties (a *ministerium*) that accorded him a dignified role within Christian society.

Chapter 6 takes up questions regarding medicine as applied knowledge that could be used both to prevent disease and to repair the sick body. It focuses, in particular, on bloodletting treatises, dietary calendars, and prognostic texts, drawing connections between these and ideas expressed in prominent computistical, astronomical, and legal texts. Such texts manifest a conviction that a logical, divine schema imbued the material universe and that a rational soul could perceive this order and was driven by its own nature to govern the body according to the temporal patterns of the cosmos. At the same time, the chapter contends that these texts betray an awareness of the impermanence of natural patterns and a belief that, if prophylactic medicine failed to protect the body's integrity, human intervention in forestalling death could still be justified with reference to an emergent discourse of "necessity." This term, utilized in penitential, legal, and medical works from the period, functioned as a means to designate exceptional circumstances and yoked the ethics of medical therapeutics to evolving conceptions of order and sin within Carolingian thought.

Finally, Chapter 7 concentrates on the intersections between Carolingian medical learning and assumptions about individual responsibility. It reveals the ways in which ninth-century compilers recognized the porous boundaries between care of the body and care of the soul and sought to promote new habits surrounding digestion and purging, connecting these restorative practices with theological discussions about the nature of the soul. In contrast to scholarship that has long employed the denigrating term *Mönchsmedizin* in order to periodize early medieval medicine, I argue that medical learning was valued outside the monastery and was advanced as a tool that lay people, too, could employ. Far from medical techniques being the purview of the few, we see a desire to popularize knowledge concerning the self-governance of the body, according to the assumption that ignorance of the inner life was a certain entry point for sin and disorder into Carolingian society.

# PART I

## An Ever Closer Union

CHAPTER 1

# The Soul

## "I Take You, Body, to Be My Lawful Partner"

At a monastery in western Francia in the late 670s, a monk named Barontus experienced a temporary heavenly journey before being returned to his earthly body. As he lay sick in bed, only half-alive (*semivivus*) and surrounded by brothers singing psalms, the archangel Raphael "plucked" Barontus's soul out of his body and carried it off to Saint Peter to be judged. In describing this unusual event, the author of the *Vision of Barontus* struggled to communicate the intangible appearance of the disembodied soul:

> I will describe how small my soul seemed to me. It seemed as small as a hen's chick when it comes out of the egg. But, small as it was, it took with it my head, eyes and the rest, sight, hearing, taste, smell and touch, though it could not speak at all.[1]

The author could offer only similes and a vague sense of difference in attempting to portray this provisional separation of spirit from matter. Questions about the soul's substance, form, and bond with the animated body were not unique to the *Vision of Barontus*, but it was not until the early ninth century that they would be addressed systematically in the first theological treatise on the subject to be composed in Francia since the fifth century.[2] Beginning with Alcuin's *On the Nature of the Soul* and ending with a cluster of texts from the 850s, this chapter considers the doctrinal arguments advanced to explain the mode of the soul's earthly existence. Alongside the works of prominent Carolingian intellectuals, it explores anonymously authored testimonies that circulated in the medical corpus of the ninth century. While not a comprehensive survey, this study of diverse material exposes the imaginative landscape of solutions to questions raised by the *Vision of Barontus* and its attempt to account for the entity hidden within the body.

In seeking clarification about the characteristics of the soul, the Carolingians were hardly engaging in new avenues of inquiry; their libraries were well supplied with writings from Late Antiquity, works by Augustine, Ambrose, Gregory the Great, and Cassiodorus, for example, offering authoritative opinions on the soul.[3] Yet, while the conversation about the soul was old, the terms of debate reflected contemporary religious concerns.[4] Indeed, councils called to stem heresy in the Adoptionist (794), Iconoclasm (794 and 825), and Predestination (847–60) controversies may well have spurred continued interest in defining the soul and its capacities. So may have evolving beliefs about postmortem punishment and the existence of purgatory.[5] Neither theological nor medical treatises were simple reiterations of earlier opinions, and a careful analysis of the differences among Carolingian authors can highlight how specific concerns about the soul-body union were brought to the fore. There was a set of points upon which most scholars converged: that the individual was bipartite—composed of a body and a soul—and that the latter could be defined by its rational nature and ability to animate fleshy matter. Consensus, however, only went so far; there may not have been demarcated factions, but ninth-century writings on the soul display clear lines of disagreement and tension.

In reflecting on the duties of an abbot, Smaragdus of Saint-Mihiel (d. ca. 840) observed that the care of souls was an onerous task because the soul "is something fine and laborious to grasp, is very subtle and precarious to ponder, and is therefore laborious and arduous to govern."[6] Authors across the first half of the ninth century sought to elucidate this distinctive subtlety of the soul, driven by the assumption that correctly ascertaining the nature of the soul was not an abstract theological exercise but was central to the practical reformation of pastoral care so important to the Carolingian elite.

## The Soul in Medical Literature

The Carolingians may never have held public disputations on the nature of the soul, as they did for doctrinal controversies such as Adoptionism, but the scientific literature in their libraries offered a dramatic (if imaginary) debate between two well-known pagan authorities on the natural world and the soul's substance.[7] The *Dispute of Plato and Aristotle*, which survives in several ninth-century witnesses, begins by setting forth the question over which the philosophers ostensibly disagreed—in which humor does the soul reside and travel throughout the body?[8] There is no prefatory information that might explain why the soul is assumed to have its home in a liquid or who these two philosophers are and what led to their quarrel. Indeed, the text seems to assume a preexisting familiarity with the arguments of Plato and Aristotle, and yet these bear little resemblance to what we now recognize to be Platonic and Aristotelian thought. The *Dispute* is not concerned with logical reasoning but rather with proving what appear to be, by the end of the interaction, self-evident truths.

The text employs direct speech and "empirical" tests to signal to the reader that these are trustworthy investigations of the natural world. Speaking first, Plato declares that there are three elements and that the soul "has its dwelling place (*mansionem*) in a humor similar to blood."[9] Aristotle responds that the human being must obviously be divided into four elements, given that the seasons and cardinal points display a fourfold division. In order to resolve the uncertainty, the two philosophers agree to a test: a man in need of bloodletting is brought forth, his arm is bound, and blood is drawn off into a container. As the blood cools, it separates into two parts, with a liquid (*humor*) floating above the blood like oil over water.[10] Plato turns to Aristotle and mockingly asks, "What good is your teaching now?" The fact that the *humor* is lighter than blood and separates from it apparently indicates to Plato that the soul cannot be blood but is a substance that travels within the blood, called spirit or *pneuma*.[11] To this, Aristotle calmly replies that Plato has not won yet—it is time for a second test! This time, the man's arm is not bound and blood is allowed to flow out unchecked, which results in the man collapsing on the floor, his eyes rolling, color drained, and limbs rigid. Aristotle does not even have to voice his point. Plato willingly concedes: "By God, father Aristotle, you have convinced me that the soul is blood!"[12] Aristotle takes on his (now certified) position as teacher and instructs Plato on the four parts of the human body, each of which is home to a specific humor that dominates during one of the four seasons of the year.[13]

As should now be apparent, the terms and theories underpinning this dispute are far from clear. The text is more concerned with drama than sequential philosophical inquiry. It promotes the idea that complex questions about creation can be deduced from simple observation: people die when they are drained of blood; hence, the soul, as the life force, must be blood. The annual cycle is divided into four; hence, humans must also consist of four parts. The principles are straightforward.

Although certain Carolingian scribes evidently believed that the *Dispute* contained information worthy of preservation, not all were willing to grant the truth of its conclusions. A revised version of the debate survives in two ninth-century manuscripts.[14] This text proclaims its distance from the original in immediately foregrounding the author as the mediator between pagan philosophy and Christian truth:

> We *read* that Plato and Aristotle, pagan philosophers, held a dispute about the human soul and the order of the elements and seasons. But in this letter, we [find] that all of Plato's reasoning was deceptive. The truthful things that Aristotle said we accept, but whatever he unknowingly spoke falsely about we do not receive but cast aside.[15]

Aristotle's teachings about the harmony among the seasons, elements, and humors are retained—because they demonstrate God's rational order—but his notion that the soul is blood is disparaged. In order to demonstrate the absurdity of this notion, the reviser employs the very same experimental "proof." This time, a man is bled, too much blood is allowed to flow out, the man dies, and dogs come and lick up the spilled blood. Again, the conclusion is self-evident: "If the soul had been blood, the dogs who lick up the blood would have been able to gulp down the soul; just consider how stupid it would be to say that. Whoever thinks this demonstrates that he is an idiot!"[16]

Although the reviser overturns the false opinions of the ancient philosophers, s/he readily accepts that humans can discover the truths of creation through analyzing phenomena of the natural world. The edited *Dispute* offers its own elucidation of human anatomy (both visible and invisible) by explaining what occurs when a person cuts deeper and deeper into the body (see Figure 2).[17] One sees, sequentially, that the skin encloses the flesh, which encloses the veins, which enclose the blood; when the veins are cut and too much blood flows out, an observer can see that the person stops breathing and then dies, from which it can be deduced that the veins enclose the blood, which encloses the breath and vital heat, which, in turn, enclose the soul.[18] The reviser avoids equating the soul with blood but cannot escape the outcome of Aristotle's original experiment. The solution is to present the body as a series of nested Russian dolls, in which the relationship between two

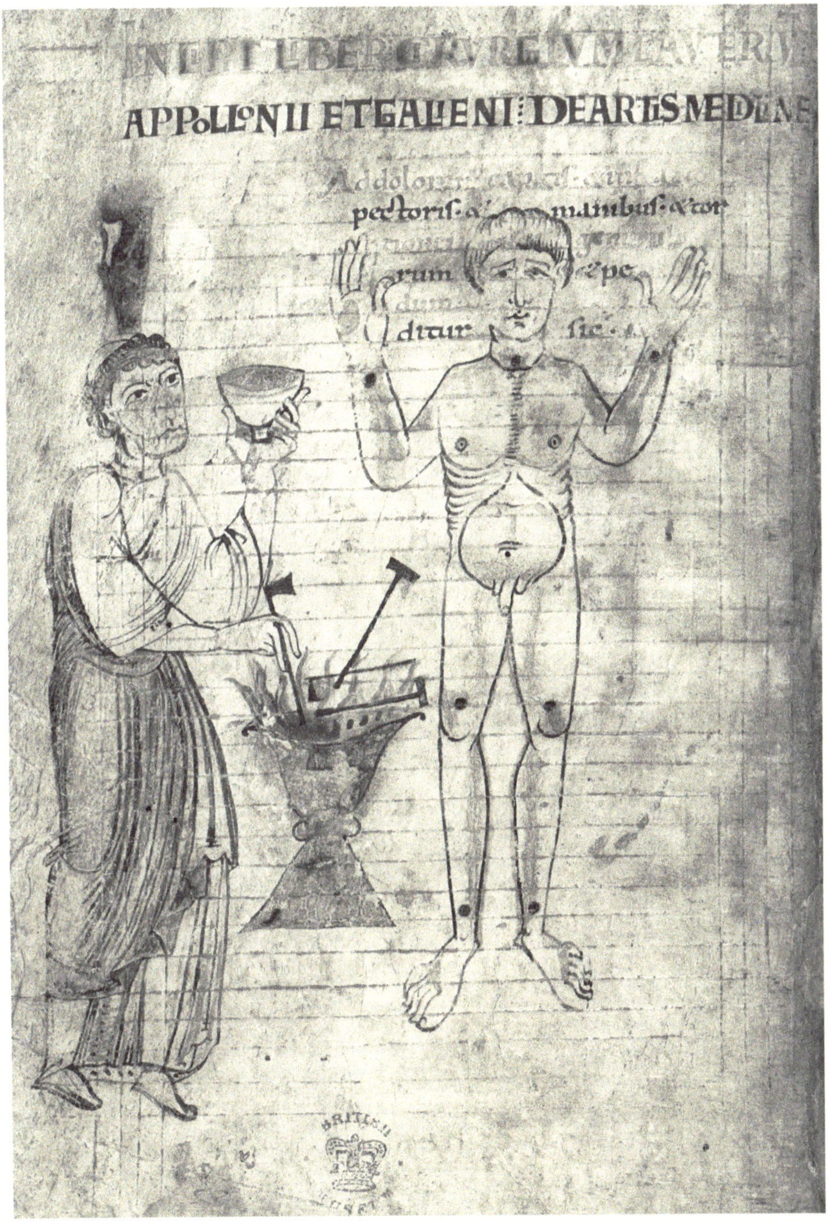

Figure 2. Cautery images are the earliest depictions of surgical operations. This one, the first in a series, shows where on the body to burn in order to relieve pain in the head, inflammation of the chest and hands, and suffering in the knees and feet; the monk-physician holds a bowl with pain relief. The manuscript here also contains the *Disputatio Platonis et Aristotelis*. © The British Library Board. London, British Library, Sloane 2839, f. 1v.

substances depends upon physical proximity and the more abstract notion of a dwelling place. Although they are hidden beneath the skin, the veins can be pictured as containers for liquid blood with relative ease, and the reviser uses this visual image to convey (but not explain) the more intangible bond between the soul and the blood.

In order to ensure that no unorthodox belief can be gleaned from the text, the reviser includes a clear doctrinal statement: "The Lord God created the soul of man in his own image, and he made it such that it would be immortal and invisible and would receive either punishments for its sins or eternal life for good works."[19] As we will see, this statement corresponds closely to definitions found in theological writings of the ninth century. It is important to note that the reviser claims that the soul is immortal and invisible but not incorporeal (a quality that would make it unable to be delimited by physical boundaries). The very capacity of the soul to be localized within the veins is what allows the reviser to explain (just as firmly as Aristotle had done) exactly *how* the soul is joined to the body, and why death is both a spiritual and physiological event.[20] Other medical texts in circulation likewise established a relationship of dependence and intimacy between blood and the soul without equating the two. A letter from "Hippocrates" to one Maecenas describes how, just as the bones support the organs, so "blood sustains the soul [and] the soul sustains life."[21] Another epistolary treatise on the humors ends with a summation that links the heart (a container for blood) all the way to God: "The heart is in the chest, the soul in the heart, the mind in the soul, faith in the mind, and Christ in faith."[22]

While we can only speculate that the author of the revised version of the *Dispute* was active in the Carolingian period, we can find clear evidence of ninth-century producers of medical manuscripts employing the act of compilation as a medium to work through problems concerning the nature of the soul. For example, a manuscript written toward the end of the ninth century, possibly at a center with Breton connections, reveals a specific agenda focused on exploring issues of generation and ensoulment. Medical material constitutes the core of this manuscript.[23] It begins with a letter purporting to be from the Evangelist Luke, which promises to set forth medical teachings appropriate for Christians. Throughout what follows, both Christian and pagan authorities (Augustine and Hippocrates, respectively) are credited as the authors of the texts. In fact, the majority of the content is drawn from works by Vindicianus, a late fourth-century proconsul and physician in Africa, and Isidore, the early seventh-century bishop of Seville. Yet it is the voice of the divinely inspired Luke that is used to frame the assembly of anatomical material, which ends with the declaration: "Luke describes this ordering of the human body."[24] To succeed this anatomical account, the compiler chose the revised version of the *Dispute of Plato and Aristotle.*

The compiler's role in organizing the medical information at his/her disposal is likewise apparent in the pattern of the anatomical content. This starts with the growth of the human body in the womb, then moves to a description of "which bones, nerves, and joints hold together the human body," before returning again to issues of conception.[25] In discussing fetal development, growth is sketched according to the mystical significance of factors of the number six, in order to prove that Christian symbolism of the six days of Creation aligns with Hippocratic theories of development. Thus, a fetus is milk for six days, blood for the next nine, coagulated flesh for the next twelve, and a perfect body for the next eighteen.[26] Whoever composed the account of the fetus that comes first in the manuscript made sure to point out that it accords perfectly with the second account by Vindicianus, which declares that in the first month, blood is generated in the womb, in the second, the expression of the body, and in the third, "the infant is conceived, as it receives a soul from God's breath."[27] Intriguingly, this is the only witness of Vindicianus's text that contains a reference to God.[28]

In addition to providing an explanation of how body and soul come together in the womb, the compiler interpolated a digression about the soul into a long description of the different parts and organs of the body from Isidore's *On the Differences of Things.*[29] After outlining the seven seats of the soul throughout the body and the various offices the soul performs (from wisdom of God to movement of the members), the interpolation ends with a doctrinal statement: "The soul was created invisible, in the image of God, possessing neither color, nor weight, but created immortal from nothing by God . . . which is not breath, or smoke, or fire, or blood, or part of the divine substance.[30] A reader of the codex would have found this definition fully in accordance with the one that appears a few folios later in the revised *Dispute.* Indeed, sections of this definition closely follow those found in Alcuin's treatise on the soul, discussed below.[31] If there remains any doubt that the ninth-century compiler of this codex was driven by a desire to elucidate the invisible bonds linking the mortal body and the immortal soul, I will note that someone several centuries later had no trouble recognizing the focus of the manuscript—at the end of the *Dispute* s/he affixed a copy of Augustine's *On the Magnitude of the Soul.*[32]

Because medical scholarship is rarely included in modern analyses of Carolingian learning, the tendency has been to cast ideas about the soul transmitted in medical manuscripts as relics from a pagan past that were copied primarily for their classical antiquity rather than for any sense of proximate utility.[33] However, this is not how the compilers of the manuscripts understood texts about the soul, including those attributed to pagans like Hippocrates or Aristotle. Even when it comes to the "uncorrected" version of the *Dispute*, nothing suggests that it was copied as a classical memento; one ninth-century witness was included in a manuscript that bears starkly Christian overtones, and another was edited by the scribe to contain a reference to the fact that God established, by his design, the fourfold order that Aristotle espoused.[34] The earliest copy of the revised *Dispute*, meanwhile, is found immediately following the unrevised version. One might assume that the compiler either composed the revision after copying the (erroneous) original or copied both together, according to the conviction that the first could not harm a Christian audience as long as the second was also present.[35] This was not at all unusual. The Carolingian obsession with orthodoxy did not entail censorship of material but focused on discernment; one could better understand correct belief if able to recognize the incorrect as well.[36]

Focusing on the ninth-century life of the *Dispute of Plato and Aristotle* enables us to identify a clear interest in natural philosophy among Carolingian intellectuals and, moreover, a belief that pagan authorities could assist in unpacking the mysteries of the human body.[37] It was not feasible to draw a clear distinction between pagan anatomy, focused on the body, and Christian theology, focused on the soul.[38]

## A Rational Soul in the Image of God

One of the reasons that texts such as the *Dispute* have been seen as peripheral to the dominant Christian culture of the Carolingian realm is that little attention has been paid to investigating understandings of the soul.[39] The scholarship that does exist has cast Alcuin as the hegemonic voice in crafting a theology of the soul.[40] However, though Alcuin's *On the Nature of the Soul* is the first extant work on the topic, it was not necessarily the definitive opinion for the generations that followed him. In the sixty years after Alcuin, members of the Carolingian elite continued to raise pointed questions about certain attributes of the soul, and in response a number of prominent scholars offered their own answers to this theological enigma. Taken together, their treatises offer glimpses of what must have been extended, wide-ranging discussions (both oral and textual) among the Carolingian lay and ecclesiastical nobility.

Shortly after the year 800, Charlemagne's cousin Gundrada approached Alcuin with a desire to learn more from him about the nature of the soul.[41] She was seeking clarification, or so Alcuin claims, because queries had been circulating among her acquaintances at court over the last year.[42] Thus, the soul was apparently a topic that garnered new and sustained interest at Aachen around the year 800. And Alcuin tailored his response to Gundrada so as to appeal to this courtly audience, choosing language that would have been appropriately evocative. He explains that "it is right that the soul be the lord and, as from the highest seat of royal power, govern what, how, when, where and in which way it should constitute the members [of the body] and contemplate assiduously what it should order each member to do."[43] The parallels between the soul's command over the body and the powers claimed by the newly crowned emperor would hardly have been lost on those gathered around Charlemagne. While Alcuin and Gundrada seem to have enjoyed a close relationship and exchanged correspondence on other theological matters, it is unlikely that Alcuin intended his letter to be for her eyes only.[44] Indeed, his *On the Nature of the Soul* appears to have been extremely popular and enjoyed a wide circulation, with over twenty copies surviving from the ninth century alone.[45]

Alcuin's decision to avoid overly technical, obscure language not only made his ideas in the letter more accessible (especially to the laity) but also reflected his assumptions about the subject matter.[46] This was a treatise about self-knowledge. It was theology at the microcosmic level of the individual. In answering Gundrada, Alcuin's very first declaration was that, despite his lack of expertise, he knew that he must possess the knowledge to address her question because "What am I, if not soul and body?"[47] He believed that this treatise was a way of furthering his contemporaries' awareness of their own identities.

Alcuin's treatise did not deal primarily in abstract concepts but explained the soul to Gundrada in terms of recognizable human impulses—the capacities of love and reason—which he showed to be interdependent. The nature of the soul is to be rational, Alcuin explains, and through reason, the soul recognizes itself to be part of a hierarchy. Above the soul is God, who imprints it with his image and gives it life; the soul, in turn, gives life to the body, which is below it. Central to Alcuin's account is the belief that once the soul has used reason to determine its place within this cosmic hierarchy, it behooves it to behave appropriately—loving what is superior to it (God) and controlling what is below it (the body).[48] Alcuin returns repeatedly to this emphasis on order and love, highlighting the connection between understanding the components of the self and leading a good life. "In sum, a person lives in an ordered way who investigates her own self (what she is and where she proceeds) and who governs the dispositions of her mind and the movements of her body with prudent reason."[49] At both the beginning and end of the treatise, Alcuin sets the body and soul in relationship to one another by comparing the soul to a powerful ruler and the body, by consequence, to a subject governed by rational laws.[50] Thus he confirms one of his key points: the soul fulfills its own nature through good governance.

When Alcuin speaks about the soul being imprinted with the image of God, he states that this image or likeness resides "in its principal part, which is called the mind."[51] However, his use of the term *mens* here is, as he later reveals, best thought of as a mode of speech. This is because Alcuin is absolutely insistent that the soul be defined as a complete unity.[52] Different terms, including spirit, sense, mind, intellect, will, and memory, are employed for the sake of human comprehension, to distinguish the manifold functions of the soul.[53] "Nevertheless, these are not divided in substance in the same way that they are by name because all of them are one single soul."[54] Similarly, Alcuin invokes a Platonic tripartite partition of the soul into appetitive, passionate, and rational functions but never suggests that these are three distinct entities.[55] He illustrates this inner unity with reference to the familiar theology of the Trinity. "The soul has as part of its nature (as we said) the image of the Holy Trinity in it because it has understanding, will, and memory. For it is the one soul, which is called mind, one life, and one substance, which has these three within it."[56] This description not only furthers Alcuin's argument that the soul is impressed by the likeness of God but also helps to elucidate how the soul can be identified in parts and yet remain essentially indivisible. Like the Trinity, the soul's nature is difficult for the human intellect to grasp completely. The important point, Alcuin emphasizes, is to *believe* in a unitary soul, just as one has sworn to have faith in a single, omnipresent God. Again, he relates the terms of discussion to concepts familiar to the Carolingian elite, building on recent courtly discussions about the Trinity to explain the nature of the soul.[57]

Augustine's *On the Trinity* and *On Genesis to the Letter* were two key sources that Alcuin relied upon in composing his treatise, and Leslie Lockett has argued that it was a Neoplatonic view of the soul, transmitted through Augustine, that Alcuin introduced to his contemporaries.[58] Although Lockett perceptively reveals the distinctions between Alcuin's Augustinian account of the soul and the non-Augustinian beliefs dominant in the Insular world from which Alcuin came, it is equally true that Alcuin did not share all of the august Father's main concerns.[59] Above all, the treatise for Gundrada called attention to the bipartite nature of the human being—composed of a rational and unified soul that itself brought coherence to the matter that formed the body and ruled it in accordance with divine order.[60] While Augustine was preoccupied with disproving Stoic convictions in a material soul, this was not of foremost interest to Alcuin.[61] When he finally offers a succinct definition of the soul (halfway through the treatise), he draws more from Isidore than Augustine: "The soul is a discerning and rational spirit always in motion, always living, capable of good and evil intention; dignified by free will according to the kindness of the creator . . . created to rule the movements of the body, invisible, incorporeal, without weight, without color, circumscribed yet whole in every member of its body."[62] There is no doubt that Alcuin adhered to a Neoplatonic belief in the soul's incorporeality, but he devotes no space to explaining this quality, preferring instead to focus Gundrada's attention on loving God through living rationally.[63]

## A Soul Similar to Its Physical Body

Given the popularity of Alcuin's treatise throughout the ninth century, his answer to Gundrada appears to have resolved some of the difficulties his contemporaries were facing. Nevertheless, while it remained influential, Alcuin's work was not comprehensive, and the issues he did not discuss became points of controversy among his intellectual successors. In particular, his relative silence on the meaning of incorporeality provoked problems. Within Neoplatonic thought, an inability to be localized in space or circumscribed by physical boundaries was deemed essential to the property of incorporeality.[64] Though Alcuin emphasized several times that the soul was not localized within the body but was fully present in every member, he did not present an explanation of how something incorporeal could be bound and affixed to a corporeal substance in a secure and lasting manner.[65] By contrast, the bond between body and soul became a prominent topic taken up by scholars at the courts of Louis the Pious and Charles the Bald.

One of Alcuin's own students, Candidus Wizo, offered an explanation for how the soul could be constrained within a material substance by tempering the extent to which the soul was, in fact, incorporeal.[66] "Just as God is the greatest spirit, thus he is also incorporeal to the highest degree. I say this for the reason that angels and souls and any other spirits that are created, although they are called (and are!) incorporeal, nevertheless in comparison to *his* incorporeality (*incorporalitatis*) and spirit-ness (*spiritalitatis*), as I call it, are in a certain way corporeal."[67] We may well accuse Candidus of being abstruse; yet, by defining God as the only *absolute* incorporeal being, he was able to offer some justification as to why God could never be restricted by time or place, but the soul, on the other hand, was *not* omnipresent.[68] Candidus clarifies that although, in the nature of incorporeal things, the soul is said to be unlocalized, in reality it is located in space because it is constrained within the material world.[69] The argument is an effort to preserve the otherness of the divinity, but it also redefines the soul as an ambiguous substance, neither fully corporeal nor utterly incorporeal.[70]

If Candidus's theology positioned the soul closer to the body along a spectrum of materiality, questions on the soul's nature answered by two other Carolingian scholars in the decades after Alcuin likewise highlighted the symmetry between these entities. Correspondence from Bishop Agobard of Lyon and the monk Gottschalk of Orbais took up a problem that Alcuin had refused to analyze in his treatise for Gundrada—namely, the soul's origin and generation.[71] Shortly before the year 830, Agobard attacked Fredegisus of Tours (Alcuin's successor as abbot) for using the phrase "when the soul reaches the body" in his writings.[72] Ever on the alert for suspicious beliefs and never one to shirk from confrontation, Agobard was determined to expose the danger inherent in Fredegisus's reckless language.[73] By stating that the "soul *reaches* the body," his opponent had implied that souls are not created for specific bodies but have an existence elsewhere in some kind of holding place before being "poured into bodies."[74] Mockingly, Agobard asks whether this holding place is in the north, south, east, or west, or if it rather lies in the heavens or even outside the cosmos? In standing by such a statement, Agobard says, Fredegisus aligns himself with the pagan philosophers, whose writings claim that the soul exists before being born into the body. Not only is there no evidence for this view, Agobard asserts, but the Fathers have taught that "the soul is not part of the divine substance or nature, nor does it exist before it is joined with the body, but it is created at the same time that the body with which it is seen to be united is created."[75]

Like Candidus, then, Agobard was most interested in underscoring the parallels between soul and body and the consequential distinction between the soul's nature and God's. While he studiously avoided offering a concrete description of *how* the soul was formed, citing the mystery of God's work, Agobard clearly was not comfortable with Alcuin's determination that nothing certain could be known about the soul's origins.[76] Instead, he implied that there was doctrinal consensus that the soul came into being when the fetus was generated and cast the shadow of heterodoxy over Fredegisus's words.[77] Fredegisus seems to have remained undaunted in his views, and others may have been equally unconvinced. However, Agobard clearly perceived a need to confirm the unity of body and soul against a theological conjecture that might be seen to endorse the possibility of a spiritual identity separate from a life lived within the body.

It was this same issue of the body and soul's common origins that surfaced in correspondence the monk Gottschalk of Orbais dispensed from his prison at the monastery of Hautvillers.[78] Confined since 849 for his refusal to recant his doctrine of double predestination, Gottschalk nevertheless maintained a reputation as a learned theologian, and the soul was one among many topics he covered in his "underground" writings of the 850s and 860s.[79] Gottschalk agreed with Agobard that the soul came into being at the same time as the body. However, he placed in doubt the assertion that the soul was a substance created in one moment by God because he completely rejected Saint Jerome's argument that the divinity was constantly fashioning new souls for every single baby.[80] This "creationist" argument did not sufficiently explain or accentuate the original sin with which every baby entered the world—a doctrine that Gottschalk believed substantiated his preaching on double predestination. While Augustine had offered no clear refutation of Jerome's position, except to speculate that original sin derived from all new souls being created from Adam's, Gottschalk laid out a detailed (if somewhat imprecise) schema in support of traducianism, the argument that every soul originates from the souls of its parents.[81] Just as human beings may cut a worm into many pieces, and each piece continues to slither about as if it were a discrete unit, so, says Gottschalk, does God cleave soul from soul to create one for every person born.[82] No one, he proclaims, should doubt that, "just as [God] creates the bodies of humans from the seeds of humans, thus also he can create and form the souls of humans (namely of small infants) from the souls of their parents (that is, of fathers and mothers)."[83]

The soul's seed is sown as a result of the sexual act and animates the body that comes into being at the same moment. However, Gottschalk is adamant that this occurs only with God's intention. "Mothers and fathers are not (heaven forbid!) creators (*creatores et creatrices*) of souls in any way, just as they are not creators of bodies, but God alone is, who is the creator of everything."[84] Each animating seed is sown in its own proper body, within which it must remain and with which it will be resurrected. To be sure, Gottschalk's behavior and writings generated extensive controversy, and he seems to have expected that this argument for traducianism would be condemned by his peers.[85] Nevertheless, the basic premise of his theory—that bodies and souls were made specifically for one another by God himself acting within the womb—was, as Agobard pointed out, central to the message of Carolingian preachers that the soul received eternal rewards or damnation for the life lived *while in the body*.[86]

## A Soul Challenged by Logic

Through writings designed to circulate to a broad Carolingian audience, the ninth-century scholars discussed above answered questions both general and particular about the nature of the soul, attempting to influence and establish doctrine by more informal channels.[87] These writings thus stand in contrast to a cluster of treatises solicited around the year 850 by King Charles the Bald. Beginning in the 840s, controversies multiplied across the Carolingian kingdoms, as Gottschalk's preaching on double predestination kicked up a theological dust storm that also came to encompass the punishment experienced by the damned, the presence of Christ's body in the Eucharist, and the beatific vision of God.[88] In this context, an issue that had been on the sidelines came more fully under the public spotlight of Charles the Bald's court, and the king solicited informed opinions, as he did with similar disputes.[89] Treatises on the soul from the 850s hardly represent a new field of inquiry, however; they may have been prompted by the Gottschalk scandal, but they stand in a direct line with Alcuin's initial treatise, likewise composed in response to questions raised at court. Historians have treated the 850s as the only debate about the soul since the fifth century, concentrating on the fact that both incidents were provoked by discussions concerning free will, grace, and Augustinian doctrine.[90] Yet this ignores the long-simmering uncertainty about the soul evident within extant writings from 800 onward.

The outlines of exactly what happened around 850 are hazy and can only tentatively be reconstructed based on three extant texts—a treatise by Ratramnus, a monk at Corbie; a letter likely written by Hincmar, bishop of Reims;[91] and a series of title headings, for which the content is now lost, in a compilation of Gottschalk's works.[92] Both Hincmar and Ratramnus indicate that their decision to compose their respective treatises was due to an external prompt.[93] Hincmar dedicates his work to Charles the Bald and declares that the prompt was the receipt of a booklet (*schedula*) of eight chapters, each of which he deals with consecutively in his treatise.[94] Ratramnus designates no recipient but begins by addressing a superior who has requested that two particular matters be resolved "by the authority of ecclesiastics."[95] Meanwhile, Gottschalk indicates that he exchanged correspondence (probably with a younger monk) on five distinct questions about the soul. The threads linking these three writings lie in the similarity of the topics addressed and the technical vocabulary employed, although there is no indication that any author had access to another's text.[96] That the tone of the treatises is not especially combative distances them from the highly vituperative treatises on predestination.[97] But we can imagine how, in the wake of discussions concerning grace and personal responsibility, Charles the Bald might, like Gundrada, have sought out information on the soul from a desire for knowledge about the self.

An explanation of the soul grounded in self-knowledge and love for God was emphatically *not* what Ratramnus offered to Charles the Bald. Unlike Alcuin, Ratramnus presented a work steeped in dialectical reasoning and the terminology of late antique Neoplatonic and Stoic debates.[98] He himself acknowledged that the work was not for the literate public, and even suggested that his arguments about the soul's nature might be dangerous to some people's spiritual health.[99] This was far from the only thorny subject that the monk of Corbie tackled at the request of Charles the Bald; he found himself at odds with his scholarly and ecclesiastical contemporaries on more than one occasion.[100] Similarly, when it came to the soul, Ratramnus stood apart from his peers and superiors. His methodology was the careful definition of terminology and its application according to logical deductions, which led to a response driven by philosophical rather than pastoral concerns.

At the very beginning of the work, Ratramnus recapitulates the two matters posed to him: whether the soul is circumscribed (*circumscripta*) and localized (*localis*). He then proceeds to define these terms, supporting his definitions with long quotations from different authorities and emphasizing, above all, a strict qualitative dichotomy between body and soul.[101] Thus, with reference to the quality of being localized, the soul is clearly the inverse of the body, Ratramnus states. The body's head, chest, and stomach do not occupy the same space, and consequently, it is divisible into parts that are not equal to the whole. The soul, on the other hand, is not contained in one part of the body but reasons, senses, wills, and remembers in every member. "It is not more in sum than in parts, nor less in a part than in whole."[102] The soul is not divisible and so cannot be localized, Ratramnus concludes.

On the subject of the soul's indivisibility, it should be evident that Ratramnus concurs with previous Carolingian scholars. Like Alcuin, he describes the soul as alive in every part of the body and performing the separate functions of reasoning, calculating, loving, and sensing without being subdivided into those functions. But, whereas Alcuin defined the soul as "circumscribed yet whole in every member of its body," Ratramnus is adamant that an incorporeal soul cannot be confined by the boundaries of the physical flesh.[103] All corporeal entities, being situated in space, Ratramnus explains, are circumscribed because they are distinguished by physical limits. In antithetical fashion, then, the utterly incorporeal soul is incapable of being circumscribed. Unlike Candidus and Gottschalk, both of whom were willing to concede some degree of corporeality, Ratramnus maintains that the soul "is contained by no limit of the body."[104] In doing so, as Gerard Mathon has emphasized, he was the only Carolingian thinker to hold rigidly to the principle that an incorporeal soul cannot be fixed in place by a body.[105]

At the same time, in order to maintain a distinction between the soul and God, who alone is omnipresent in the universe, Ratramnus is forced to acknowledge that the soul both is and is not defined by circumscription. He resolves this problem by arguing that the soul "is circumscribed by its own qualities and not by the border of the body."[106] Similarly, in order to maintain the absolute incorporeality of the soul, Ratramnus declares that it governs by means of "an incorporeal nod," such that the soul "commands the body through a precise intention *not* by material force."[107] Although the nod moves the body through space, the soul itself, being fixed like a hinge or joint, does not move in any way. Both Alcuin and Ratramnus cited the same work by Augustine to explain how the soul directs and interacts with the body, but in choosing different passages they conveyed distinct theological points.[108] Not being as concerned with a strict definition of incorporeality as

Ratramnus, Alcuin allowed the finer materials of light and air to act as mediums between soul and body (thus suggesting that the immaterial and material could still "touch" in some fashion).

In the manner that Ratramnus sought to highlight, above all, how the "essence of the soul and body is not the same," he significantly departed from the model set by Alcuin, who preferred to stress the soul as intermediary between God and body.[109] By refusing to accept the notion that the embodied soul was bound within the physical limits of the body by anything other than its own spiritual characteristics, Ratramnus essentially severed the innate links between body and soul that other ninth-century scholars were concerned to maintain. The suggestion that, aside from a vague inclination to inhabit the body's space, the soul was under no compulsion to remain within it, treated the body as an accidental container, one animated by the life of the soul but otherwise holding little import.[110] This very divergence from the other soul treatises examined here should highlight for us the way in which *most* Carolingian thinkers prioritized a framework that upheld the coherence and integrity of the bipartite individual.

## A Soul Firmly Bound to Its Home

In contrast to Alcuin, Agobard, and even Gottschalk, Ratramnus framed the soul primarily as a logical problem that was best approached by way of dialectical reasoning rather than a reliance on specific moral and doctrinal principles. That his work should not be taken as representative of ninth-century solutions to the soul-body enigma is best seen by comparing it to two contemporaneous soul treatises. As noted above, the first was written around 850 by Hincmar, bishop of Reims, as a response to King Charles the Bald's queries. The second was composed in 856 by Hrabanus, bishop of Mainz, for King Lothar II of Lotharingia.[111] Both these treatises were crafted by prominent bishops who judged it their duty to teach and advise Carolingian rulers; both were designed to be accessible to a wider audience; and both assumed that knowledge about the soul was important in order for a ruler to be able to govern his subjects correctly. Not only do they return to the style of Alcuin's letter to Gundrada, but they also share Alcuin's emphasis on the soul as mediator. In this case, Hincmar and Hrabanus situate the soul in a kind of middle ground, theoretically incorporeal but practically possible to localize and enclose within a corporeal home.

Hincmar opens his treatise by praising Charles for cherishing "those parts of philosophy that are known to reach toward the pinnacle of true and singular wisdom" and by linking the search for wisdom with the soul's ability to seek, approach, and perceive the divine.[112] The preface draws explicit links among divine favor, successful rulership, desire for education, and knowledge of the soul. In emphasizing that Charles ought to study his treatise because no one can know God "who does not take care to know himself," Hincmar underscored in bold terms that an accurate understanding of the soul was critical to the prosperity of self and state.[113] Despite the initial similarity with Alcuin's work for Gundrada, after the preface Hincmar's treatise diverges from his predecessor's to tackle many of the same problems addressed by Ratramnus on corporeality, localization, physical boundaries, and movement through time and space.[114] At first glance, indeed, Hincmar appears to reiterate the same doctrine as Ratramnus, defining the soul as a spirit that is a simple substance, impossible to localize, and moved through time but not space. Hincmar even quotes some of the very same selections from patristic authorities that Ratramnus employs.[115] However, such parallels belie a stark disparity in how the two intellectuals viewed the essential nature of the soul—a disparity that has been overlooked by scholars focused on the Carolingians' faithfulness to Augustinian Neoplatonism.[116]

As to whether the soul is corporeal, Hincmar weaves an ambiguous answer that defines the soul as a "life-giving spirit" (*not* a body) but ultimately fails to classify it as an incorporeal being. He begins by stating that the soul seems "the least corporeal" to humans because it is not made from the four elements (earth, air, fire, water).[117] However, while the soul is a simple (indivisible) substance compared to the composite body, Hincmar observes, compared to the immutable God, the soul is a complex and versatile substance, since it is beset by ever-changing feelings and impulses. Consequently, the soul cannot be called simply "spirit" because God and the angels are proper spirits, and the soul is not the same as them. Furthermore, although the soul does not depend upon the body for thought and is not perceived by bodily sight, Hincmar claims that it "perceives and is perceived with the semblance of a body" when it contemplates various matters in sleep or in ecstasy.[118] Augustine had used the fact that the soul often envisions itself in bodily form in dreams to argue for the soul's incorporeality—the dream images drawn from memory could not possibly be corporeal, he states, and only an incorporeal soul could hold incorporeal images within itself.[119] Hincmar includes none of this rather complex discussion, and his loose adaptation of Augustine's words on the matter suggest the very opposite of what the Father argued. Without ever declaring the soul to be *incorporea*, Hincmar concludes this section on the soul's quality by stating that "even if [the soul] is not understood to be a body, which it is not, nevertheless it is believed to possess a corporeal likeness (*similitudinem corpoream*)."[120] He effectively leaves his reader with an understanding of the soul that situates it somewhere between an elemental body and an incorporeal spirit.

Hincmar sets up arguments throughout the treatise in a similarly equivocal fashion. He includes quotations from the Fathers that define the soul as incorporeal but never employs this term himself—except when he repeats the doctrine espoused by Candidus Wizo approximately fifty years earlier that "those things, which are by nature incorporeal, in comparison to him [God] should be considered just as if they were corporeal."[121] With similar ambiguity, Hincmar cites Gregory the Great's declaration that, "although the soul is incorporeal, nevertheless because it clings to the body, it is recognized to be localized (*localis*) on account of that very quality of itself which is detained to carnal places."[122] This seems to endorse Ratramnus's belief that the soul is constrained to the body by its own qualities and not by physical boundaries, but Ratramnus strenuously and consistently denies that the soul can ever be defined as *localis*.[123] Hincmar, on the other hand, freely applies the terms *circumscripta* and *localis* to the soul.

If Ratramnus's primary concern was to preserve the soul's incorporeality, the emphasis within Hincmar's treatise is "the incomprehensible bond (*copulam incomprehensibilem*) with the body."[124] The longest assembly of scriptural and patristic quotations in the treatise is used to support Hincmar's assertion that "although it is a spirit, the soul is contained by the body in a miraculous and ineffable way."[125] He is convinced that the soul cannot separate from the body according to its inclination; it can withdraw from the senses in sleep or in ecstasy, but it can leave the body only in death, with the assent of God.[126] Indeed, in answering the question of "whether the soul is held spatially in the body," Hincmar seems to grow increasingly incensed, finally erupting: "Look how many and what types of proofs (not mere arguments) show us that souls are clothed by, joined with, and bound to bodies! It seems dangerous to us to oppose their authority."[127] If anyone does not believe these proofs, Hincmar continues, that person should be banished from the communion of the *ecclesia*. While there is no indication that Hincmar had Ratramnus in mind here, it is certainly the case that this work for Charles the Bald was designed to highlight the soul-body union above all else.[128]

In many of the same ways that Hincmar positioned the soul as a spirit that was not entirely incorporeal, Hrabanus, too, embraced a vision of the soul that made it tangible within the body. Like Hincmar, Hrabanus opens his treatise by praising Lothar II's desire for knowledge and suggesting that this work will assist him in his various duties as king.[129] Lothar had just succeeded to his position after his father's death in 855, and Hrabanus was in many ways continuing a relationship that he had forged with the father, who had requested a series of biblical commentaries from this renowned scholar.[130] Just as Hrabanus offered Lothar I exegesis that he could carry with him on campaigns, so did he compose for Lothar II a work that summarized a range of essential topics: the soul, the four virtues, the body, and, finally, a few chapters on Roman military training.[131] The eclectic nature of the topics highlights how knowledge about the soul was deemed practical, not an abstract theological exercise. As an advisor, Hrabanus supplied information to protect the kingdom and to secure the salvation of its subjects, writing succinctly so that the work might be committed to memory.[132] This may have been the last text ever written by the bishop, who, at the age of seventy-six and after several years of ill health, would that same year experience the separation of his own soul and body.[133]

The definition of the soul that Hrabanus supplies in many ways resembles that found in Alcuin's treatise: "The soul is created by God, a spiritual and individual substance, vivifying its body, rational and immortal but changeable both to good and to evil."[134] Like those before him, Hrabanus equates the soul with both reason and life force and proclaims that it is made in the image of God and thus shares in God's immortality but not in his divine substance. Only humans have a soul (*anima*) that animates the body and lives on after its death, Hrabanus explains, whereas animals have a spirit (*spiritus*) that dies with an injury to the physical body.[135] Reiterating the same terms put forth by Ratramnus—that the substance of the soul is spiritual and simple—Hrabanus emphasizes much more than Hincmar that the soul's spirituality means "it has nothing in it that is corporeal," and that this incorporeal nature allows it to contemplate divine and invisible matters.[136] Similarly, he includes no statement that the soul should be considered corporeal relative to God's incorporeality. In absolute contrast to bodies, which are solid, palpable, and demarcated, souls are incorporeal, formless, and uncontainable within a delineated space (*spatio linearum*), Hrabanus asserts.[137]

Even as Hrabanus seems to fall closer to Ratramnus in how he defines the substance of the soul, his descriptions of how this spiritual substance exists in a physical body bring him more in line with Hincmar. Though the soul lacks height, width, and depth, Hrabanus speaks about it being "weighed down by the mass of the body."[138] He explains how the soul "is a unique substance because no other spirit takes up matter in such a way that it feels pain or rejoices with the experiences of its own body."[139] Here, the soul is not only the instrument (*organum*) of the body's members, regulating and governing them, but it is also depicted as dependent upon those members, being directly affected by their physical state or constitution. In children, Hrabanus affirms, "on account of the smallness of their members, the power and reason of the soul is impeded," and in youth and elderly people "it is suppressed by a certain irregularity of their parts or thickness of their humors (*humorum crassitudine*)."[140] In allowing for the power of the soul to be affected by the bodily elements, Hrabanus implies a physical connection between two substances that he has elsewhere defined as divergent—the one, a solid, delineated form composed of the elements, the other a formless spirit, containing nothing corporeal within it.[141]

Despite his logical exposition on why an incorporeal soul cannot possess a form, Hrabanus concedes a major point that undermines the soul's inability to be spatially delineated. Whereas Alcuin, Ratramnus, and Hincmar underscored that the soul is fully present in all parts of the body, Hrabanus argues for the existence of a principal seat of the soul.[142] "Although the soul is diffused throughout all the members of the body," he begins, "nevertheless, as is evident by tangible signs, it does not preside equally in all the members."[143] According to the bishop, others have argued that the seat of the soul is the heart because they believe that good and evil thoughts arise in the place where the purest blood and vital spirit are found. Hrabanus, however, favors those who see the head as the soul's principal residence. His proof is scripture's statement that God, although omnipresent, holds a seat in the heavens—likewise the soul, made in the image of God, sits in the pinnacle of the body.[144] He adds that the roundness of the skull mirrors the heavenly sphere, which is where the soul desires a permanent home.[145] Furthermore, because finer elements like fire tend upwards, so does the delicate substance of the soul tend toward the highest part of the body. The bishop's final point of evidence is the fact that all five senses are found in the head and that changes in the soul's emotions are immediately signaled in facial expressions.

With every detail in this argument, Hrabanus endorses a soul that can be localized within the body, thereby seriously undercutting its incorporeal and indivisible nature. If he is prepared to compare the soul's behavior to that of the elements, his willingness stems from a desire to present the body as the perfect residence for the soul. Asserting that the nature and state of the soul can actually be mapped onto the physical form and read therein, Hrabanus forges an interdependent relationship between the soul and its own little home.[146]

## Back to Blood and Barontus

The book of Leviticus declares that "the soul of every body is in the blood."[147] Despite the apparent relevance of this passage to developing theologies of the soul, only the treatises of Hincmar and Hrabanus take up the question of the soul's relationship to blood. Both authors drew on Cassiodorus's explanation that this passage refers exclusively to animals, whose life ends when blood is lacking. The human *anima*, by contrast, takes its very name from *anaema*, meaning "distinct from blood." While the human soul animates its own proper body, which is nourished by blood, it lives on after the death of that body.[148] Clarifying the distinction between the death of the soul and the death of the body, Hrabanus explains that "it is one thing to desert a home at the appropriate moment and another thing to make an end with that home."[149] Thus, as a spiritual substance, the soul cannot be destroyed by an effusion of blood, and yet, a lack of blood prompts the soul to abandon its home. Here, we can see ninth-century theologians grappling with the same problem faced by the reviser of the *Dispute*: how to relate the physiological processes of dying to the life of an invisible, incorporeal entity?

Why did these two bishops deem it necessary to address a topic that no other Carolingian treatise on the soul included within its orbit? The answer may lie in a greater familiarity with Cassiodorus's *On the Soul*, in a newfound interest in exegesis of Leviticus (Hrabanus and Claudius of Turin composed the first commentaries on this book since the fifth century), or perhaps in the more widespread circulation of texts such as the medical material discussed above.[150] In contemplating when a coagulated substance in the womb is first animated, for example, Hrabanus observes that "investigators of nature (*naturarum investigatores*) assert that the mortal and human breast receives the soul on the fortieth day of conception, and this is verified because then [the fetus] begins to move in the womb."[151] Both he and Ratramnus invoke the theories of "philosophers" and "men of expertise" in their treatises, Hrabanus with the aim of proving that Christian knowledge confirms and improves these theories.[152] Whether the bishop had read texts such as those by Vindicianus is not clear.[153] However, it is entirely possible that the medical tradition copied within Carolingian scriptoria formed a kind of "background noise" that subtly shaped the composition of treatises on the soul.

We can say with more certainty that the ideas found in ninth-century medical codices are by no means as divergent from beliefs expressed in the soul treatises as they may first appear. Both genres display a concern with demarcating a soul that clings to the body, one that is corporeally grounded while still distinct from temporal matter. To be sure, no theological treatise argues that blood is the seat of the soul; yet, despite avowals of incorporeality, works by Candidus, Hincmar, and Hrabanus favor imagery and language that ascribe some material presence to the soul, make it more tangible in space, and render it more accessible through its counterpart, the body. The rational soul, as all of the treatises emphasize, needs to be incorporeal in order to bear the image of an incorporeal God. But for that soul to act as mediator between God and matter, it needs a touch of corporeality to be capable of governing its physical home.

This chapter has sought to highlight the different approaches taken by various Carolingian authors in their attempts to present a concise account of the soul's nature. Given that many of these authors share a similar vocabulary and cite the same Church Fathers, there has been a tendency to see these ninth-century discussions as mere repetitions, especially as another iteration of the fifth-century clash in southern Gaul between Platonic and Stoic theories of the soul.[154] However, as Lockett elucidates, our conception of distinct philosophical positions may well have been invisible to the Carolingians, in part because Stoic doctrines on the soul sometimes circulated under the name of Neoplatonic thinkers like Augustine, and in part because authorities like Gregory the Great and Isidore of Seville themselves expounded an "eclectic psychology" of the soul.[155]

Instead of classifying Carolingian soul treatises according to their varying adherence to late antique philosophical sects, it is more illuminating to compare the treatises to one another. In doing so, we find that Ratramnus was the only intellectual to set the matter of the soul's incorporeality above all other considerations. Compared to his dense, philosophical language, the other treatises spoke about self-knowledge in terms that were accessible. And, we can assume, accessible to both men and women, as *no* treatise indicated that gender had any influence on the soul-body relationship, and Alcuin's

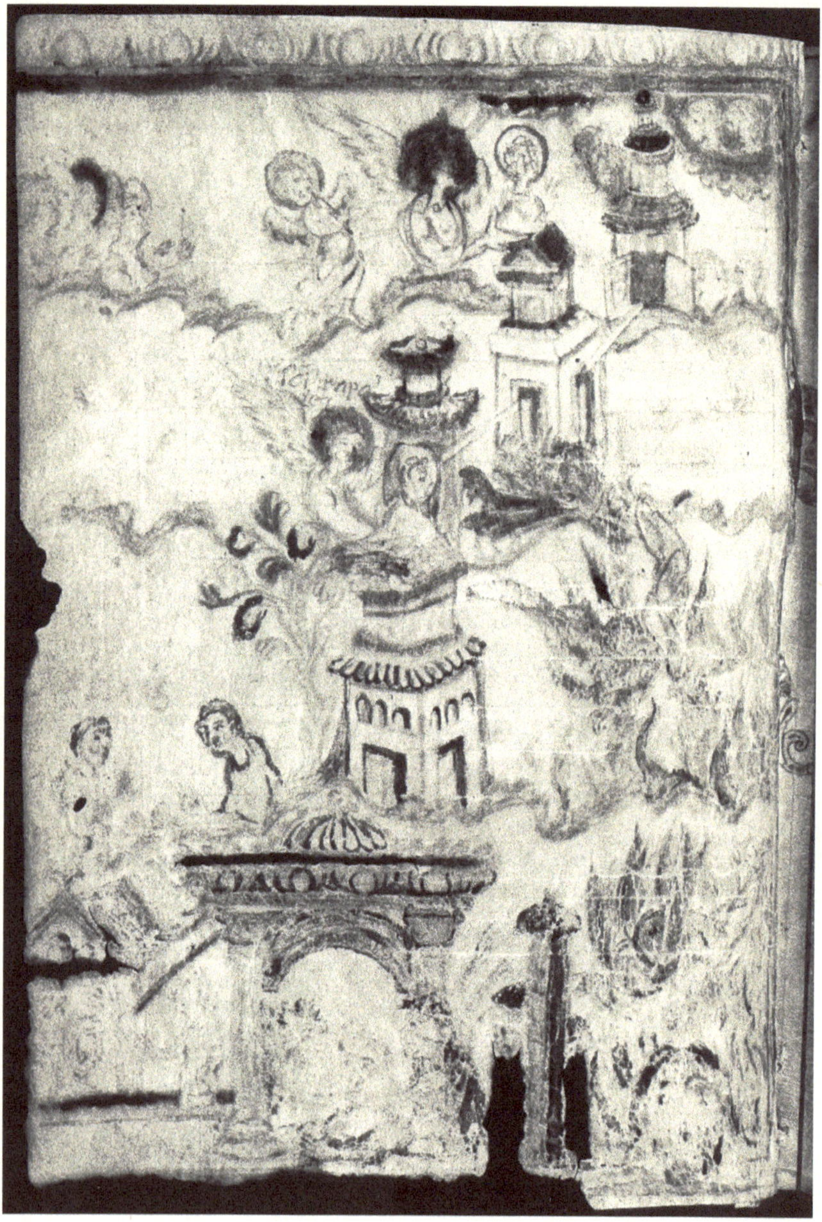

Figure 3. Frontispiece to the *Vision of Barontus* in St. Petersburg, National Library of Russia, lat. O. v. I. 5, f. 1v. Photo credit: Lawrence Nees. By kind permission of the National Library.

treatise, in being dedicated to Gundrada, explicitly drew attention to the unsexed nature of the soul.

The first-person description of the soul found in the late seventh-century *Vision of Barontus*, with which we began this chapter, seems to have appealed to a Carolingian audience as the text survives in multiple copies from the ninth century.[156] Among these was one illustrated version, found in a codex produced at Reims, possibly for Charles the Bald himself.[157] The frontispiece depicts the scene where the monk's tiny soul (with its five senses) is carried off to heaven: we see the archangel Raphael bearing aloft a sculpted bust of Barontus's head, of normal size but without any functional capacity (see Figure 3). There is a distinct correspondence between the illustrator's choices and Hincmar's and Hrabanus's declarations that the soul has "a corporeal likeness" and resides in the head, where it maintains a connection with the bodily senses and facial expressions. Given that this illustrator was working around 850 and displays connections with artistic and theological trends at Charles's court, can we associate this unique set of images with debates about the soul's nature active at the very same moment?[158] If so, as Charles was reflecting on Hincmar's and Ratramnus's answers to his queries, he may well have had before him a picture of his own tiny interior soul, molded in his physical likeness, guiding his actions from its bodily pinnacle.

# CHAPTER 2

# The Self

## "To Have and to Hold from This Day Forward, for Better, for Worse"

In the early 840s, as civil war shattered the empire and divided the nobility, Dhuoda, the wife of the former royal chamberlain, set to work on a handbook for William, her teenage son. William was then being held as a hostage at the court of Charles the Bald, as surety for the continuing loyalty of his father, Count Bernard of Septimania. It was a pressing concern for William's safety that, Dhuoda states, drove her to put her thoughts down in writing.[1] From her husband's estate in Uzès, over the course of two years, Dhuoda composed her *Handbook* (*Liber manualis*) as a replacement for her physical presence in William's formative years. It was a mother's memory book, a courtier's etiquette guide, and a spiritual instruction manual brought together in one compact form.[2]

If the world around Dhuoda appeared to be fracturing as various members of the imperial family turned against one another, it is in contrast—or, we might speculate, in reaction—a message of harmony that pervaded Dhuoda's *Handbook*. This affirmation of concord is witnessed in Dhuoda's description of the strong bonds of love infusing her family (in direct contradiction to the tales of infidelity that were circulating about Count Bernard). It is also evident in her conviction that the loyalty owed to God, father, and lord could be fulfilled without conflict (although the current internecine struggles among the Frankish aristocracy might have suggested otherwise).[3] Thirdly, and most importantly for our purposes, the message of harmony is attested in Dhuoda's remarkable emphasis on the indestructible unity of body and soul. This is a theme that recurs throughout the pages of the *Handbook* and yet has been consistently overlooked by modern scholars.[4] It must, however, have been one of the most important lessons that William was meant to imbibe because it was the foundation upon which he could construct both his spiritual and social identity.

As the only lengthy text by a Carolingian laywoman to survive, the *Handbook* is often treated as an exception. But, when it comes to the body, if we trace an arc across the advisory texts that preceded Dhuoda's, it becomes clear that her perspective and agenda are less exceptional than they may first appear.[5] Her outlook is simply an especially evocative signal of a broader imaginative and intellectual shift, in which imagery of the "self as battleground" was gradually supplanted by language evoking the partnership of body and soul.

## Advisory Literature for the Laity

The previous chapter explored ninth-century assumptions concerning the soul's embodiment—the connections, at the individual level, between matter and spirit. This chapter confronts the moral aspects of that relationship. How was the rational soul's dominion over the body to be exercised? And how did a consideration of identity through these binary entities encourage a certain type of inward reflection? These questions will lead us into medical writings in Chapter 7, but before it is possible to analyze modes of bodily care, we must assess the value ascribed to such care. Here, then, we are pursuing the question of *salus* (understood primarily as spiritual health) as a negotiation between body and soul, in order to illuminate the status of the flesh within Carolingian ethics.

The body has a tendency to fade away beneath the constant references to the soul and its welfare in Carolingian didactic literature. Yet behind every movement and habit stood the body, and the authors explored here assumed that its regulation was essential to ethical living—where they differed, I argue, was whether the goal was to punish or protect the flesh's own well-being. In order to maintain a grip on this ubiquitous but ill-defined "body," I focus on a detailed analysis of texts within a single genre; I then shift attention to similar developments in a wider range of contemporary works. The aim is not only to illuminate the key concepts and metaphors that different authors employed in their models of the virtuous life but also to reveal the chronological patterns suggested by comparing the various works.

At the heart of this chapter are four texts that were written for the Carolingian lay elite as guides to assist them in navigating the temporal world with their attention fixed on eternal salvation.[6] These are Bishop Paulinus of Aquileia's *Book of Admonition* for Duke Eric of Friuli (ca. 795); Alcuin's *On the Virtues and Vices* for Count Wido of the Breton March (ca. 800); Bishop Jonas of Orléans's *On Lay Instruction* for Count Matfrid of Orléans (ca. 825); and Dhuoda's *Handbook* for her son William (ca. 843).[7] Because both Jonas and Dhuoda refer to their works as a "mirror," in which their readers should be able to see a reflection of their souls, these are often known as the lay *specula* (mirrors), although here I will refer to them as the lay manuals or handbooks.[8] The four texts have typically been cast as a subcategory within the larger genre of "mirrors for princes," advice written for medieval and early modern rulers.[9] However, as Rachel Stone observes, the first such "mirrors" were directed to the Carolingian laity and actually predated those for royalty.[10]

While Paulinus, Alcuin, and Jonas were important churchmen at the courts of Charlemagne and Louis the Pious, what groups these works together is not the characteristics shared by the authors but the audience for whom each text was written.[11] As Andrew Romig has illuminated, Paulinus's and Alcuin's mirrors were revolutionary for how they espoused a model of "elite discipleship" for the laity grounded in the same performance of charity that the ascetic male embodied.[12] All four authors—abbot, bishops, and mother alike—acted from a sense of pastoral responsibility when they composed their manuals. They deemed it necessary to guide others on the path toward salvation and to correct faults they perceived in contemporary society.[13] This was a paternal as well as a pastoral charge, and one that Dhuoda, assuming the spiritual authority of a father, evidently believed herself compelled to shoulder in regard to the younger generation.[14] Not only do the manuals evince a common ideological agenda, but, to the extent that the authors demonstrate an awareness of the others' works, they also share an intellectual genealogy.[15] While each of the four texts was explicitly composed for one individual, the authors seem to have been convinced that they were contributing to the welfare of the general populace.[16] Paulinus and Jonas both re-edited their original compositions with the intention that they circulate more widely.[17]

And Jonas and Dhuoda overtly refer to the possibility that Matfrid and William might share the works with their peers.[18] Of all the manuals, however, Alcuin's *On the Virtues and Vices* was the most popular, with several dozen copies extant from the early Middle Ages and an audience that encompassed laity and ecclesiastics.[19] Such fluidity is often witnessed among Carolingian didactic texts—despite a prescriptive insistence that different "orders" within society should follow a distinctive way of life, one finds a remarkably porous boundary between works ostensibly tailored to a secular versus ecclesiastical reader.[20]

Given the strong ideological ties among the four texts, this chapter treats the handbooks by Paulinus, Alcuin, Jonas, and Dhuoda as part of a semicoherent textual group.[21] It focuses in particular on these extant manuals for the very reason that they were deemed by their authors to be broadly applicable to diverse members of society (and I include the possibility that women as well as men might have been part of their intended audience).[22] It is the works' shared fundamental sense of a spiritual mission that allows for a greater appreciation of the subtle but significant contrasts revealed in a chronological comparison.[23] And so, while other scholars have concentrated primarily on the similarities among these four works, this chapter pursues, above all, the points upon which they diverge. Certainly, there are a number of superficial differences among the manuals in terms of length, structure, citations, and personal details.[24] But it is the authors' varying assumptions about the body-soul union that interest us here.

Although their specific advice differed, the four authors worked from the same conviction—that readers needed to be taught how to develop a mode of self-reflection.[25] With the lay manuals, unlike monastic handbooks, we are not dealing primarily with rules for the operation of a community (although they certainly offer concrete instruction on the duties of judge, spouse, and parent, for example).[26] Rather, the manuals present the belief that correct behavior and communal welfare will spring from an accurate knowledge of the mechanisms by which an individual operates in the world—above all, through the interplay among soul, body, external stimuli, and divine contact. The laity were not being taught the importance of obedience (as with monks to their abbot) so much as the practice of monitoring their own inner existence. In this way, the turn of the ninth century brought a new insistence on the value of rigorous mindfulness. And yet, in encouraging certain patterns of reflection, these authors utilized different terminology and imagery, which itself must surely have influenced the disposition of those who sought to follow the handbooks' advice.

## From Conflict to Harmony

In the earliest of these spiritual manuals, Paulinus, bishop of Aquileia, fashioned an approach to individual identity that established a strong dichotomy between body and soul.[27] Paulinus begins the *Book of Admonition* by explaining the constitution of Eric's very own self, highlighting the most important part of his being, the image of God in his soul. This soul with its wondrous image is, Paulinus explains, Eric's *interior homo*, and it consists of three parts: intellect, will, and memory.[28] It is essential that Eric be able to picture his soul because that is where his true identity lies, and it is the only path by which he can draw closer to God. The opening thus recalls the soul treatises discussed in the previous chapter—a point that evinces the threads consistently (if invisibly) connecting theoretical outlines of the nature of the soul and hortatory discussions of the moral life.[29]

Paulinus's worldview is dominated by a sense of opposition. It is not simply that the material world and the body are the sources of sin; it is that the body appears irredeemable, and the most the soul can do is subdue it. Paulinus explains that "it is the flesh that ruins the soul," because it is there that the devil inserts his influence.[30] It is no symbolic or metaphorical insertion that Paulinus invokes; his entire scheme of the individual person rests upon a belief in a strict binary between the body, which can come under the sway of the devil, and the soul, which cannot. Though demons with their goads are the ultimate cause of the soul's ruin, Paulinus is clear that these demons affect the soul only because they control it through the body. "The soul does not sin except through the flesh," Paulinus explains succinctly to Eric.[31] There is no distinction between sins of the body and sins of the soul, as we will find in other Carolingian manuals, but instead all of the blame is rooted in the essence of the contrary body. The body is hardly a participant in Eric's search for salvation, and little allusion is made to its eventual redemption or resurrection.[32] Instead, it is a burden on the soul, suffocating it, dragging it down to hell. The relationship between body and soul can never, Paulinus implies, be a harmonious one while on earth. "Our body fights daily against the soul; and daily we ought to fight against our body."[33]

Eric, a layman, is here presented with a vision of his life as a direct battle with the devil and his minions. Like the Egyptian Fathers in the desert, Eric is supposed to fend off the constant attacks of demons seeking to undermine his spiritual progress toward God. Just as the fifth-century ascetic Evagrius had designated the vices as eight different demons, so was Eric taught by Paulinus to confront sin as a demonic force.[34] The *interior homo* may be protected within the shell of the body, the *Book of Admonition* suggests, but if that body is penetrated by the devil's presence then the soul's image of God, in turn, is corrupted by the impure body housing it.[35] The struggle against evil takes place within the individual, but it is fought against external forces constantly pressing on the body in their attempts to corrupt the soul.[36] "It is the flesh that receives the devil, for the devil sows his seeds in our flesh."[37]

As Paulinus begins his work with a description of the soul, he ends it with "a prayer of the soul to God against the evils of the body," a tirade that encompasses nearly a tenth of the entire handbook.[38] Ending the text with a first-person narrative of the soul was an evocative and persuasive stylistic flourish. Presumably, Eric and other readers were supposed to envision this as the voice of their own soul and be moved, consequently, to carry out the dictates of the text with more fervent devotion. The soul is asked how it would respond to the evils described of the body and replies: "Because the flesh with which I live always wishes to lead me to sin, because it wishes to be crowned with me but it does not want to struggle [for eternal life] with me, I suffer no worse enemy than my body in which I live."[39] Since the body and soul are irrevocably yoked together in the earthly world, Paulinus clarifies for Eric that one of his constant concerns must be the management of his own "worst enemy," his body. The language that Paulinus uses to characterize the nature of this managerial relationship is telling: the body, he asserts, should be subjugated to the soul "just as a domestic slave should serve her mistress."[40] The handbook is teaching Eric how to think about his identity, in terms of how the self is originally constituted and how it is constantly reconstituted through the dynamics of the battlefield.

In addition to his comparison of the body to a slave, Paulinus invokes an ancient metaphor of the soul as charioteer in order to shape his readers' perceptions of how they must strive for salvation. He draws this metaphor from one of his chief sources, a late fifth-century spiritual manual addressed to young monks.[41] The image is intended, again, to present the soul and body as bound but opposing forces and to impress upon readers the necessity of strictly disciplining the flesh.

> Just as bridles must be set on horses, thus our bodies must be bridled by fasts and prayers. For in the same way that charioteers, if they loosen the bridles, are drawn precipitously downward, thus also the soul, with its body, if we do not set a bridle on it, will fall into the precipices of hell. Therefore let us be good and learned charioteers of our bodies.[42]

Eric had probably never witnessed a chariot race, but in northern Italy he may well have seen surviving depictions of ancient Roman races, where charioteers looped the reins around their bodies to better control the horses (see Figure 4).[43] This technique made any fall that much more dangerous, as an experienced warrior and horseman like Eric would have recognized. The soul, as the metaphor urged, had to be constantly aware of the instincts of the body and manage them appropriately, thereby ensuring the temporal stability and purity of the individual while also drawing itself toward its own eternal salvation. As the final monologue makes clear, it was essential for the soul to

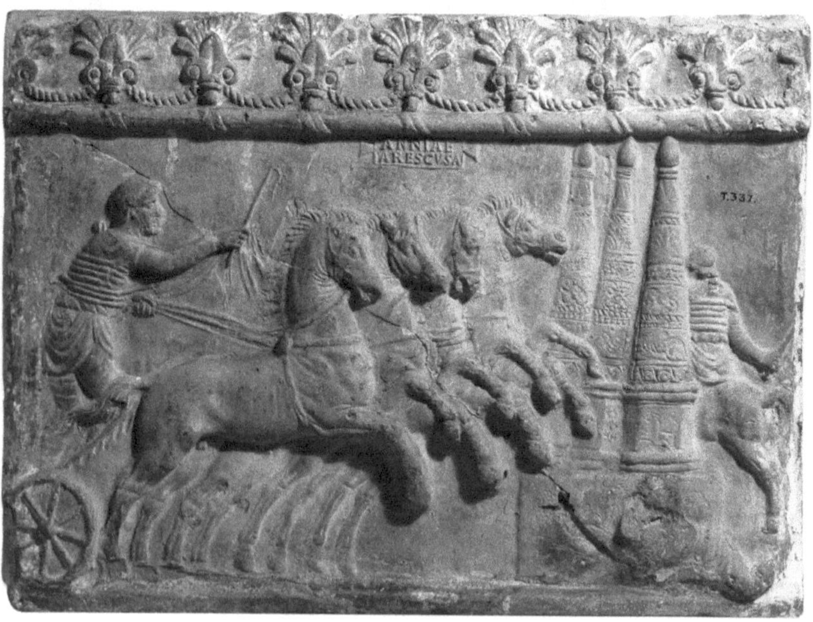

Figure 4. A four-horse chariot approaches the turning post, driven by a charioteer who has the reins wrapped tightly about his body. Terracotta plaque, Italy, first century C.E. © Trustees of the British Museum. All rights reserved.

implore Christ's help in cultivating the virtues and discerning rationally (*discernere rationabiliter*) how to keep the body away from evil so that it could successfully perform good deeds in life.[44]

* * *

Paulinus may have been the first to offer a written guide for the Carolingian layperson, but while others took up a comparable duty, they apparently were not constrained by the model he put forth. Similar themes and injunctions reappear, but the tone and style of the later works are distinct. Comparing Paulinus's work to Dhuoda's, the last of the extant lay manuals, highlights in particular a radical divergence in their treatments of the body.

Dhuoda informs William at the opening of her work: "Know that everything, through it all, in it all, is intended entirely for you, for the health of your soul and your body."[45] This is a point that she returns to again and again. At the close of the work she reiterates: "I have dictated these little verses, above, here, and below, as well as many other things, for your soul and body."[46] Throughout the *Handbook*, Dhuoda uses the phrase "soul (*anima*) and body" or "mind (*mens*) and body" over twenty times; just as in the theological treatises (from Chapter 1), she does not seem to distinguish between the terms *anima* and *mens*. She instructs William to read and reflect in his soul and body, to be loyal in soul and body, to be humble and pure in soul and body, and to cultivate patience and gentleness of soul and body. She calls God the governor of one's soul and body; similarly, she calls priests the guardians of one's soul and body. William must love God in his soul and body; he must carry the yoke of Christ in his soul and body; he must pray for the soul and body of his relative Theoderic; he must fix the virtues and the gifts of the Holy Spirit in soul and body. If William follows his mother's advice and seeks God constantly, he will (she assures him) receive "all that is necessary for the enjoyment of [his] soul and [his] body" as well as "attain the salvation not only of his body but of his soul."[47]

Sometimes Dhuoda uses the pair soul and body in a metaphorical sense, as a way to compare rewards and securities granted in the earthly life to those granted for eternal life.[48] Her worries for William encompass the practical—land, honors, political influence—as well as the spiritual, so it is not surprising to find an emphasis within the *Handbook* on temporal affairs.[49] While the other three lay manuals tend to be somewhat wary about the accumulation of temporal goods, since they draw the mind away from spiritual reflection,

Dhuoda emphasizes that obedient and devoted service to God will necessarily yield material wealth.[50] Just as she accepts without angst the temporal goods bestowed by God, so does Dhuoda cast the body as an inherently good part of God's creation. The parallels between the earthly and heavenly life that anchor Dhuoda's thought may have encouraged her to invoke the relationship between body and soul as representative of the two spheres of individual pursuit.[51] And yet, one cannot say that it was simply her dual concerns for William's eventual salvation and his current safety that caused her to turn constantly to this pairing.

Through her continual repetition of the phrase "soul and body" Dhuoda implicitly argues for an understanding of identity that is harmoniously singular. In this way, her account of the relationship between soul and body is a pronounced example of a discursive shift in talking about the self.[52] The *Handbook* never refers to the need for the soul to govern the body, unlike the other three advisory handbooks, but rather assumes that body and soul *can* work together, and *ought* to work together, to cultivate virtue and reject vice.

Only twice does Dhuoda suggest that soul and body might not act in concert and harmony. The first time is in quoting Paul's dictum that "the flesh lusts against the spirit, and the spirit against the flesh [Gal 5:17]."[53] Yet, even here, she mitigates the antagonism implied in this statement with her ensuing explanation that the ancient Fathers fought this passion with a spirit of gentleness and leniency.[54] The second time is in a section on fornication, where she observes that, as a result of the devil's persuasions, "a sting of the body" (*stimulus carnis*) may stir William to sin.[55] This same phrase is found in Paulinus's *Book of Admonition*, but unlike Paulinus, Dhuoda attributes to the devil not solely the power of attacking the body but equally of assaulting the soul. The root of fornication can come from the devil stinging the body or slapping the mind, she asserts.[56]

Dhuoda's model of the virtuous life is one in which "the soundness of the soul rests secure through all things and guides its body, unharmed, to a lofty end!"[57] Her example of this life is the prophet Moses, who was at peace in his mind and enjoyed a healthy and intact body—to the extent of preserving all his teeth up until the end of his life.[58] The language and images employed throughout the *Handbook* present physical health and old age as the natural corollaries to a life of devoted prayer and charitable action in the world. Dhuoda's anxiety about her son's dangerous situation—her tangible concern for his physical existence—may well underlie her elevation of the healthy body as a sacred ideal. Nevertheless, even for the privileged in the premodern world, physical well-being was *always* precarious, and children's lives especially were recognized to be fragile and often fleeting. We fail to take Dhuoda's teaching about the body seriously if we attribute it merely to maternal angst about her son's political circumstances.

Dhuoda was educating her readers in a specific theology of the body, not naively writing in haste or out of a motherly desire to comfort her beloved son. This is manifest most clearly in the sections that follow the title *Counsel of Singular Usefulness* (*Admonitio singularis utilissima*), which Janet Nelson has pinpointed as the "fulcrum of the whole work."[59] Drawing on Ovid and Augustine, Dhuoda outlines a twofold definition of birth and death that represents her dual concern for William's temporal and eternal health while simultaneously justifying her own role as spiritual advisor.[60] Every Christian has a physical birth from a mother's body and a spiritual birth in Christ, she explains. Although no human can escape a first death in "the migration from the body," those who cling to Christ can avoid a second death of the soul to eternal damnation. Weaving parallels and intersections among these sets of two, as she does throughout the entire *Handbook*, Dhuoda emphasizes not the denigration of being born into a body and passing out of it but rather the fundamental harmony that properly exists between the physical and the spiritual layers. Although the second birth is "nobler" than the first, "the one cannot be reckoned beneficial to the human race without the other."[61] And from this state of affairs, the mother draws implications as they relate to her own body: whereas Augustine had contrasted the biological parents who "beget for death" with ecclesiastical parents who "beget for life," Dhuoda establishes her physical nurturing of William as the basis of her ability to guide his spiritual progress.[62]

By way of such multifaceted interpretations, Dhuoda's text stands in utter contrast to Paulinus's, where the health of soul and body operate in an inverse relationship. According to the bishop, the more the body is mortified, the weaker it becomes, and the stronger the soul grows as a result. Conversely, the more the body is nourished, the greater the chance that the soul will lose its battle. Despite his military duties to the kingdom, Eric ought to embrace physical weakness, for "so long as we fear the infirmity of the flesh, we neglect the health of our soul."[63] In support of this agenda for mortifying the body, Paulinus cites the Apostle's dictum, "Do not take care of the body in your desires [Rom 13:14]," a quotation that we will return to repeatedly throughout this book as we survey its various adaptations in the ninth century.[64] If Paulinus's firm dichotomies between inner and outer, impermeability and corruptibility, and soul and body led him to dismiss any concern for the latter's needs, Dhuoda, on the other hand, resolutely declared that bodily health might be expected to accompany devoted service to God.[65] Just so, she held out to her youthful son the image of virtue embodied in Moses with his perfect teeth.

## Conflict Abstracted

There are many ways to interpret the discrepancy between Paulinus's and Dhuoda's handbooks of moral advice. One could see it as an issue stemming from clerical versus lay authorship, as a divergence rooted in gender, or as a reflection of the more personal relationship between author and addressee in Dhuoda's case. Yet another answer could locate the contrast in shifting assumptions about the body over the nearly fifty-year time span that lies between the production of the two works.[66] I argue for this final possibility based, in part, on the gradual changes apparent when the other two lay manuals, composed in the interim, are brought into the discussion. This chronological comparison suggests a general shift (far from absolute) in attitudes toward the soul-body relationship over the first half of the ninth century. Though Paulinus's handbook continued to be popular, those Carolingian intellectuals who imitated his general outline distinctly shifted the tone of the conversation.[67]

Despite the bonds of friendship between Paulinus and Alcuin, as well as multiple quotations of Alcuin's writings in the *Book of Admonition*, no allusions to Paulinus's work for Eric appear in Alcuin's guide for Wido.[68] This, regardless of the fact that Alcuin almost certainly knew of Paulinus's endeavor according to correspondence between Alcuin and Eric exchanged after the two had met at Aachen in 795 and while the duke was in the midst of leading a campaign against the Avars. Eric had apparently asked Alcuin for a text about the "duty of Christian piety," but the master deferred, instructing the duke to turn to his own adviser, Paulinus, for guidance.[69] We can assume that the *Book of Admonition* was completed over the next two years, as Eric died in 799. Around the same time, in 798, Alcuin addressed a request from Charlemagne to answer a layman's confusion about an apparent contradiction in the Gospels; in his reply, the scholar promoted the ability of wise noblemen in high office to preach and to model good behavior to their subordinates.[70] One assumes there must have been some association in Alcuin's mind between this decree and the precepts he composed, at Wido's behest, only a few years later (perhaps after they had met in Tours when Wido served as *missus* there in 802).[71]

These networks of textual exchange and personal relationships speak boldly to Romig's argument that we must finally cast aside the entrenched assumption that the lay manuals are but a Carolingian example of classic unsolicited (and unwanted) advice.[72] Rather than insistent clerical voices speaking to a heedless laity, we see the desire of the laity *to be trained* in Christian leadership. Eric and Wido were warriors, both undertaking risky military operations at the frontiers of empire; they wanted to feel assured about their eternal prospects.

If the recurrent theme throughout Paulinus's description of the spiritual life was the daily battle between soul and body, Alcuin's manual for Wido instead recharacterized this struggle as one between the virtues and vices. Military metaphors are employed by Alcuin only in reference to the opposition between these two forces, which encapsulates the exertion against sin within every individual.[73] Becoming aware of the constant internal battle between the "dukes of impiety" and the "warriors of Christ" is the key to understanding the self and achieving salvation.[74] Alcuin may well have read Paulinus's manual for Eric, and yet he chose not to focus his arguments on the dichotomous constitutions of body and soul.[75] He borrowed the concept of a list of chief vices from earlier Christian Fathers, such as John Cassian (d. 435) and Pope Gregory the Great (d. 604), who had utilized the schema in works written for monks and those holding clerical office.[76] However, he brought this internal battle outside of the monastery, making the virtues and vices common forces with which all individuals across society (not exclusively the spiritual elite) had to grapple (see Figure 5).[77]

Like Paulinus, Alcuin concentrates on the need to know oneself, a theme that we saw was also prominent in his treatise for Gundrada, where he relates self-knowledge to the soul's possession of the image of God. He entreats his patron Wido to consult his little work frequently "so that the soul, harried by external distractions, may find a return to its own self, in which it rejoices."[78] He emphasizes the need to purify the soul (through the reading of scripture, the confession of sins, and patience during tribulation), but his manual does not draw attention to the body as a dangerous entity. This refusal to disparage or vilify the body immediately sets *On the Virtues and Vices* within a register that diverges from Paulinus's worldview.

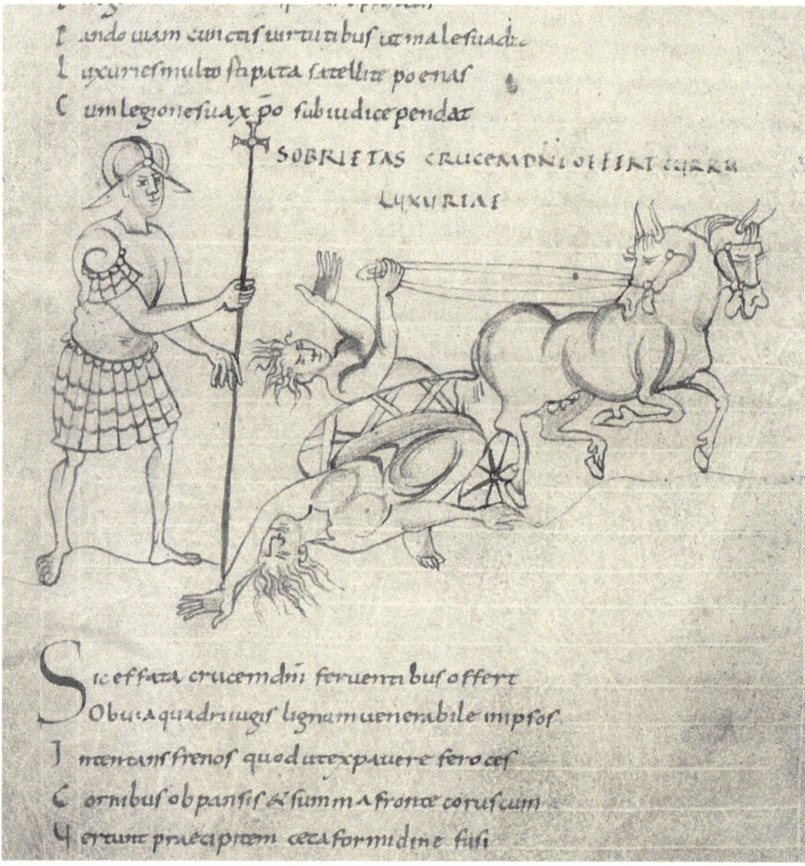

Figure 5. The war between vices and virtues was personified in the fifth-century *Psychomachia* of Prudentius, often copied with illustrations of matched warriors engaged in combat. Here *sobrietas*, employing the assistance of the cross, faces off against *luxuria* in a ninth-century copy of the text. Brussels, Bibliothèque royale MS 9987-91, f. 114v. Copyright KBR.

"Perfected is the fast," Alcuin explains, "that occurs alongside almsgiving and prayer."[79] Referencing Adam and Eve's fall through the act of eating, he posits fasts as "mighty spears against the advances of demons" because it is much easier for demons to insert themselves in a person who is already marked by overindulgence in food or drink.[80] This is one of only a few references to the indwelling of demons in *On the Virtues and Vices*, a fact that highlights the threads connecting Alcuin's work to Paulinus's but also evinces the nuances differentiating the two manuals. Like Paulinus, Alcuin signals that a feeble body is indicative of a more virtuous state, praising abstinence for how it "weakens the body but strengthens the soul."[81] He implies that uncleanliness is connected with the entry of demons into the physical person and that the body's inclinations are not conducive to the health of the soul. However, when an individual abstains from food, in conjunction with avoiding bad deeds and pursuing prayer, Alcuin asserts that that person, "having been made spiritual, is joined with the angels and united more fully with God."[82] His choice of words conjures an image of all-inclusive human redemption, in which the body, too, is refined and purified during its time on earth. Similarly, defining chastity for Wido as sexual relations between husband and wife at the right time and for legitimate reasons, Alcuin declares that the chaste live "an angelic way of life on earth."[83] In comparison with the *Book of Admonition*, then, *On the Virtues and Vices* gives more space to the body's participation in heavenly pursuits.

While Paulinus's work is marked by binaries of opposition, such that the body's nature works against the soul's well-being, Alcuin is far more inclined to stress binaries that set the body and soul in parallel. So, for example, in fasting, he explains that the only effective approach is to pursue twofold abstinence—of the body, from food and drink, and of the soul, from desire for power.[84] A similar section by Paulinus on twofold fasts urges Eric to abstain from anger, drunkenness, murder, and other sins. Yet here, the bishop defines these vices as those things that "nourish the body and kill and oppress the soul."[85] Of the two writers, then, only Paulinus goes so far as to categorize sins as things that nourish and sustain the body—suggesting that, just as one can never entirely escape the need to eat, so is the body inherently disposed toward evil actions.

Although Alcuin eschews casting the body as an enemy to the soul, by no means does he posit as active a role for it in the pursuit of salvation as Dhuoda.[86] Indeed, his most negative comments regarding the body are identical to phrases found in Paulinus's manual. In discussing the vice of fornication, he declares that "the soul should be the mistress and rule over the body, and the body should be the slave, obedient to its mistress, the rational soul."[87] That said, even here, small differences between the two ecclesiastical authors may be observed in their choice of language: while Paulinus refers to the need for the flesh to be "subjugated" (*subiecta*) to the soul, Alcuin states the need for the flesh to "obey" (*obedire*). Alcuin's description of fornication as a foulness of the body resonates with themes in Paulinus's manual. However, in a style discordant with the *Book of Admonition*, Alcuin locates the impulse to fornicate in the soul as much as the flesh: the vice occurs "from incontinence of desire and softness of the soul, which conspires with the body to sin."[88] His aim here (in the same section where he invokes the metaphor of the slave) is to make clear to lay readers that there is a certain divine hierarchy among the components of the self, just as there is among members of society, and to invert this hierarchy is to reject the order of the created world. In the same way that the manuals sought to confirm a role for the laity within Christian society, likewise, they aimed to show that each "member" had its place at the level of the individual.[89] The soul's rational nature, Alcuin emphasizes repeatedly, must be honored by using reason to command the body and restrain vice.[90]

The battle between the virtues and vices in Alcuin's manual displaced the conflict between body and soul in Paulinus's. In the *Book of Admonition*, the vices are equated with the body's reception of demonic suggestions, while Alcuin classifies the eight principle vices and their offshoots as manifold iniquities not only of an "unchaste body" but also of a "corrupt soul."[91] Whereas Paulinus attacks the body for driving the individual into sin, focusing Eric's attention on the divinity of his soul, Alcuin is far more inclined to distribute blame ambiguously between body and soul. His sources, Cassian and Gregory, had divided the vices into two categories (the natural or extranatural in Cassian's case, and the carnal or spiritual in Gregory's case) and moved sequentially from one to the next.[92] Alcuin begins, like Gregory, with pride, which he names a spiritual vice, then moves to gluttony and fornication, identifying the former as a sin of the body.[93] But none of the other five vices he treats is characterized by a clear label. Given how Alcuin purposefully changed the definition of certain sins in order to make them more relevant to the life of a lay noble, as Alain Dubreucq has illustrated, one can see his decision not to group the vices into carnal and spiritual as a conscious choice.[94]

The crucial difference between Alcuin's and Paulinus's manuals is that the former shifts the generation of sin away from the external pressure of the devil and his demons toward the inner, invisible life of the individual.[95] However, in doing this, Alcuin does not divide the individual against himself, teaching Wido to hate his own body. Rather, he suggests that a greater degree of harmony can exist within the self (or between its two components of body and soul) than Paulinus had envisioned. By abstracting the battle against sin onto the scheme of the eight virtues and vices, Alcuin extended the possibility for the vices to be conquered. This is clearly a more optimistic position. In Paulinus's grimmer worldview, the human individual can never escape the battle against his/her fundamentally flawed body.

* * *

While the dominant binary in Paulinus's work is between the soul and body and, in Alcuin's, between the virtues and vices, in Jonas's manual, much of his advice to Matfrid is framed according to a dichotomy between necessity and desire. Jonas does not speak at length about the need to subdue and punish the body, nor does he recurrently invoke the battle against the vices as a way for Matfrid to think about sin. Rather, *On Lay Instruction* addresses the question of how the necessities of life can be managed in an appropriate fashion.[96] For Jonas, moral behavior hinges on the difference between divine design and personal pleasure, and sin is understood primarily in terms of excess, luxury, or desire.

The chapters on the eight vices in Alcuin's text for Wido were known to and used by Jonas in one section of his own manual.[97] Given his direct citation of *On the Virtues and Vices*, Jonas was evidently aware that he was participating in a tradition (albeit a relatively recent one) of offering a behavioral guide tailored to the Carolingian lay elite.[98] Like Paulinus and Alcuin, Jonas initially composed his mirror for the lord of his diocese—Matfrid of Orléans, who, like Eric and Wido, was also fighting on the frontiers around the time that he requested the work.[99] Yet, many of the ideas Jonas formulated in the 820s for one member of the court, he clearly deemed applicable for society at large, given that he reused passages from *On Lay Instruction* in multiple other hortatory and regulatory texts and produced a longer, revised version of the manual after Matfrid's political downfall in 828.[100] As a leading intellectual and firm supporter of Louis the Pious, the bishop was responding to royal initiatives, flagging, as Francesco Veronese has argued, the importance of a pious domestic life for those exercising public office, an issue that took center stage in the years around 820 as the new emperor encouraged criticism of his father's sexual misconduct.[101]

Although he clearly found Alcuin's depiction of the eight vices a useful concept for pursuing the health of the soul, proportionally Jonas devoted significantly less space in his work to the conflict between the virtues and vices than did his predecessor.[102] Jonas and Alcuin both tend to portray sin as occurring primarily from a lack of internal awareness and rational judgment, rather than from the body's antagonistic efforts to corrupt the soul, as in Paulinus's treatise. However, while Alcuin maintains Paulinus's emphasis on conflict, Jonas lets martial imagery fade to the background, instead drawing increased attention to the theme of balance. Moderation is a virtue that appears in Paulinus's and Alcuin's works, but as a standard for daily life it takes on a much more integral role in *On Lay Instruction*.

Paulinus and Jonas both utilized the ancient metaphor comparing the relationship between soul and body to that between a horse and its rider. However, whereas Paulinus evoked the image of a charioteer barely restraining the instincts of a wild racehorse, Jonas presented an entirely different scenario. Comparing the two authors' deployment of this metaphor vividly highlights the divergent attitudes with which they approached the soul's control over the body. Instead of a chariot race, Jonas suggests a metaphor from daily life, that of the spent and chastened workhorse. Inverting Paulinus's image, he states that "the exhausted body is a type of bridle on the soul that desires luxuries."[103] His point is that fasting is most useful as a reminder to the soul to abstain from vices. Certainly, the image implies that a physically weaker body acts as a deterrent to sin, but the impulse to err is located firmly in the soul's longing for luxury. This metaphor falls within a section of the manual devoted to hunting, wherein Jonas chides nobles for the great sin they commit when they care more for their hunting dogs than for the poor.[104] He implies that there are many who believe abstention from food gives them license to pursue their other desires, not realizing that acts that tame the body are meaningless when the soul does not follow God's will.

We can see how Jonas shifts the conversation away from a topos of combat toward an ideal of measured conduct. He encourages Matfrid to imagine sin residing in his thoughts and decisions rather than his flesh. Lay people were (purportedly), for example, expressing to Jonas the view that it must be licit to use their genitals as they pleased, given that God was the creator of those genitals. While Jonas emphasizes his displeasure at hearing his congregants' arguments, he does not seek to counter such views by disparaging the genitals or the body in general; rather, he explains that God created all members of the body but expects them to be used in an "ordered manner," according to divine law.[105]

As in the example above, much of what drives the advice in *On Lay Instruction* is Jonas's depiction of the laity as an ignorant and lazy bunch.[106] Early in the first book, he rebukes them soundly:

> A deplorable custom has crept in among certain lay people, who do not observe the divine laws to which they submitted themselves through faith, as is fitting, but instead set as law for themselves not only what is pleasing and not lawful but also that which is permitted yet not advantageous; and they believe that they are able to live blamelessly according to that which is pleasing.[107]

Not only is this a self-reinforcing justification for his own text, but Jonas's characterization of the laity also introduces a framework for understanding behavior and sin. The problem lies with not recognizing the difference between personal whim and divine design, excess and moderation, luxury and necessity. Jonas borrows heavily from Augustine in setting out this framework of thought, which he undertakes as part of his detailed discussion of marriage. Augustine had outlined three ways that humans could use necessary things, each with different ethical ramifications. Jonas concentrates on two of these formulations—first, when humans use necessary things for the sake of something other than their defined end, they sin; second, when they use necessary things for the sake of their defined end, they act well and do not sin.[108] In trying to explain the rules of sex to the laity, Jonas cites Isidore of Seville: "When, therefore, anyone lives luxuriously, beyond whatever the necessity of procreation demands, it is a sin."[109] One could replace the word "procreation" in this quotation with a range of other activities and thereby encapsulate Jonas's approach to the moral life.

Procreation is certainly one of the most important subjects in the handbook; most of Book Two is devoted to a discussion of marriage and its rules.[110] Quoting from Augustine's *On the Good of Marriage*, Jonas classifies marriage with food, drink, sleep, and sex as a necessary thing—that is, a thing necessary for the sake of a defined end rather than an end to be sought unto itself.[111] Although this does not exalt the conjugal life, it is no feeble declaration. Virginity is a blessed state, but, Jonas counters, marriage is a "great good," created by God, modeled by Job, and capable of giving birth to "sacred and humble virginity."[112] This is dependent, however, on husbands and wives maintaining a chaste union by strictly following specific rules and restrictions regarding their sexual activities.[113] At base, as Jonas repeatedly emphasizes, marriage remains a sinless state by using the "mixing of the flesh" judiciously, for the purpose it was intended.[114] The bishop reassures his readers that it *is* possible for the laity to maintain a conjugal life free from pleasure and luxury. Engaging in sex within marriage for the sake of children, Jonas explains, is an act governed by reason.[115] Yet, "the [sex] which proceeds beyond that necessity [of generation] is pursued not with reason but with desire."[116]

As he does in his treatment of sexual relations, so does Jonas deploy a dichotomy when he turns to the problem of eating and the vice of gluttony.[117] He borrows quotations from Julian Pomerius's *On the Contemplative Life* (ca. 500) in order to draw a distinction between food that is permitted "for the necessity of sustaining life" and food that is taken "for the desire of [the] flesh" and is thus prohibited.[118] He refers to the opinions of "many," who claim to themselves that because God gave food and drink for human use it cannot be sinful to consume these things according to the demands of their pleasure.[119] Just as he does when referring to the laity's beliefs about the use of the genitals, Jonas seeks to shift the concept of what is natural from that which accords with personal urges to that which accords with God's original intentions. He makes clear to these foolish people that "without doubt they err when they take [food and drink] indiscreetly, either before the proper time or at the proper time but beyond moderate measure."[120] It is when desire overreaches need that sin takes root. "It is obvious that the intake of food and drink ought to be employed moderately for those practicing abstinence, not for the sake of enjoyment but for the necessity of the body, and that it is not the intake of those substances but rather the immoderate delight in them that is sinful."[121]

The health of the soul, as Jonas presents it, depends less on waging a constant war than on meticulously following the rules. He gives allowance to the necessities of life in order to contrast them with the temptations of luxury. Yet, in doing so, he encourages a discourse in which the physical world appears less dangerous, in part because little is classed as evil unto itself. It is not that sin is located in a particular place—demons, or the body, or forces of armed vices—but rather that sin is rooted in excess and abuse. While Paulinus is more prone to speak of bridling and mortifying *the body*, Jonas tends to emphasize the mortification of *desires* (*voluptates*).[122] While Paulinus argues that the only means for the devil to attack the soul is through the body, Jonas avoids language that describes the body at war with the soul.[123] Lastly, while Paulinus ends his manual with a diatribe against the evils of the body, Jonas ends his work with a chapter on the care that ought to be shown toward dead bodies and a chapter on the resurrected body.[124] He explains how the physical flesh will assume a spiritual (yet still bodily) form at the resurrection and will retain all the special features distinguishing individual identity.[125]

Throughout, *On Lay Instruction* draws attention to God's creation as innately good and useful. It challenges its readers to think more meticulously about how they engage with said creation, warning them that God made everything to meet one's needs but not to satisfy personal desires. It is, in the end, not a far leap from Jonas's acceptance of necessity to Dhuoda's interest in the well-being of the body. If God intended the body's needs to be met, then it was only proper for William to respect the health of his body—in protecting a body designed perfectly by God he would, in turn, be cultivating the health of his soul.

## Beyond the Lay Mirrors

An evaluation of the lay manuals produced in distinct locations across the realm and addressed to a broad audience suggests that discourse concerning the relationship of soul to body shifted noticeably along a spectrum over a nearly fifty-year period. At one end of this spectrum was warfare, and at the other, collaboration. The question, however, is to what extent these lay manuals are representative of general trends. A thorough survey is beyond the scope of this book, but here I touch briefly upon three further, distinct textual traditions in order to highlight analogous shifts in thought: first, guidelines regarding the ascetic life in Carolingian commentaries on the Benedictine Rule; second, understandings of human creation in Carolingian exegesis of Genesis; and, finally, attitudes toward material reality in the Carolingian debate about sacred images.

In his commentary from 817 on the Benedictine Rule, Abbot Smaragdus of Saint-Mihiel begins by outlining the need to chastise the body and its desires through vigils, fasts, and tearful confession.[126] Although his emphasis on bringing the body into subjection parallels the tone of Paulinus, the metaphor that he chooses to illustrate this process is starkly different. In place of a charioteer lashing his horses or a master demanding a slave's submission, Smaragdus urges his peers to compare the soul's relationship with the body to that of a king exercising dominion over his subjects or God watching over the created world.[127] The monks of Saint-Mihiel, then, were inspired to undertake the ascetic disciplining of their bodies, according to the dictates of the rule, with the same kind of merciful justice that (ideally) the lord of the Carolingian realm meted out for transgressions of fidelity.

On the one hand, we are reminded of Paulinus's dualistic approach in Smaragdus's repetition of passages from Galatians on the conflict between the flesh and the spirit (5:17) and the need to crucify the flesh with its vices (5:24).[128] Yet, on the other hand, the abbot tempers such dualism in his interpretation of Benedict's own image of Jacob's ladder, with its sides representing the body and soul and its steps the ascending path of humility. Here, Smaragdus invokes the necessity of cooperative progress, in a style similar to that of Dhuoda. The monk must do "what good he can in each part of him"—in both body and soul—"in order that in the glory of the resurrection he may receive the rewards of his labor in each part of him."[129] It was not escape from or repression of the body that was required, but, rather, the physical had to strive alongside the spiritual in this imperfect life in order to obtain the ultimate reward of a new eternal body, free from vice.

A second commentary on the Benedictine Rule from the 840s (contemporaneous with Dhuoda's *Handbook*) struck an even more moderate tone than Smaragdus's.[130] Hildemar of Civate's exposition of Benedict's Rule consistently recognized a need for balance, granting more latitude and flexibility to the needs of the body in the routines of the monks.[131] "In chastising the body," he emphasizes, "great discretion is necessary, so that it is neither chastised too little nor too much."[132] Like Jonas, Hildemar relies on a conceptual dichotomy between necessity and desire in crafting guidelines for the monks. He does not present the body as a dangerous weight on the soul but instructs the monks to render what is due to the body, as Jesus told his followers to render unto Caesar that which was owed to him (Mt 22:21).[133] Whereas Smaragdus interpreted the Rule's "having our loins girded" as restraining "the luxury of the flesh and of the mind," Hildemar preferred to read Benedict's directive as a reference to subduing luxury, bridling vainglory, or simply eliminating vice.[134] His tendency to look beyond the body for the root of sin is evinced in how he references the earthly battle—he says nothing about a conflict between body and soul but speaks about a battle of effort to keep the inner man focused on God while the outer man is occupied by necessary earthly affairs.

If Hildemar and Dhuoda represent a strain of Carolingian moral thought that highlighted the tractability of the body, recent studies of ninth-century exegesis have uncovered similar propensities. While commentators on Genesis generally assumed that God's creation of Adam in his own image referred exclusively to the rational part of the soul (as we saw in Chapter 1), this did not preclude several commentators from emphasizing the goodness of the "complete person" (*totus homo*).[135] As Raffaele Savigni elucidates, they drew attention to the nobility imbuing the body as a result of its upright stature, to Christ's decision to assume the flesh (rather than appear in a heavenly body), and to the humility embedded in the body as a result of God creating it from earth, not spirit.[136] According to the exegesis of Angelomus of Luxeuil (ca. 850), this *homo plasmatus* (sculpted Adam) into which God breathed a living soul was following an eschatological process whereby the earthy body was spiritualized through obedience.[137]

In similar fashion, the writings of Claudius of Turin (d. 827) presented the image of God as residing in the soul but as being only fully restored (from its deformity through sin) when the body had been spiritualized through the work of the Holy Spirit. As Pierre Boucaud has shown, Claudius set his exegesis apart with his decision to cite the second-century Greek Father Irenaeus and his belief that humankind was formed in the image of the incarnate Christ, not the incorporeal God.[138] Another mid-ninth-century reader of Irenaeus, Paschasius Radbertus of Corbie (d. 860), even went so far as to locate the image of God in *both* body and soul.[139] Although he sometimes included references to the body as weight, prison, or burden, Paschasius was nevertheless committed to affirming its participation in an individual's reformation, as David Appleby has argued.[140] He spoke of spiritualization, not as detachment from the body, but as the body's perfection on earth, advancing a controversial argument that, when partaking in the Eucharist, not only "is the soul fed by this mystery . . . but also our body is repaired to immortality and incorruption."[141] These specific exegetical examples illustrate, for Boucaud and Appleby, the tempering of a strongly Augustinian theological outlook with more optimistic approaches toward the body among ninth-century thinkers.[142]

The affirmation of Adam's flesh within certain biblical commentaries aligns closely with changing attitudes toward the physical world, as elaborated in the decades-long controversy over the religious value of images and icons.[143] The *Libri Carolini*, written by Bishop Theodulf of Orléans and edited by Charlemagne himself over the early 790s, set forth the first Carolingian response to Byzantine Iconoclasm.[144] It argued that images could contribute nothing particularly valuable to Christian worship because no relationship existed between a material object and the spiritual reality that an object referenced.[145] In formulating this position, the court drew strict boundaries between the visible, physical world and the invisible, spiritual world, declaring that material objects were unable to act as conduits to the divine.[146]

As Celia Chazelle concludes, at the level of the individual, Theodulf's work assumed that a person's own material and spiritual spheres of existence were alienated from each other just like an image was alienated from its spiritual referent.[147] The body had no role to play in striving for the divine.

However, if this was the consensus reached at court toward the end of the eighth century, by 825, the Carolingians were much more willing to condone the belief that material objects could direct the worshipper toward divine realities and that God could be reached through the visible, physical world.[148] Drawing on the writings of Pseudo-Dionysius, the 825 Colloquy of Paris declared that "it is impossible for our mind to reach incorporeal things (the imitation and vision of the celestial hierarchy) unless we are able to advance *through the visible beauty of the elements* to the most beautiful invisible form; visible, sweet-smelling images beam forth the invisible in rational instruction."[149] Here we see leading scholars under Louis the Pious explicitly asserting that matter created by God is able to be processed by the body's senses and abstracted by the mind to invisible realities. There is no chasm between matter and spirit but rather an innate and sanctified relationship between the two.[150]

While the long-lasting Iconoclasm debate may well have acted as a spur to rethinking the devotional value of the physical world, this brief sketch does not propose that there was a single catalyst driving a transformation in attitudes toward the body. Indeed, some of the scholars surveyed above were driven in different directions by the response to Iconoclasm. And yet, even those with opposing beliefs about icons and paintings, such as Claudius and Jonas, both inclined toward a more positive model of the soul-body relationship than that espoused in earlier texts of a similar genre.

## Self and Society

Whether in the lay manuals, in exegetical remarks, in conciliar proceedings, or in reflections on monastic regimen, the early decades of the ninth century appear to have witnessed a growing assumption that the body had a valuable role to play in the path to perfection and that concord rather than dissension should set the tenor of the soul's governance over its body. Despite the startling shift in how identity and virtuous conduct were presented to the Carolingian laity, what remained constant across all the lay manuals was the style of awareness that they advocated. Each insisted that the soul ought to contemplate its own activity and to meditate on its relationship with the body in a regular fashion. The terms in which the authors idealized that relationship changed, but the very idea that it was necessary to reflect on the state of the self did not change. Alcuin urged Wido to treat the manual as a "kind of solace" by which he could return to himself.[151] Paulinus ordered Eric to "extend yourself always to interior matters," while Jonas insisted that Matfrid learn to "to return to the soul often, as if to one's customary seat."[152] All four authors repeated this basic refrain so that their Christian audience could recognize the good within and cultivate an orientation to the divine. Even as manuals like Jonas's admonished the laity to submit themselves more frequently to external monitoring in the form of priestly penance, the overriding message was the individual mandate to monitor oneself. The turn of the ninth century thus brought to the Carolingian elite a new insistence on the value of mindfulness.

Yet, as Romig explains, this act of turning inward was never disassociated from the goal of establishing bonds of charity between the self and society.[153] Alcuin consistently indicated that only "he who begins from himself and guards himself diligently" could demonstrate those same virtues toward others and thereby contribute to the construction of a stable, peaceful society.[154] In 802, two years after assuming the title of *imperator*, Charlemagne commanded that every man age twelve and older take an oath of fidelity to him according to his new title (as they had taken an oath previously to him as king). Included in the instructions sent out with the *missi* was the message that "each individual person should strive to preserve himself completely in the holy service of God, according to God's command and his own pledge, because the lord emperor himself is not able to show the necessary care and discipline to every person individually."[155]

It was individual self-governance that was set forth here as a requirement of inclusion within the newly constituted empire.[156] Charlemagne's aim to establish an orthodox society could only be realized if each person recognized the role s/he had to fulfil in cultivating a disciplinary attitude toward the self. This acknowledgment is also articulated by the authors of the lay manuals, who framed their mandates in more gender-inclusive language than that suggested by the oath of 802.[157] These texts made clear, albeit by means of a diverse set of metaphors, that the logic of God's creation demanded that the soul and its rational capacities exert constant governance over the physical body.

Twenty years after the capitulary of 802, reflecting on his ministry as emperor, Louis the Pious would circulate his own admonition to his subjects:

> But although the essence of this ministry is seen to rest in our person, nevertheless, by both divine authority and human arrangement, it is understood to be divided into parts in such a way that each one of you in your place and order (*in suo loco et ordine*) is understood to hold part of our ministry. And consequently, it is apparent that I ought to be an admonisher (*admonitor*) to you all and all of you ought to be assistants (*adiutores*) to us.[158]

This message functioned as a stern reminder that the members of the realm could not abdicate responsibility for the well-being of the community. Not only did they need to maintain themselves in a virtuous condition, but they were also required to recall constantly the way in which care for the self extended outward to encompass appropriate social relations. We can discern a disparity between the language employed by Charlemagne and that chosen by Louis—the first emphasized individuality, the second, mutual accountability. Similarly, the manuals by Paulinus and Alcuin focused more on the behavior of each individual, while the manuals by Jonas and Dhuoda drew attention to how personal responsibility intersected with communal ties and obligations.[159]

As the structure of society and its ministries might be divided into various orders, so was there an intensifying interest in demarcating the respective roles of soul and body within the person. We observed in the previous chapter how the soul was often compared to a ruler, overseeing the workings of the body from the highest point, the head. In the above legislation from the 820s, Louis depicted himself as the *locus* from which all order stemmed, just as the soul was intended by God to be the *admonitor* to the body, and the body was supposed to be the obedient *adiutor* to the soul. It was this same division of the whole into parts that was addressed by the authors of the lay manuals. They were concerned not simply with outlining a ministry proper to the laity, as other scholars have argued, but with setting forth a way of understanding the duties proper to the divisions within the self. They encouraged laymen (and women) to be aware not only of their habits and dispositions but also of the internal mechanisms by which those habits and dispositions were fostered. And they admonished them strenuously to act on this knowledge in performing their daily duties. The participating actors—body and soul—were to have their own distinct places and roles (*loci et ordines*), and, just as within the empire, as Dhuoda makes clear, they had to work together to achieve the goal of salvation.[160]

CHAPTER 3

# The Body

## "In Sickness and in Health, Until Death Do Us Part"

In the summer of 813, bishops, abbots, and lay nobles convened in five separate regional synods across Francia, called together by Charlemagne to discuss the sweeping religious reforms outlined in the *Admonitio generalis* of 789.[1] With a sense of urgency propelled by the recent deaths of three of his children, ominous natural phenomena, and a series of military upsets, Charlemagne encouraged his ecclesiastical leaders to institute stricter penitential practices.[2] The realm and its subjects appeared in critical need of correction.

Those reformers gathered at Chalon-sur-Saône that summer gravely emphasized the work still required to instill an unwavering orientation toward God in the inner mechanisms of the individual. They painted the current situation in hyperbolic terms, declaring that some people "suppose themselves to be purged from sin by the simple sight of holy places."[3] These foolish people, the council implied, did not understand that purgation depended on a change in the condition of the soul: the external eyes of the body might take in a sacred site, but without an additional transformation in the interior state, no purification could occur. At base, as the ecclesiastical leaders explained, Christian subjects did not fully understand how sins were generated and the tools available to rectify their accumulation.

> Because it is apparent that a human being consists of two substances (namely the soul and body), and sometimes sin results from the movement of the soul and sometimes from the fragility of the body, those sins ought to be scrutinized through a rigorous investigation, so that a full confession may occur from both [body and soul]. . . . For as the creator and dispenser of salvation and health (*salutis et sanitatis*

> *auctor et largitor*), God demonstrates this [purging of sin] many times through the invisible workings of his power and many times through the operation of his physicians (*medicorum operatione*).[4]

The close correspondences between the language of the council and the lay manuals examined in Chapter 2 should be apparent. Indeed, the reformers drew directly on Alcuin's handbook for Wido when they recommended the schema of the eight vices as the best guideline for recognizing sin.[5]

This chapter carries the previous analyses of the soul-body relationship into discourses about health, as the imagery chosen by the council suggests. In doing so, it contemplates the ways in which metaphors, terms, and processes constantly crossed the boundaries of the physical and the spiritual. The chapter begins by considering the inside of the body as a space that was, to some extent, knowable as a material entity and yet never fully grasped given its concealment from observation. Ninth-century accounts of the soul explained that the perceptible animation of the body's members and senses was due to the internal workings of the soul, although that spirit itself remained invisible to human detection. If the soul was incorporeal, as many treatises stated, it was also (as we have charted) constrained within the physical limits of the body. Thus, the presence of the soul "within" overlapped with the material space beneath the skin, occupied by the internal organs, bones, and fluids that constituted the flesh. How exactly this space was configured remained uncertain due to the instability of the material elements, and this obscurity endowed the hidden cavity with that quality of mystery more typically associated with the spiritual world.[6]

The health of both the invisible soul and the unseen body depended on powerful opposing forces. As the second section of the chapter demonstrates, terms such as virtue (*virtus*) and vice (*vitium*) appeared in the medical texts that began to be copied with increasing frequency at the turn of the ninth century—just as, simultaneously, Carolingian pastoral texts began to popularize the notion that the moral life was a battle between the virtues and vices. These writings assumed that external signs pointed toward an underlying internal condition, but, because of the hidden nature of the interior realm, there remained a high degree of ambiguity in interpreting such signs.

The lack of alignment between internal and external states was particularly apparent when writers turned to the question of illness, since it was widely acknowledged that the outer, physical appearance of health did not necessarily correlate with the inner, spiritual health of the soul. As at the

Council of Chalon-sur-Saône, Carolingian ecclesiastical authorities often employed physiological and medical metaphors as a means to convey the damaging effects of sin on the religious purity of the social body. The language of revealing moral corruption, purging pollution, and applying penance as medicine suggested that physical health and spiritual well-being ran together. However, it was also assumed that a lack of bodily health—including consciously engaging in activities such as fasting and mortification—was a primary mechanism of eradicating sin and thereby correcting the ill health of the soul. From this perspective, one of the many paradoxes of Christian thought was the belief that it was the sick and damaged body that was truly to be understood as "healthy."

As the third section of this chapter illustrates, the meaning of illness remained fundamentally opaque in the Carolingian world and might be read in diametrically opposing ways depending on the context. Early medieval intellectuals inherited from late antique sources various possibilities for interpreting sickness, and it was in large part the conventions of genre, I suggest, that determined which interpretation would predominate. Furthermore, in decoding the truth of illness, scale mattered greatly. The sickness of one individual might be read as an indicator of holiness and divine favor, but epidemics or widespread diseases were deemed incontrovertible signs of human sinfulness and God's displeasure. Thus, disability and infirmity in large numbers, like the many who flocked to the sites of relics to obtain healing, were generally seen to reflect pervasive spiritual disorder in the polity rather than discrete, individual sin. Along these lines, Carolingian writers evaluated the natural world as if performing a diagnosis of the body, reading events and phenomena as symptoms that stemmed from a hidden vice within the religious collective, one that required immediate correction. Such arguments are manifest in Einhard's account of his translation of ancient relics from Rome to Francia. The chapter ends with a study of this influential ninth-century miracle collection, with its particular attention to the boundaries between internal and external and the capacity of divine power to turn the hidden and indeterminate into the visible and known.

If the Council of Chalon-sur-Saône derided the simplistic belief that the sight of the sacred could cure sin, it was nevertheless widely accepted that the sacred could illuminate what was concealed and make it comprehensible to human vision. Relics held out the possibility of making the internal manifest and thus subject to definitive knowledge.[7] Indeed, the very alignment between inner truth and outer appearance was itself an indication that sin, with its disruptive and deceptive potential, had been purged. Just so, running throughout each section of this chapter is the Carolingian conviction that binaries are a product of human knowledge, while divine knowledge perceives everything equally. It was within this disjuncture between the seen and unseen that both pastoral care and medical expertise assumed a unique power to affect the health of soul and body, respectively.

## Internal Anatomies

At the very beginning of his letter to Gundrada, Alcuin sets out what he takes to be common sense: "The body is that which is known to all those who understand themselves to be human beings."[8] Unlike the soul, which few understand and which consequently requires a detailed explanation, the body is accepted as straightforward and uncomplicated. If Genesis made clear that God formed Adam's body from clay, most Carolingian writings aligned this scriptural proof with the ancient philosophical belief that the body was constituted by the four elements of the material cosmos: air, water, earth, and fire. In his didactic, elementary dialogue for students, Alcuin answers a question about the origins of the body with the following response: "The flesh is formed from the four elements . . . for earth is in the flesh, air in the breath, water (*humor*) in the blood, fire in the vital heat; every element has its own part in us, which is owed [back] when the fastenings [of the body] are loosed."[9] In his encyclopedic work intended to complement Isidore's *Etymologies*, Hrabanus similarly states that the body is composed of all four elements, even if the term for human (*homo*) comes from the fact that God created the first human being from soil (*humus*), as noted in Genesis. When the soul departs the body, and the body decays, the four elements composing it return to their places in the cosmic configuration. Fittingly, Hrabanus elucidates, the term for body (*corpus*) comes from its corruptible nature (*corruptus*), in the sense of both its eventual physical dissolution and the spiritual imperfection of the human race.[10]

Among Carolingian intellectuals, Bede was the great authority on the natural world, and he had declared "the entire universe, which consists of heaven and earth" to be "rounded out of four elements into the appearance of a complete sphere."[11] His *On the Nature of Things*, a text that circulated widely in the Carolingian realm over the course of the eighth and ninth centuries, outlined the order of this universe according to weight, with earth, being the heaviest element, at the center, followed by water, then air, and finally fire.[12] Thus, both the body and the cosmos might be defined as having "zones" appropriate to one particular element. Yet at the same time, elements were never found only in their particular places but, being inclined to merge, were always creating new substances in various combinations.

As Isidore summarized in his *Etymologies*, this constant merging meant that the four elements that composed the world and the four humors that composed the body were most likely to be found "comingled into a single disposition."[13] Reiterating Isidore's teachings in his own *On the Natures of Things*, Hrabanus explained that the elements and humors were not simply comparable but were equated with one another in pairs, such that "each humor resembles its element: blood resembles air, bile fire, black bile earth, and phlegm water."[14] Their fluctuations within the body ensured health or brought forth sickness. Correspondingly, Carolingian authors, closely following Isidore and Bede, alternately described the body as an ordered entity, with different elements constituting distinct parts, and as a disordered, unstable amalgam, subject to erratic internal and external reconstitutions of its cosmic building blocks. In a dissection of Hrabanus's poem *In Honor of the Holy Cross*, Lynda Coon demonstrates how he linked the volatile disposition of the human will with the constant mutability of the elements: the ability of earth, air, fire, and water to alter one another, to intermingle in new associations, and to escape and return to their proper domains.[15] These dynamic processes were the natural way of the world, but they also explained why the material universe was corruptible. The body maintained some stability as a result of the direction and animation of its own soul, but at death, the bonds holding its elements together were "loosed," and these reentered the cyclical patterns of the cosmos.[16]

* * *

As the previous two chapters have made clear, Carolingian intellectuals firmly upheld the notion of a bipartite individual. Indeed, in the same pedagogical dialogue as above, Alcuin is asked whether a human being is simple or double. He replies that it is double because it is composed of interior and exterior, with the interior person being the soul and the exterior, the body.[17] In just this way, the dual nature of the self reflected larger cosmic divisions between the material and spiritual, the corruptible and incorruptible, and the visible and invisible. Within this synoptic model, the body was supposed to represent the visible world; it could be known through sight and the other senses in a way that the spiritual world could not. During earthly existence, it was the exterior surface and the physical movements of the body that gave clues as to the life of the soul within, as discussed in Chapter 1.[18]

However, just as Carolingian conceptions of the soul resisted a definition that was utterly incorporeal, so did assumptions about the body escape the strict binaries mapped onto the microscopic-macroscopic universe. For the body itself also had its invisibilities. The internal workings of the body were neither evident to the senses nor entirely knowable. Rather, they remained in many ways inscrutable, not unlike spiritual mysteries about the soul. In his treatise for Lothar II, for example, Hrabanus made clear that he believed the formation of a fetus in the womb to be only partially knowable. He was certain that "human seed coagulates into vital substance" early in this process and that infants begin to move within the womb around the fortieth day but remained doubtful about how these physical changes related to the merging of soul and body within that inner, unseen space.[19]

In this same work, Hrabanus included a chapter detailing the perfection of the human form. If the body is examined according to each of its members, he asserts, "great mysteries are revealed in it by those who dedicate themselves to investigating such things."[20] The head, he states, resembles the heavenly sphere, and the eyes, the two great lights in the sky (sun and moon). He proceeds to praise all of the members that are found in twos (ears, nostrils, lips, arms, hands, sides, legs, and feet) and the members that balance these pairs with their dignified neutrality (nose, mouth, throat, chest, stomach, belly, and genitals). While Hrabanus's summary effectively divides the body into discrete parts, each with a distinct function, his ultimate aim is to emphasize how all members are bound together "with such charity" that they miraculously cling together and harmoniously operate as a unity.[21] If, here, he focuses on the external members visible to the eye, *On the Natures of Things* goes into much greater detail on the many internal parts and reveals how each has a spiritual meaning that relates to divine truth.[22] The kidneys, for instance, he defines as producers of a polluted liquid when warmed by lustful heat; drawing on biblical citations, he associates these organs with the need for internal constancy and restraint in guarding against luxurious dissolution.[23] In general, Hrabanus relies on Isidore for his anatomical information, but by elevating his moral explanation of anatomy above a mere physical description, he emphasizes the divine order pervading the body, such that its members emulate the unity of the "holy and elect of God who are the members of the body of Christ."[24]

Just as Hrabanus moved from head to toe in his account of the human body, so was this the approach found in the anatomical texts that circulated in ninth-century medical manuscripts.[25] The most popular anatomical guides of the early Middle Ages were two texts that now go under the names the *Gynaecia* and the *Epitome altera* and have been attributed to the fourth-century African physician Helvius Vindicianus.[26] These works were included in numerous Carolingian and Beneventan codices produced in centers ranging from northern Francia to Montecassino, although their titles and contents vary widely in the different witnesses (with Hippocrates or one Accius Iustus sometimes listed as the author rather than Vindicianus).[27] Despite their different emphases—the *Gynaecia*, as the title suggests, devotes more space to conception and fetal development—both texts follow a similar pattern in moving through the external appearance and inner space of the body.

The prologues of the anatomical treatises promise to break down the human body into its constitutive parts (with more attention to the differences between men and women in the *Gynaecia*). So the *Epitome* begins with a frank question: "From which joints, from which junctures, from which bones, veins, sinews, and combinations of various members does a human being come into existence?"[28] The answer is that fourteen different materials constitute the components of the body—sinews, veins, arteries, bones, blood, air, flesh, fat, cartilage, nail, humor, hair, marrow, and skin.[29] The *Gynaecia* observes that information about the insides of the body and the causes of death was known to earlier medical investigators who were permitted to dissect the dead; yet, because such customs are presently forbidden, the mysteries of internal anatomy must be passed on in written texts.[30] As if to remedy this absence of knowledge-through-observation, both works move systematically from one organ or body part to the next, painting a mental picture of the inner physical space enclosed by the skin and hair. For example, after detailing the head or skull, Vindicianus next describes the brain, then the hair, eyes, ears, nose, and neck, followed by the teeth, lips, tongue, palate, uvula, the two shafts (windpipe and esophagus), the epiglottis, and the lungs.[31] Certain of these anatomical parts can, of course, be viewed externally, but the text draws on what is visible to make sense of the invisible—the cavities behind the nostrils to the brain, the way in which air and food travel down the correct canal by means of the smooth functioning of the epiglottis.

With organs such as the stomach, heart, lungs, and liver, these anatomical treatises offer greater detail. They explain, for example, that "the heart has four veins, two with air and two with blood. The ones with air attach to the lungs. The ones with blood connect to the liver; when a contraction of these occurs, blood is discharged throughout the entire body."[32] However, it would be a mistake to assume that the primary purpose of these treatises was to define all organs according to their function or furnish specific information on the configuration of each individual part. Rather, the focus of the texts is on the organs' relationships to each other, their positioning within the whole. Thus, instead of learning about the operations of the spleen, the reader is told simply that "the spleen is situated on the left side, longish and near the stomach, lying next to a thin membrane containing fat, which covers the intestine and warms it."[33] Through such language, a kind of physical chain is created among the various pieces of the body. Under and to the left of the fatty membrane are found the kidneys; under these, the intestine; under this, the small intestine; and, finally, under this, the colon and rectum; in close proximity to the rectum is the bladder, which is held between the two kidneys and is connected by sinews to the testicles.[34] Not unlike Hrabanus's celebration of the body, the implicit message in the two anatomical treatises attributed to Vindicianus is one of physical harmony, with each part fitting into another like a perfect puzzle. Almost no illustrations of anatomy were available in the ninth century, but works such as these constituted a kind of mental map of hidden internal spaces.[35]

## Vocabularies of Health

Exegetical texts produced by prominent Carolingian intellectuals and anatomical treatises copied within Carolingian scriptoria offered a textual diagram of the external and internal components of the human body. Yet much of the ninth-century language of health and disease focused not on the functionality of multi-organ systems but on the powers of different virtues and vices at play within the bodily cavity. This language was not unique to Carolingian medical developments but was inherited from the herbals and encyclopedias of late antique Greek and Latin medicine. Nevertheless, it acquired a new significance as the language for the moral training of the soul increasingly conceptualized the spiritual life as a battle between the virtues and vices.

The Greek word *δύναμις* was employed in certain Hippocratic writings to convey an entity's specific qualities, its capacity to affect things in the world and thereby reveal its own essential nature.[36] As ancient Greek medical works were translated into Latin, this concept generally appeared in its transliterated form, *dynamis*, or as the Latin word *virtus*.[37] As a result, the medical texts that circulated in early medieval Europe (whether originally written in Greek or Latin) were peppered with the terms *virtus* and *virtutes*, which might variously signify the powers, properties, or merits of particular plants, geographic locations, winds, medications, foods, or bodily elements.

Early medieval intellectuals also introduced a new technical word for classifying information about the virtues of natural substances. *Dynamidia* (which was never used in classical texts) first appeared in Isidore's *Etymologies* and was defined therein as "the power of herbs, that is, their force and capability. In herbal medicine, potency itself is called [*dynamis*], whence also the books where herbal remedies are inscribed are called *dinamidia*."[38] As Loren MacKinney has demonstrated, *dynamidia* did not deal solely with herbs but could be employed for material that dealt with vegetables, environmental conditions, and all types of *materia medica*.[39] Indeed, one tenth-century medical codex stated that it was "the description of the virtues of all medicines."[40] This definition makes clear the close connection that existed between *virtus* and the new subgenre of *dynamidia*. Just so, MacKinney found that *dynamidia* was used as a title in early medieval manuscripts but *only* for texts in which the term *virtutes* appeared frequently.[41]

Earlier scholarship proposed that Isidore's invention of *dynamidia* was grounded in his desire to clearly demarcate medical from moral "virtue."[42] Yet, even if this was Isidore's original intention, it was the inverse situation that resulted. Early medieval scribes clearly favored a medical language that evoked parallels with the spiritual discourse of the time—Carolingian medical codices are suffused with the term *virtus*.[43] Scribes apparently preferred *virtus* over *dynamis*, even as they (sporadically) adopted *dynamidia* as a label for dietetic and pharmaceutical texts, and despite the fact that they often devoted substantial space to explaining Greek medical vocabulary.[44] This is precisely because the idea of *virtus* resonated with a Christian audience. The early Middle Ages did not introduce *virtus* to medical thought; nevertheless, the particular historical context called forth a Latin medical tradition reliant on a term that crisscrossed important genres of the moment.

Herbals and remedy collections that circulated in the early Middle Ages offered the *virtutes* of a range of natural substances that could be employed against the pains suffered by various parts of the body. The most popular herbal of the time, attributed to Apuleius Platonicus and often transmitted alongside four other *materia medica* texts, included the term over thirty times in its descriptions of various plants.[45] On the herb artemisia (wormwood, tansy, or mugwort), for example, Pseudo-Apuleius offers a brief etymological history: "It is said that Diana [in Greek, Artemis] discovered these three types of artemisia and their *virtutes* and relayed the remedies to Chiron the Centaur, who first prepared medicine from these herbs" (see Figure 6).[46] The implication here is that the herb's virtues are both hidden and powerful; they are not equated with remedies but rather are the properties that must be known in order to produce effective treatments. The instructions

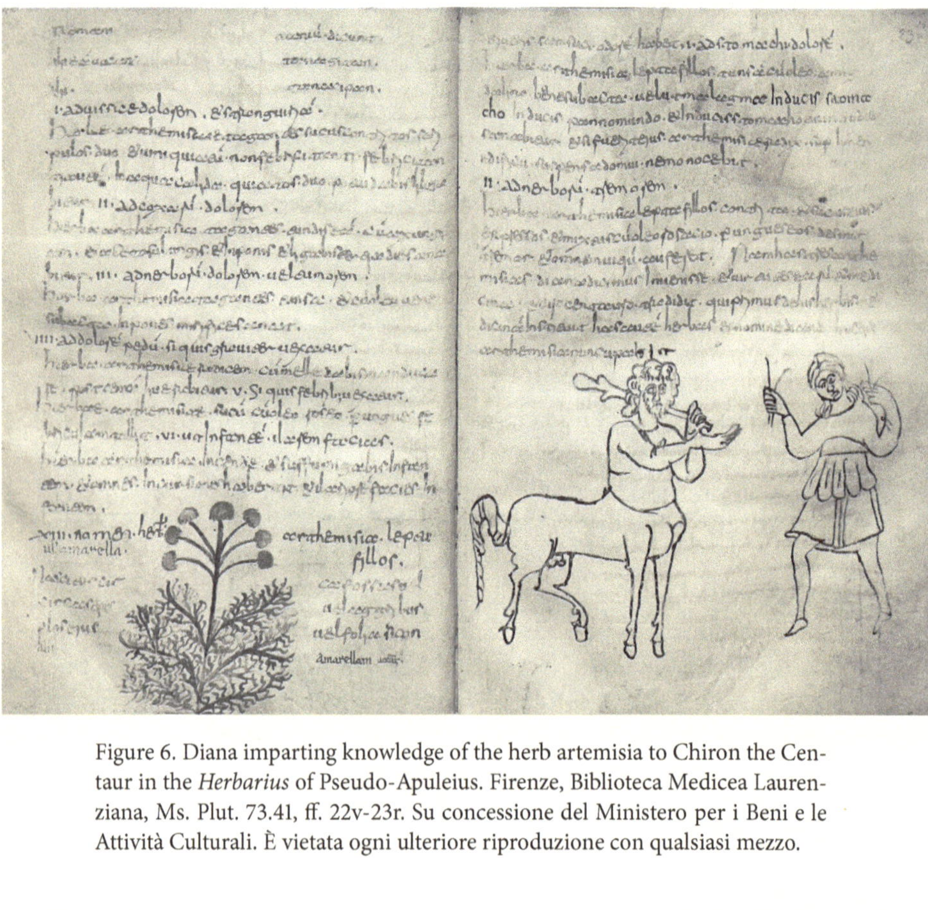

Figure 6. Diana imparting knowledge of the herb artemisia to Chiron the Centaur in the *Herbarius* of Pseudo-Apuleius. Firenze, Biblioteca Medicea Laurenziana, Ms. Plut. 73.41, ff. 22v-23r. Su concessione del Ministero per i Beni e le Attività Culturali. È vietata ogni ulteriore riproduzione con qualsiasi mezzo.

listed under the illustration of the herb outline how to draw out the *virtutes* with specific steps for treating pain in the stomach and muscle tremors.

A manuscript produced in the middle of the ninth century (with contemporaneous marginalia), at a center closely connected with Charles the Bald's court, contains an herbal ensemble that includes the Pseudo-Apuleius *Herbarius*.[47] At the start of the ensemble, the scribe has inserted two tables, the first with a numbered list of the various herbs mentioned in the codex followed by the number of *virtutes* that each herb possesses.[48] In this case, *virtus* refers to an ability to treat one specific ailment. Thus *camepitis* (ground-pine) is listed as having two virtues, and under the illustration of the herb are found two cures, one for wounds and the other for twisting abdominal pain.[49] The marginal notes throughout the *Herbarius* draw even more attention to the term *virtus*—although every herb has its own large title in red ink, beside almost every illustration, someone has written "On the virtues" and then the name of the plant again (see Figure 7). Each folio, then, repeats this word as a substitute for remedy or capacity. Furthermore, another treatise in the ensemble, *On the Herb Betony* attributed to Antonius Musa (see Figure 11), makes clear that the *virtus* of the plant is itself bolstered by the power of God.[50] The preface provides an (ambiguously pagan) invocation to be said while gathering betony, which entreats the herb to be effective in the forty-seven cures it provides; beside this invocation is a marginal note "a prayer for this herb through the *virtus* of our Lord Jesus Christ."[51] There can be no doubt that *virtus* has a strong religious valence here, a fact that underscores the constant interplay between medical and spiritual language.

The precise meaning of *virtus*, however, was slippery. It did not always denote a remedy but could also refer to a substance's particular qualities. An early ninth-century manuscript from Saint-Germain-des-Prés is suffused with the language of the virtues, consisting primarily of a series of four texts that promise to reveal the *virtutes* of herbs, drugs, foods, and drinks.[52] Here, for example, mint is described as possessing a "cooling *virtus*," which refers to both its own properties and its effects on the body when ingested.[53] A list of various types of meat associates their virtues with qualities such as heaviness, lightness, moistness, and amount of blood, while also relating these characteristics to their powers to dry the body, nourish it, provoke thirst, and stimulate urine.[54]

Texts generally treated both ingested substances and the material of the body itself (produced from digested food and drink) as consisting of different *virtutes*. Descriptions of the four different humors often used the term

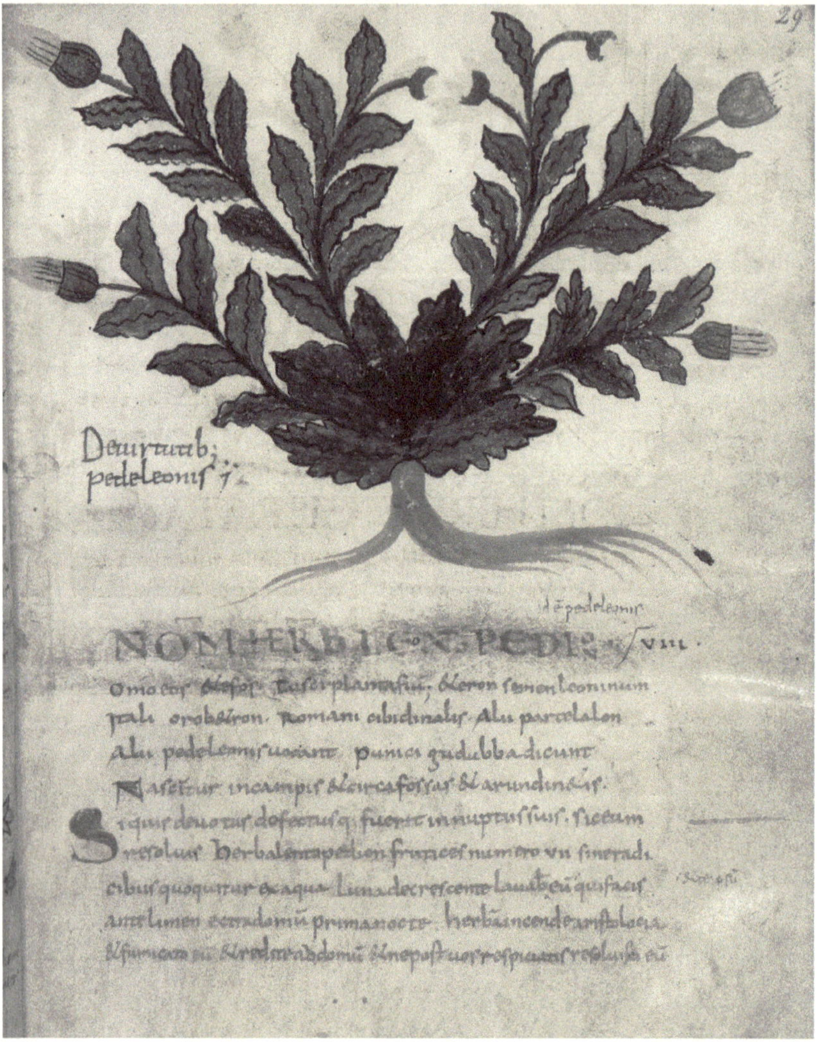

Figure 7. The herb lion's foot (*Alchemilla vulgaris* or *Leontice leontopetalum*) from the *Herbarius* of Pseudo-Apuleius. Paris, BnF lat. 6862, f. 29r. By kind permission of the Bibliothèque nationale.

*virtus* to indicate the qualities specific to each humor. For instance, a popular treatise entitled "On the four elements of the body" outlines each of the humors, in turn, beginning with phlegm, which has a cold and wet *virtus*; then blood, hot and wet; next yellow bile, hot and dry; and finally, black bile, characterized by its cold and dry *virtus*.[55]

As a remedy, as a property, or as a power, the concept of "virtue" assumed a greater spiritual valence simply because the term *vitium* (vice) was also part of the medical language of the early Middle Ages.[56] Alongside herbals and *materia medica*, the bulk of an average Carolingian medical manuscript typically consisted of *receptaria*, long lists of relatively short recipes arranged according to the condition they treated (often in a general head-to-toe pattern).[57] It is in these types of texts that the idea of "vices" surfaces most often. There were many possible Latin terms for sickness and disease (including *morbus, aegritudo, infirmitas, valetudo, causa, passio*), for suffering and pain (including *dolor, vexatio, labor*), and for debility (*debilitas, imbecillitas, languor*).[58] But, alongside these, *vitium* surfaces often and indicates some vague malady or hurt.[59] The tables of contents that sometimes preface remedy compilations immediately display the recurrence of the term. So a compilation entitled *Tereoperica* (*Therapeutics*) uses it five times in the first thirty entries, promising to treat vices of the head, eyes, ears, nose, and mouth.[60] A poem of medical remedies popular with the Carolingians includes the term *vitium* in over ten of its sixty-four chapters.[61] The *Antidote of Theodorus*, a more complex recipe transmitted in several ninth-century manuscripts, vows to "purge most thoroughly all internal vices."[62] And a dietary treatise attributed to an envoy to the Merovingian court speaks of the ability of raw bacon to cure the *vitia* of the intestines and of the hazards vinegar and cheese bring to those who suffer from *vitia* of the kidneys.[63]

Again, "vice" was not a new term in medieval medicine but was found in late antique Latin texts like the poem just mentioned or Caelius Aurelianus's *On Chronic Diseases*, which claimed that the Greek god Asclepius, famed for his healing, "was the first to excel in the treatment of obstinate diseases [*vitia*]."[64] Although the words *virtus* and *vitium* are not equally present in all of the herbals and recipes that circulated in the Carolingian period, they are sufficiently common to be recognized as a window onto early medieval imaginings of the powers affecting health and illness. These terms did not necessarily possess the same moral resonance as they did when found within spiritual treatises: *virtus*, especially, had a more neutral connotation in medical texts. However, the expectation that both the physical self and spiritual self could be represented in terms of the dominance of particular virtues or vices in the body or soul, respectively, forged a common link between medical and theological thought. The preface to the *Tereoperica* recalls such parallels to the reader's mind when it declares that (according to Aristotle) "medicine cures those things that are *vitia* of the body, while philosophy cures those things that are *vitia* of the soul."[65]

If vice was something to be purged, or at least counteracted, by the *virtutes* of specific herbs and foods, this worked to configure the body as a site within which different forces engaged in contestation for control of the individual.[66] Of course, this same dynamic of struggle underpinned the moral literature on the virtues and vices, portrayed by Alcuin as "the eight dukes of every impiety and their armies . . . who are easily vanquished by the warriors of Christ through the holy virtues, with God's assistance."[67] Alcuin himself described several of the vices as diseases, which could be cured by the cultivation of an appropriate virtue—as avarice was opposed by mercy and charity.[68] By doing so, he drew on a long tradition of late antique Christian thinkers, such as John Cassian and Gregory the Great, who had themselves turned to classical medicine and appropriated theories such as "cure by contraries."[69] The theory held that a disease could be overcome by employing a substance whose qualities were opposite: for example, a fever could be treated by cooling herbs, an excessively moist organ by a drying remedy.[70] The basic principle was employed loosely by theologians to illuminate dense doctrinal points. Thus, in his sermons, Augustine explained humanity's fall as an incurable spiritual disease, a great tumor of pride; against this, Christ was sent as an antidote, with his humility counteracting human pride just as Hippocratic medicine cured by contraries.[71]

A medicalized approach to the virtues and vices, then, was not novel at the turn of the ninth century, but Alcuin's simplified schema of eight pairs, as presented in his exceedingly popular manual for Wido, amplified a language that was already "trending" in the Carolingian realm as a result of changing beliefs about penance.[72] Insular penitential handbooks, introduced by eighth-century Irish and English missionaries and monks, might be structured according to the cardinal vices and often included references to the priest, as spiritual physician, curing sins by the "remedy of penance" (*poenitentiae remedium*).[73] Such expressions were adopted by Carolingian authors when they composed their own "authoritative" penitential treatises.[74] Halitgar of Cambrai's "Roman" penitential (820s) began by urging priests to fast and pray on behalf of those to whom they assigned penance, lest they remain distant from their flock like a physician who refuses to come into contact with "stinking" parts of the flesh.[75]

It may be coincidental that this intensifying concern with enforcing proper confessional practices (as evidenced in conciliar decrees from 813 and 829 and Louis the Pious's own penances in 822 and 833) occurred alongside the copying of a significant amount of medical literature. However, shared language and metaphors between these two genres surely drew them closer together in the minds of readers. Hildemar of Civate described the conversion to monastic life as "the eradication of vices and the planting of virtues," a relatively generic instruction, but one that alluded to a botanical landscape of natural *virtutes*.[76] In 802, Alcuin composed a treatise for the youth at the monastery of Saint-Martin, wherein he compared confession to a priest with the act of a patient exposing hidden wounds to the physician's gaze.[77] Individuals believe "with false hope that [their] sins are concealed within the walls [of a house]," when, in truth, Alcuin emphasizes, nothing can be concealed from God.[78] Confession was a salutary opportunity to accuse oneself before the final judgment. So, he urged the youth in provocative language, "if you do not conceal the wounds of your conscience from a physician," you will be healed instantly, but "if you blush to uncover your many painful sores to the physician," you will perish from "the festering wounds."[79]

This imagery clearly builds on the notion of the body's interior as hidden and thus only partially knowable. The conscience is likened to an inner organ, the wounds of sin are compared to embarrassing sores in private areas. Abigail Firey has highlighted how Alcuin's treatise sets up a "therapeutic model" centered upon the internal psyche—shame should not drive a Christian to conceal sin but to confess quickly and openly, so as to receive a penance capable of purging the offense.[80] The model depends upon a dichotomy between blushing (the physical effect of shame) and confessing (exposing the concealed wound). As Courtney Booker elucidates, this very idea of blushing as a superficial sign of a suppressed sin assumes that the body reflects the soul's moral impurity.[81] A blush across the face signals something that the sinner wishes to keep secret but inadvertently communicates.[82] The outer appearance reflects the inner state of sickness.

According to the logic of the blush, the confessor acts like a physician not only in having access to private parts of the person but also in relying on his expert knowledge to probe the body's surface for clues to the cause of disease. The Council of Aachen in 836 referenced just such a conviction when, in calling priests spiritual physicians, it declared, "for who does not know that interior wounds are more obscured than the wounds of the organs?"[83] The confessor must, like a physician, play the role of a detective in using techniques of observation to determine the deeper disorders beneath the flesh. Only thus can a spiritual condition partially known to the patient be fully understood and corrected by the priest.[84]

Firey observes an intensifying interest in discussing the conscience in the ninth century. Although it did not take one concrete form but was conceived in various guises (as a book, a house, a courtroom, for example), descriptions of the conscience often overlapped with characteristics of the soul—an interior space, a place to which one returned, a private site known fully to God, an invisible entity contained within the boundaries of the body.[85] Similarly, processes that denoted the discovery of internal vice were shared across the body and soul. As Alcuin intimated in his manual to Wido, identifying sin was a matter of reading backward from visible signs to the underlying condition.[86] The *vitium* of indifference (*acedia*) he compared to a "pestilence" that "infects" the soul. "From this," he asserted, "is born sleepiness, laziness in good work, instability of location, wandering from place to place, a lukewarm attitude toward labor, anxiety of the heart, murmuring, and empty speech."[87] These *effects* are, at the same time, *symptoms* that enable a Christian to trace behavior to a root cause or corruption.[88] In like manner, a treatise on teaching the art of medicine (transmitted in several ninth-century manuscripts) laid out instructions for a physician visiting a patient for the first time. Taking the patient's pulse is one of the first investigatory activities because, we learn, "by touching her pulse, you may discover what fault (*vitium*) lies within."[89] Just as with the blush, bodily signs could relay (albeit obliquely) the truth of the interior, spiritualized space, and both the confessor and physician had to hone their abilities to read these patterns.

## Illness as Unstable Sign

If many stories in the Old Testament presented long life and robust health as the just dispensations for a righteous life, such a correlation between vigor and virtue was also prominent within the classical Greco-Roman tradition and became an influential trope within Christian hagiography.[90] The lives of early Christian ascetics (both male and female) offered heroic histories of human endurance in the desert, where individuals battled demons and deprived themselves of even basic necessities yet emerged unscathed.

Here, Athanasius of Alexandria's fourth-century *Life of Anthony* set a model for future hagiography in describing the saint's body appearing perfectly healthy after twenty years of harsh living and scarce sustenance.[91] The ascetic's flesh was a mirror for his unblemished soul, signaling the recovery of prelapsarian stability and the promise of the resurrected body to come.[92]

Such ideas regarding the imprint of holiness on the physical body surfaced in early medieval Latin hagiography primarily through the topos of the incorruptibility of the dead. Saints' intact and sweet-smelling remains testified to the virtuous life they had lived and the peaceful rest their souls currently enjoyed.[93] When Jonas of Orléans was asked to document the 825 translation of Saint Hubert's body to the monastery of Andain, he accentuated the miraculous state of Hubert's corpse, even reworking the description of an earlier transfer of the relics according to this agenda.[94] When the saint was first dug up in 743, those assisting assumed that "in the custom of mortals that most sacred body had broken apart, lost its solid structure, and returned to dust," but instead they discovered "his most glorious corpse suffered from no detriment, unharmed from dissolution and putridity."[95] Hubert even appeared youthful, his face glowing with dew and his hair beautiful with volume and color—a clear validation, according to Jonas, of God's promise that "not even a hair of your head will perish [Lk 21:18]."[96] The exact same body was found by Jonas's contemporaries when they moved Hubert's relics again in 825. The bishop adamantly reminded his peers that they should understand from this sign that the saint had overcome "the transgression of the first parents" and that God had freed his body from its subjection to natural laws.[97]

Of course, if the physical beauty of the dead was believed to radiate the soul's purity, the reverse was also true. When Charles the Bald died in 877, those critical of his reign described in vivid detail the speed with which his body rotted and gave off such a noxious smell that a rapid burial became necessary.[98] In a letter from 858 to King Louis the German on the need to respect ecclesiastical property, Hincmar likewise deemed it useful to detail an incident from a century earlier regarding the king's great-grandfather, Charles Martel. He recounted how a certain bishop had had a vision of Martel's soul twisting in purgatorial flames for his sins (the seizure of church lands) and had informed his peers that proof of the vision's truthfulness could be seen in the state of Martel's corpse: when his coffin was unearthed, it was found empty and scorched inside as if burned by fire.[99] Evidently, those wishing to convince contemporaries of the iniquity of particular royal family members found a persuasive rhetorical tool in images of bodily integrity (or the lack thereof).

Nevertheless, if dead bodies could sometimes be taken as transparent indices of individuals' otherworldly fates, the bodies of the living were caught up in an acutely equivocal relationship between sin and sickness.[100] As Andrew Crislip has demonstrated, the *Life of Anthony* offered one model for endowing physical health with divine significance, but Christian hagiographers from the following centuries advanced competing archetypes of sanctity, with texts like the Great Coptic *Life of Pachomius* presenting chronic illness, persistent infirmity, and an early death as markers of the devout ascetic.[101] It is by now well established that, in contrast to long-standing Greco-Roman philosophical tenets, early Christian writers treated bodily suffering neither as an indication of moral inferiority nor as a neutral circumstance to be born with equable acquiescence but as a spiritual good with profound benefits.[102] The belief that Jesus's painful death was key to his salvific grace and that the continued imitation of his suffering (whether through martyrdom or asceticism) constituted the apogee of Christian faith introduced a radically new dynamic to understandings of duty and piety in Late Antiquity. However, there emerged no stable interpretation specifically of sickness within the Christian tradition. Rather, as Crislip argues, a dialectical tension governed the meaning of illness: perfect health was associated with spiritual purity even as infirmity realized the Christian message. Similarly, sickness was understood to shift attention to the eternal life and act as a spur to humility, but it was also known to give weight to temporal needs and undermine the soul's absolute control over the body.[103]

Carolingian writers, no less than late antique Christians, acknowledged a diverse set of causes for why both the sinful and the saintly might fall ill. A clear pattern that emerges from the extant texts, however, is that genre played an important role in determining the lens through which bodily infirmity was construed and discussed. In epistolary exchanges, for example, the elite emphasized, above all, illness as a divine trial that aided in purifying the soul, drawing comparisons with the scourging of the righteous Job and invoking (if only implicitly) the Pauline dictum "whenever I am weak, then I am strong [2 Cor 12:10]." Within the corpus of Alcuin's letters, sickness is a subject that recurs often, especially over the last decade of his life when he complained frequently of the fevers and infirmities that kept him from certain duties.[104] Alcuin acknowledged that age brought with it a physical depletion—but such weakness reminded one to focus on the eternal, he insisted. Thus, we hear much about the spiritual benefit of illness from his letters and little about any attempts to remedy such ailments.[105] Setting illness within the framework of earthly struggle, Alcuin tacitly denied any suggestion that his fevers might be read as punishment for sin and instead compared his "tribulation of the body" to the sufferings of the saints.[106] Six years before his death, he wrote to Bishop Arn of Salzburg: "We are prosperous, thanks to God, except that fever and infirmity keep me tired. Nevertheless, he who is weaker will be stronger, according to the Apostle. And often corporeal infirmity is beneficial since it causes faith to grow stronger in the soul."[107] Running throughout Alcuin's correspondence is this reassurance—to himself, to his friends, to the elite of the empire—that just like the refining of gold, "man is cooked in the pain of the body so that a purer soul may spring forth from its place of imprisonment."[108]

Starting in the 820s, based on purported visionary journeys to the afterlife, there was a surge of textual descriptions of the purgatorial torments that might be inflicted for sins not fully expunged at the time of death.[109] As it became easier to imagine in vivid detail the cauldrons of scalding water, the whips of demons, and the frigid temperatures that awaited an imperfect soul, earthly sickness of the body held out the possibility of a purification *now* that might lessen the necessary purification *then*. In just this vein did Einhard offer consolation to Bernharius, bishop of Worms, regarding his illness: "I still take some comfort from knowing that this suffering will help you, for it is part of the purgation of your soul."[110] Although, Einhard clarified, one should remain hopeful for a cure, sickness was a salutary reminder to prepare for the certainty of death. Indeed, allusions to one's own ailments in correspondence served as indirect prompts for the solicitation of prayers. Lupus of Ferrières wrote to another monk that a potentially fatal abscess in his groin "produced such an abundance of prayers wherever the report of my illness spread that I make bold to suggest that this was brought about by divine favor."[111] In her *Handbook*, Dhuoda also frequently linked references to her weakness and frailty (alongside language suggesting she was ill) with requests that she be remembered in readers' prayers.[112] Just as physical suffering created a kind of bridge between the temporal and eternal phases of life, so were prayers and alms deemed essential to easing the soul's passage out of the body and alleviating the gravity of purgatorial punishments.

The body humbled by illness proved a popular image by which to evoke and reference oneself in epistolary exchanges among Carolingian peers. These writers were, for the most part, average Christians—sinners, attempting to lead a repentant life, not saints. When the Carolingians turned to the lives of the saints, they found therein examples of those who suffered bodily tribulation with patience and those who inflicted severe agony on their bodies as service to God. Although sometimes this mortification manifested as perfect health (as with Anthony), in other cases, it was the visibly broken body that was configured as saintly. Anthony's near contemporary, Symeon Stylites, was renowned not simply for his life atop a pillar but for cultivating a body covered in bug bites, with ulcers oozing pus and lacerations dripping blood.[113] By no means were these paradigms of extreme asceticism located only in eastern realms or the distant past—the sixth-century *Life of St. Radegund* by Venantius Fortunatus, for instance, praised the Abbess Radegund for the manner in which she shackled and burned her body, leaving it bloody, scarred, and putrefying.[114] And the style of sanctity introduced to the Frankish elite in the seventh century by the Irishman Columbanus and his disciples prized a particularly harsh attitude toward the body and an austere mode of life modeled on that of the Desert Fathers.[115]

Yet, while hagiography of both the early Christian age and the more recent Merovingian past continued to exert a strong influence on the development of monasticism across eighth-century Francia, the favor shown to the Benedictine Rule by Charlemagne and his successors tilted the scales in favor of a less severe ideal of sanctity than that modeled in the lives of Anthony, Symeon, Radegund, or Columbanus.[116] Although Carolingian councils actively discouraged the recognition of new local saints, *vitae* continued to promote the cults of recently deceased holy men and women.[117] The *Life of Benedict of Aniane*, composed by Ardo (a monk at Aniane) around 822, charted a path from excess to moderation for this prominent reformer of Benedictine monasticism under Louis the Pious.[118] When Benedict first became a monk, as Ardo describes, he sought to "damage his body with incredible fasting . . . endangering his own flesh as if it were a bloodthirsty beast."[119] His limbs wasted, his face gaunt, and his skin crawling with lice, Benedict was reprimanded by his abbot and instructed to reduce this regime of mortification, but he refused to comply with what he deemed the spineless Rule of Benedict of Nursia.[120] He left that first community to pursue a more abstemious way of life, until divine grace gradually taught Benedict to love the Rule, and he learned to become an exemplar to all monks.[121] Representing Benedict as the catalyst in the push for uniform monastic practice across the empire, Ardo connected these reforms with the manner in which the saint "turned away little by little from the rigor of his first way of life."[122] Ardo's work of hagiography offered no endorsement of an ascetic life that involved "choosing" illness.[123]

Rudolf of Fulda's *Life of Leoba* (d. 799), composed around a decade later than the *Life of Benedict of Aniane*, displays clear parallels to the ideal of sanctity elevated by Ardo. Here, Leoba, abbess of Bischofsheim and confidant of the missionary Boniface, is praised for the moderation she consistently exhibited in her habits.[124] As an example of how she acted according to the demands of reason, not excess, Rudolf draws attention to her insistence that the nuns not keep lengthy vigils for fear that fatigue would dull their attention to divine study.[125] In stark contrast to Fortunatus's Radegund, Leoba's holiness is shown to spring primarily from imitation of Christ's obedience and humility, not his physical suffering.

The same ascetic norms endorsed in ninth-century portrayals of Benedict and Leoba feature as significant concerns in contemporaneous prescriptive sources, like the commentaries on the Benedictine Rule by Smaragdus and Hildemar.[126] These authors made absolutely clear that the willful pursuit of infirmity was not an option for those seeking a cenobitic life. As they reflected on the Rule's directives about the treatment of sick brothers, the commentators were seemingly more concerned with those who willfully neglected their health and refused treatment than those who malingered in pursuit of special accommodations like meat and baths. While listing the accommodations that were to be granted to the sick, Smaragdus summed up the issue with discretion: "The healthy ought to accept those who are ailing, but the sick should not doubt that those who are healthy and those who are working are valued ahead of them."[127] Hildemar, by contrast, bluntly stated how the abbot should respond to a brother who refused to attend to his health by eating meat (the Rule allowed meat only to the very sick): "Brother, do not act thus. For it is better to eat meat and to recover from your sickness and to practice obedience than to not eat meat and to fall into greater sickness. . . . And, in the end, there will be a greater penalty, because you ought to have been a servant to your brothers and you were not."[128] If illness was frequently interpreted as a sign of divine testing—even of divine favor—among the Carolingian elite, these guides to the ascetic life in no way countenanced a response to sickness that privileged resigned suffering over active amelioration.[129] The lives of the Desert Fathers were not to be imitated in specifics by these Benedictine monks. Poor health was unfortunate because it prevented the monk from participating in the common schedule that bound the community together, but choosing illness through mortification was a dangerous vice because it stemmed from a will that had not been properly subjected to the abbot's authority. Hence, in contrast to the epistolary evidence, the ascetic literature suggests that illness could be a sign of disobedience or pride in ninth-century readings of the body.

## The Purgation of Sin

On an individual level, the ill and suffering body was a potent symbol—but an ambiguous one. Just as the Bible contained contradictions that could be decoded only with an advanced knowledge of signs and their multivalent interpretations, so did health (or its lack) only sometimes signal with transparency the state of the soul within. Sickness could be read as sanctity, as purification, as pride, or as selfishness, and Carolingian authors clearly recognized this inherent obscurity as they made efforts to categorize their subjects within one of these traditions.[130] Sickness could also be understood as a direct manifestation of sinfulness, whereby God or his servants punished an offense in an immediate and perceptible fashion. However, early medieval sources only rarely ascribed personal illness to personal sin.[131] Instead, sin and sickness were most directly correlated when discussing larger collectives, not individuals. To the extent that mortality, disease, and pain were consequences of the fall from paradise, illness on a broad scale reflected the sinfulness of humanity.[132] It was in this vein that Carolingian writers assumed widespread disease within the population indicated retribution from an angry God.

The annals and chronicles that documented the affairs of king and kingdom were particularly likely to embed reports of disease within implicit references to divine judgment. As Paul Dutton has illuminated, the author of the *Royal Frankish Annals* did not simply record natural phenomena like eclipses, earthquakes, famines, and epidemics but—especially between the years 820 and 829—shaped these disasters into a statement on Louis's rule. The annalist, as a "reader of patterns of disorder in the Carolingian empire," interpreted these events as responses to the king's fall from righteousness and the ensuing escalation of sin within the populace.[133] Thus, the entry for 820, which associated a deluge of rain with a failure of major crops and a pestilence that struck both humans and cattle, can be situated within the tide of criticism that resulted in Louis and his court performing a public penance in 822.[134]

This chain of connections between sin–weather–disease–reparation was nothing new, as Charlemagne had responded to famines and epidemics with a call to all subjects to fast and pray as a means to restore divine favor.[135] In 805, for example, learning that disease had broken out in certain regions and anticipating a dangerous famine as a result of bad weather damaging crops, the emperor ordered all people to observe three sets of three-day fasts (with accompanying litanies and masses).[136] For, as he announced, the realm was suffering such calamities "on account of our deserts," and thus it was necessary to seek help from God who had promised, "Ask, and it will be given to you [Mt 7:7]."[137] Indeed, just as the confessor-physician needed to peel back the external layers to expose the hidden sin, so did Charlemagne deduce the origin of the problem by reading the signs: "From these earthly (*exterioribus*) events we are able to infer with absolute certainty that we, who are compelled to suffer such great evils *externally* (*exterius*), are not pleasing to God *internally* (*interius*) in all respects."[138] With a similar mentality, when composing the entry for 869 in the *Annals of Saint-Bertin*, Hincmar criticized King Lothar II not only for bringing an epidemic upon his men, as retribution for his sinful attempts to secure a divorce, but also for failing to recognize the epidemic as a judgment of God and take immediate penitential action.[139]

The same assumptions about widespread sin undergirded early medieval miracle compilations. Over the course of the ninth century, holy relics were increasingly disseminated across the Carolingian countryside, establishing little pockets of concentrated divine power within local communities.[140] Here, at the shrines to the saints, simply by displaying their devotion to God and his servants, the sick and disabled could anticipate a spontaneous cure. In documenting and summarizing these cures, Carolingian stewards of the relics followed the paths laid by such popular texts as the *Miracles of St. Martin*.[141] Yet ninth-century accounts did not necessarily emulate the tenor of Gregory of Tours's descriptions. Gregory was comparatively explicit in linking the healing miracles of Martin with the alleviation of individual sin, suggesting that every cure on earth manifested forgiveness of iniquity in eternity: "Just as they [the saints] cleanse the horrible ulcers of ghastly leprosy here, so through their intervention they obtain relief for the blemishes of sin there."[142] In composing his vignettes, Gregory often detailed the specific fault that precipitated the illness or disability.[143] By comparison, in a presentation of the cures effected by relics under *his* protection, the Carolingian courtier Einhard favored a looser association between disease and personal sin.

As one of the earliest narratives detailing the transferal of martyrs' relics from Roman crypts to Frankish churches and monasteries, Einhard's

*Translation and Miracles of Saints Marcellinus and Peter* established a model for future medieval *translatio* accounts.[144] Not only did it shape a new genre of hagiographical writing, but it also deployed miracle stories as commentary on the troubled state of the realm in the late 820s.[145] Like the *Royal Frankish Annals*, the text depicted the empire suffering under a mounting tide of disorder left unchecked because of the inaction of those responsible for its safekeeping.[146] Einhard attributed culpability primarily to Emperor Louis and implied that the ill health of souls under his care was visibly manifest in the disabled bodies flocking to the relics for aid.[147] Indeed, the text offers a relatively concrete etiology for sickness: the demon Wiggo (speaking through a possessed girl) explains that he and eleven other demons have been divinely ordered to devastate crops, infect cattle, spread pestilence, and stir up other evils because the people have not kept their promises to God or atoned for their sins.[148] While Einhard is clear that pervasive sinfulness is the cause of disease, only once in the entire text does he name a particular, personal sin as the trigger for a disability.[149]

Rather than a small-scale relationship between inner sin and outer disease, Einhard highlights the large-scale relationship between a sinful realm and dysfunctional bodies—a situation of turmoil that makes the saints' help urgently necessary. And it is here, in his descriptions of the cures themselves, that sin is made tangible to the senses. Einhard's saints purge the realm by purging bodies of corrupt matter. The work is not a series of accounts of liminal individuals being restored to their communities; it is a series of individual testimonies that fuse into one account of the realm being healed from its deep-seated disease.[150] The emphasis is on the hiddenness of sin being exposed in vivid, bodily terms.

Within the *Translation*, there are a total of seventy-two healing miracles (including three exorcisms), most of which concern physical impairments obvious to an observer.[151] Of this total, the majority are brief entries (with no specifics apart from the date, name, place of origin, and illness), but among those entries that are longer, ten miracles involve a moment when some type of fluid gushes out of the afflicted individual.[152] This is important because of the disruption it causes and its role as signifier of invisible divine action. In most instances, this fluid is blood and runs out of the nose and mouth, but phlegm, bile, and sweat are also mentioned, and in one case, blood runs out of the toenails of a woman with contorted muscles.[153]

One of the first of these miracles occurs upon the arrival of the relics at Einhard's property in Seligenstadt. As Einhard narrates, just as a Mass was coming to an end, two healing miracles occurred nearly simultaneously, one inside and one outside the church. Beside the doors to the sanctuary, a paralyzed woman lay on the ground and called out to the martyrs for help. "And soon, in front of all those who had been standing around watching, she began to be shaken, with her internal organs moving about as if she were going to be sick, and then, vomiting, she began to spew forth a huge amount of phlegm and bile."[154] Once these substances had been shaken out of the poor woman, she was able to drink some cold water, hobble inside the church, and worship the relics.

On another occasion, a blind man who suffered from a severe trembling that prevented him from carrying out basic functions received a cure from the saints at the very moment that the Gospel was being read out. This man cried out to the saints, fell to the ground, and lay prone on the floor of the church. Rushing over to him, witnesses found his "chin and chest soaked with blood running out of his nose." After drinking some cold water, the man proclaimed that he thought "someone had struck him in the neck with a fist." However, it was all for the best, Einhard observes, because that blow was "so health-giving" (*tam salutaris*) that he never suffered any trembling again.[155]

These two examples evince many of the elements common to the longer miracle accounts in the *Translation*. The miracle almost always occurs during a divine service, particularly the Mass. The sufferer typically falls to the ground as if dead or asleep and then rises, cured. In addition to (and often in conjunction with) the outpouring of fluids, it is common that the saints heal through violent force—shaking, striking blows, vigorously stretching out contorted muscles.[156] Rather than suggesting that the saints bestow healing only on those willing to suffer further bodily pain, Einhard implies that the saints act thus because they are still bound, in some way, by the constitution of the physical world. They must induce a reconfiguration of the fluids and structures of the body by purging harmful substances, rupturing blockages, and reshaping anatomical frameworks. The saints do not punish but release.[157] Their methods leave the floors of the church covered in blood, like a room in which a physician has recently performed phlebotomy. Given the timing of many of the miracles in Einhard's narrative, there is a powerful symmetry between the ingestion of the body and blood of Christ in the Mass, "by which the populace is restored to the health of their souls," and the discharge of blood from the bodies of the infirm.[158]

The purgation effected by Einhard's relics is an eradication of sin, made possible by the bloody sacrifice of Christ and the martyrs Marcellinus and

Peter. It is a sign that bodies have not been made "temples of the Holy Spirit" (1 Cor 6:19), but whether those bodies were singularly exposed to risk on account of their own iniquity is not made clear in the text.[159] Certainly, one finds parallels with Paulinus's manual for Eric in the idea that demons have the ability to penetrate the flesh. The line between illness and possession is blurry, since both are in some way attributable to demonic influence yet not to a specific fault of the victim.[160] Composed in the 840s, Rudolf of Fulda's account of relic translations includes many examples of exorcisms, several of which follow Einhard's model of equating purification with violent bodily processes.[161] A woman who had suffered demonic possession over ten years, for example, was led to the church by her parents, and as the priest was celebrating Mass, Rudolf explains, "suddenly she vomited forth something foul and fetid (I do not know what), and together with the vomit the demon exited, and she was cured and became sound in mind."[162] There is no suggestion that a particular bodily constitution is more prone to demonic entry (as Nancy Caciola has found for the later Middle Ages).[163] However, there is a strong connection between cosmic disorder and bodily matter—particularly, internal, hidden matter that needs to be expelled, externalized, and made visible. Blood and putrid substances flow forth from the body as part of the healing process, and a humor with the color of blood also miraculously drips forth from the relics themselves.[164] Just as the latter manifests the living soul that continues to animate the dead bones, so can we see the former as proof of the "unblocking" of the inner soul, its freedom to move through the body unrestrained now that evil has been overcome.[165]

## The Difficulties of Diagnosis

Carolingian *translatio* texts emphasize repeatedly that those cured by the saints receive "the most complete health of mind and body," being restored to a "pristine" state (*prima sanitas*).[166] This pristineness evokes images of Adam and Eve in Eden while also pointing toward the future resurrected body, as manifest in the integrity enjoyed by the uncorrupted bodies of dead saints. Just as we saw above that the language of virtues and vices crossed between the physical and moral spheres, so in these miracles do the *virtutes* of the saints (or divine *virtus* channeled through the saints) overcome the disorder within and return the body and soul to a harmonious and purified existence.

Among the instructions to her son William, Dhuoda included a short section devoted to explaining the meaning of bodily illness and the appropriate response to it. She urged her son neither to give up nor despair if he were struck by infirmity because sickness was not necessarily a punishment from God. To assist William in decoding sickness, she laid out a tripartite schema: some people suffer "simple" illnesses as chastisement for minor sins; some (like Pontius Pilate) endure "double" torments in body and soul for their wickedness; and some (like Lazarus) become infirm on no account of their own but as a means to glorify the healing power of God. Dhuoda expressed the sincere hope that William would receive bodily health from God as recompense for his faithful service. Yet she wavered in declaring this a certainty by acknowledging that illness could also serve as a spiritual benefit and, consequently, might be bestowed by God as a demonstration of divine love. Ultimately, the only conclusive message this spiritual advisor could impart to her reader was that "health and illness have various effects in this world, as is often the case in human affairs."[167]

Dhuoda's uncertainties about bodily health (especially in the face of the certitude and confidence with which she pronounced on other religious matters) reflected her society's doubts regarding the right way to construe fluctuations in the state of the soul's home or container. We have seen that the sick body could be presented as both an indication of sanctity and proof of punishment for sin. In referencing their own illnesses, the Carolingian elite played on both possibilities, asserting that their ailments testified to a process of purification (for sins that would otherwise be cleansed in purgatorial punishments) and presenting themselves as weak sinners in need of others' prayers.

At the same time, despite this range of interpretations, I have suggested that writers associated with the Carolingian *correctio* did not favor the ideal of the sickly saint. Hagiography was a particularly conservative genre, in which late antique models played a powerful role. Thus, Ardo's and Rudolf's decisions to present their male and female saints in terms that frowned on the willful pursuit of sickness point toward a shift in Carolingian priorities, one also evinced in monastic prescriptive literature that discouraged extreme asceticism.

At base, illness could never be definitively categorized because it was implicated in twofold obscurity—the hidden space of the body's interior and the invisible nature of the soul. The virtues and vices that competed for dominance were concealed within these entities, and thus a diagnosis of the *salus* (health/salvation) of body and soul was subject to misinterpretation. A response to illness, however, did not necessarily depend upon determining its spiritual significance. What mattered was the religious orthodoxy of the response itself—and so the next chapter takes us into Carolingian theories of medical intervention.

# PART II

## Medicine for the Body and Soul

CHAPTER 4

# Christianizing Bodily Cures

Around the year 800 at the monastery of Lorsch, an anonymous group of scribes put together a manuscript of just over one hundred folios replete with a variety of medical texts: a poem on the earth's salubrious bounty, a short history about medical authorities, a description of the humors, lists of herbals recipes, and dietary recommendations, to name but a few.[1] Yet, in the eyes of modern historians, by far the most intriguing part of this codex has been its opening text.[2] Of unknown origin, it conveys an animated mood of righteous authorial indignation in its very first lines:

> I am forced to respond to those people who say that I, inanely, have written this book, and who declare that there is very little truth contained in it. But I, *like a deaf man, did not listen* to their words [Ps 37:14], because I considered the need of those suffering more than the denunciation of those in a frenzy against me. Hence, I will respond to them, not in my own words but in the words of sacred scripture, that human medicine ought not to be completely cast aside, since it is apparent that it is not unknown in the divine books. Therefore, let us now describe what [scripture] says, with the Lord's support.[3]

Not only is this a particularly self-assured declaration in an age dominated by the standard humility topos, but it is also the only such "apology for medicine" written in Latin from the early Middle Ages, and the Lorsch manuscript preserves its sole witness. What significance should be attached to this unusual text and the circumstances surrounding its production at Lorsch in the years around Charlemagne's assumption of the imperial title?

The *Lorscher Arzneibuch* (as this codex is now called) has figured most prominently in nationalistic arguments for German contributions to Western medicine.[4] This chapter, by contrast, situates the Lorsch codex, particularly its opening preface, within the evolution of Christian theological and pastoral problems foregrounded by the impulses of the Carolingian *correctio.*[5] The ways in which medical texts were presented (including how they were prefaced, decorated, and framed) in numerous extant manuscripts suggests that medicine as a field of study and practice was subject to intensified scrutiny around the turn of the ninth century. Against unnamed detractors, the Lorsch apology claims that medicine is useful, a pagan heritage that can be turned to Christian ends, an art contributing to the pursuit of wisdom, and a bodily treatment that is endorsed and overseen by God. This chapter follows the lines of these arguments through other medical manuscripts as well as exegesis, encyclopedias, handbooks, capitularies, and liberal arts curricula produced by Carolingian scholars over the late eighth and ninth centuries. I hope to demonstrate that the act of defining what constituted medicine was a gradual process that exposed and reflected a network of interrelated concerns: the dangers of what were classified as "lingering pagan practices," the presence of so-called magical elements in late antique medical texts, and the continuous negotiation of Christian identity across a realm of diverse traditions. In this way, discussions about medicine's benefits and risks stood alongside other rites and customs that came under urgent scrutiny in the ninth century. Just as the Saxon conquests triggered questions about the conversion mechanisms of baptism, so did new interest in the Roman liberal arts and anxieties regarding subversive paganism encourage the Christianization of medical care.[6]

To be sure, herbal, dietetic, and surgical medicine were already part of the Frankish world before the Carolingians came to power.[7] The herbals of Pseudo-Apuleius and Dioscorides and the Galenic synopses of Oribasius seem to have been available in at least some Merovingian libraries, and over the seventh and eighth centuries monasteries such as Corbie may well have been key participants in the translation of Greek medical texts.[8] There is also every likelihood that Visigothic manuscripts supplied the Carolingians with some of their exemplars.[9] I am not arguing that medical techniques were forbidden before the development of Carolingian strategies to legitimize them. Rather, I am proposing that, during the reigns of Charlemagne and Louis the Pious, the religious and intellectual environment was one that encouraged the elite to critically assess the value of medicine.

The concept of a Christian medical art assumed form through repeated scholarly endeavors to demarcate the orthodox beliefs of the present from the pagan learning of antiquity. Such endeavors impinged not only on the uses of medical literature but also on theological understandings of the care of the body. The act of restoring a suffering body to health through medicine rather than miracle raised a variety of thorny, interconnected questions about the value of ascetic practices, the divine meaning of sickness, and the carnal indulgence of medical treatments. Thus, to justify treatment as a necessary and worthy skill in a Christian society was to encourage a more positive attitude toward physical health than certain early medieval ascetics seemed to condone. Determining the ways in which knowledge of medical cures *should* be part of a Christian lifestyle was especially problematic because late antique Latin authorities offered little guidance on these matters.

Although Carolingian scholars relied heavily on the writings of the Church Fathers in determining matters of orthodoxy, no Latin Father had offered a precise, prescriptive statement on the legitimate uses of medicine.[10] The Greek Fathers engaged the issue of classical medicine explicitly—Bishop Nemesius of Emesa (fl. 390), for example, attempted to reconcile Galenic anatomy and physiology with Christian teachings on the soul, and Bishop Basil of Caesarea (d. 379) answered at length the question of whether the medical art was compatible with norms of ascetic piety.[11] But there was no Latin text comparable to Nemesius's, and Basil's section on medicine did not make it into the Latin translation of his *Rules*; in general, the works of Greek theologians were less well known in the western kingdoms of the former Roman Empire.[12] To be sure, between the third and early eighth centuries, prominent Latin theologians from North Africa to England indicated a familiarity with classical medical ideas and texts but did not see a need to pronounce on the legitimacy of medicine as a discrete discipline.[13] The most revered Latin Fathers (Ambrose, Jerome, and Augustine) are not mentioned or cited in the Lorsch apology; the only authorities called upon by name are Pope Gregory the Great, Isidore of Seville, and Bede the Northumbrian monk.[14]

Of earlier Latin writers, it is two in particular—the sixth-century Roman official Cassiodorus and the seventh-century Bishop Isidore of Seville—who furnished the apologist with examples of Christianity's adoption of medicine. The apology recommends that the reader consult Isidore's encyclopedia, the *Etymologies*, and cites, without attribution, his *Sentences* and *On the Differences of Things*. In his encyclopedia, Isidore devoted an entire book to medicine's history, the humors, various ailments, and general remedies; by including such information, he implicitly classified it as something essential for future Christian societies.[15] He offered no theological justification for medicine's presence but appealed to an ancient trope that it was like a "second philosophy" because it required education in all of the liberal arts to understand the body (as philosophy did the soul).[16] Cassiodorus, meanwhile, in his *Institutes*, a study guide for the monks at his own southern Italian monastery of Vivarium, encouraged the brothers to read and copy works by Hippocrates, Galen, Caelius Aurelius, and Dioscorides.[17] Cassiodorus not only framed medicine as a component of Christian education but also advocated a devotional angle to medical endeavors, emphasizing the eternal rewards granted to those who charitably heal the sick. Of all Latin writings prior to the ninth century, then, the *Institutes* offered the most explicit endorsement of medicine as a Christian practice and, not surprisingly, was the one patristic work quoted at length in the Lorsch apology.[18]

Still, nothing resembling the defense of medicine can be found among the writings of earlier Latin authorities. The circumstances of the *Lorscher Arzneibuch*'s production were determined by the paleographical work of Bernhard Bischoff, who assigned the manuscript to the scriptorium of Lorsch between the 780s and the early ninth century.[19] The numerous corrections and marginalia throughout the codex show that it was continually used and edited across the ninth and tenth centuries, although there is no evidence that the manuscript was ever copied.[20] Its clear organization, with the preface and a series of short pedagogical texts followed by five chapters of cures for different ailments, suggests that the scriptorium considered this an important undertaking, not a hasty assignment.[21] While the apology itself may have been composed by a single person, the complete finished codex reflects the effort of several individuals, as witnessed in the many scribal hands.[22] Additionally, although a first-person voice structures the apology (and I refer to this voice as the Lorsch author or apologist[23]), the composition should surely be read as a consensus of opinion among a particular group within the scriptorium or among the monks at the monastery. Given that much of the work involved selecting and ordering remedies from earlier collections (such as the *Physica of Pliny*), some scholars have suggested that the prefatory apologetic text was most likely a copy of an existing work, too.[24] To be sure, the five books of cures may well have been copied from an earlier exemplar, and it is plausible that the apology was too, but the most likely scenario is that the first section of the codex was composed at Lorsch. The manuscript produced there contains the only extant copy of the apology, and later library catalogues from Lorsch indicate the possession of several works utilized in its composition.[25] Furthermore, the apology mentions "Bede the priest" by name and cites a work he composed in 710—evidence that it must postdate the early decades of the eighth century.[26] By midcentury, certainly, Bede's reputation was already well established on the Continent thanks to English missionaries like Boniface, and it would continue to grow under the influence of Alcuin and his students.[27]

The Lorsch author positions the text as a defensive rebuttal.[28] If his words are to be taken seriously, the apology assumes a context in which medical material was already circulating and had attracted criticism from certain factions within the Carolingian elite.[29] Such a perspective is confirmed by the survival of a handful of Carolingian medical codices produced around the same time as the *Lorscher Arzneibuch*.[30] Recent scholarship has begun to overturn the narrative that open-ended debate ceased with the Christianization of the Roman world, and it is within this newfound appreciation for generative dialogue in the early Middle Ages that we should set the Lorsch apology.[31] There is no reason to read the combative stance of the apologist as merely formulaic, especially in light of the fact that public discussions on theological matters occurred frequently at Aachen in the years around 800.[32] Nor, indeed, should we assume that debate about medicine's status concluded in the early ninth century, given that declarations about the legitimacy of medicine continue to be found in manuscripts produced over the century. With the *Lorscher Arzneibuch* as a guide, it becomes easier to see these as ongoing attempts to build consensus about the definition of a Christian medical art.

## The Usefulness of Human Medicine

As promised in the opening lines of the apology, the author brings together an impressive array of quotations from scripture (citing approximately fifty distinct passages from the Old and New Testaments) to support his claim that the Bible recognizes the legitimacy of medicine. Alongside scriptural references, the one constant that runs through the apology is the recurrent declaration that "human medicine should not be opposed" (*medicina humana non est refutanda*). With some variations that include "earthly medicine" (*medicina terrena*) and "human comforts" (*solacia humana*), this declaration is reiterated five times in different contexts.[33]

Although the concept of *human medicine* occurs in patristic writings, it exists there either as a general term denoting, broadly, all human endeavors or, alternatively, as a specific reference to medical practice, in which case it is encumbered by negative associations. When, for example, Jerome refers to it in discussing Job's trials, he does so in order to contrast the futility of human medicine with the healing efficacy of Job's patience and faith.[34] By contrast, every time that the Lorsch apology invokes the idea of human or earthly medicine, it underscores the efficacy of medical remedies and the divine sanction that they enjoy. *Human medicine* signals a defined realm of human ingenuity—namely, the cures and recipes discovered by earlier medical authorities and transmitted in the rest of the codex. The very recurrence of the phrase assumes the existence of a clear (if contested) discipline of medical practice, and the string of biblical proofs employed to endorse this discipline, in turn, emphasizes its authoritative position within the sphere of earthly human labor.

Evincing a familiarity with the hermeneutic of layered biblical exegesis, the author turns to two Old Testament events with the aim of illustrating how they can be read as God's validation of the medical art.[35] When, according to God's commands, Moses immersed wood into bitter water and Elisha sprinkled salt into corrupted water in order to make it drinkable, they represented the practice of medicine, the apologist proclaims. At the historical or literal level (*iuxta hystoriam*), these holy men imitated the actions of doctors mixing honey and garlic into bitter medicines. At the mystical level (*mysticus sensus*), they symbolized the divine physician: that is, God's own act of healing humanity's corruption through the wood of the cross and the salt of Christ's wisdom.[36] Although a certain degree of creative flexibility was inherent in biblical exegesis, the Lorsch author takes a particularly expansive view of the literal sense in interpreting a miraculous cure for water as a medical custom (*medicinalis mos*) of compounding remedies. This enables him to find scriptural validation for the work of real, human physicians by likening it to God's spiritual act of healing sin.

The apologist frequently undertakes this rather unusual literal interpretation of the Bible. For example, the Apostle Paul's statement, "Let him who is weak eat vegetables [Rom 14:2]," was typically construed as a metaphor about gradations of spiritual faith and the need to adjust teachings according to the capacity of the audience.[37] In the apology, however, Paul's saying is taken as a straightforward dietary recommendation.[38] Similarly, when Jeremiah employs figurative language to recall the sins of the Israelites ("Though you wash yourself with lye and frequently use the herb soapwort, you are stained in your iniquity [Jer 2:22]"), the apologist asserts that substances like lye and soapwort should be understood as the names of drugs and that the presence of drugs in scripture is proof of divine approbation for the medical art.[39] His exegesis moves fluidly between metaphorical phrases, literal interpretations, and the moral meaning of scripture in order to showcase how the Old Testament prophets and Christian disciples proclaimed the utility of physicians and their remedies.

The contention that human medicine is useful (*utilis*), and that this is reflected not only in direct scriptural references but also in the bounty of the material world, is one of the very first arguments articulated in the apology.[40] What impelled the author to compile this book against those who would criticize it was the need of the sick—a need, he shows, that is addressed by God's creation and God's written word in the Bible. Here, the argument moves between demonstrating *practical utility*, in that natural substances are medically efficacious in healing the body, and *spiritual utility*, in that healing the body can be a means of worshipping God. Citing Psalms on the fact that God made everything in the heavens and on earth, the apologist concludes that all created things are good due to God's goodness. He later elaborates that God's creation of man from the earth was complemented by his dispensation of earthly medicines to heal the body's infirmities.[41] Just so, the Gospel anecdote about Christ healing a blind man by rubbing a mixture of earth and spit on his eyes becomes, in the apology, proof of the healing properties of the earth rather than of Christ's miraculous spit.[42]

In this discussion, the apology relies heavily on the biblical book of Sirach or Ecclesiasticus, which includes a long discourse on the respect and honor owed to physicians because their healing skills come from God.[43] Sirach declares that "the Most High created medicine from the earth and a judicious person will not scorn it," an idea that the apology emphasizes repeatedly.[44] Given the biblical affirmation that the earth's substances are to be used, those who would criticize treatments made from nature are "foolish and ignorant" (*insipiens et inprudens*).[45] The apologist even provides a list of exemplary men from the past who made use of medicine and were nevertheless recognized as holy and favored by God (Germanus of Capua, Gregory the Great, Luke the Evangelist, and Saints Cosmas and Damian). Of course, the Lorsch author focused on those aspects of scripture that supported his agenda; his opponents could well have called up the example of King Asa of Judah, who sought the skill of physicians, not the help of God, for his diseased feet and died in his stubbornness (2 Chr 16:12–13).

The Lorsch apologist was not the only Carolingian scholar to highlight these particular passages about medicine in Sirach. A medical manuscript produced in western or northern Francia some decades after the *Lorscher Arzneibuch* contains a text entitled *Letter of Solomon*, which turns out to be the first nine verses of Sirach 38.[46] That the compiler ascribed the biblical passage to Solomon was not at all unusual, but that s/he chose to frame it as a letter and inserted it among other medical letters attributed to Hippocrates, Galen, and Vindicianus was unique. Evidently, the agenda of the compiler was to lend a Christian authority and justification to the copying of the other medical treatises, and the most effective means to do this was to turn to scripture.

Around the same time that this manuscript was produced, Hrabanus Maurus completed the first Christian commentary on the book of Sirach, which he dedicated to Archbishop Otgar of Mainz.[47] Like the *Lorscher Arzneibuch*, Hrabanus's exegesis focused on the belief that all of God's creation was good, and it was the duty of humans to use these gifts prudently—"From the things of the earth, God provided comforts for human sicknesses, so why would anyone wise and sensible dare to condemn and despise these?"[48] Indeed, many of Hrabanus's comments show a remarkable resemblance to the declarations of the Lorsch apologist. Both authors concentrate on the usefulness of human medicine and the mandate not to reject divine benefaction: "We should not spurn those things that we know that our Creator produced for our utility and health, but with thanks we ought to receive them and turn them to our uses."[49] When composing his Christian encyclopedia, *On the Natures of Things*, a few years after his commentary on Sirach, Hrabanus chose to reemphasize these same themes. As part of his attempt to establish *On the Natures of Things* as a complement to the more secular *Etymologies*, the bishop employed Sirach to elaborate on Isidore's declaration that "the cure of medicine should not be spurned." For, he added, "we read that holy men utilized it and in Ecclesiasticus the following is written about it: *Honor the medicus on account of necessity because the Most High created him* [Sir 38:1]."[50]

While Hrabanus relied on Isidore's text primarily as a foundation upon which to build his own spiritual interpretation of various diseases and cures, his encyclopedia did not dismiss or overlook the value of classical medical learning, as the *Etymologies* had summarized it.[51] He retained much of Isidore's prefatory information regarding the history of medicine, the framework of the humors, and the aims of medical care, and he sought to strengthen the *Etymologies*'s message that pagan medical learning was a gift from God.[52] That he turned to Sirach as a means to endorse medical practice should draw our attention to the discursive lines connecting Hrabanus with the *Lorscher Arzneibuch* and the *Letter of Solomon*.[53]

This interest among Carolingian authors in the book of Sirach correlates closely with a viewpoint that considers God's provision for human illness through the bounty of the material world. Such a view is on display in a set of verses composed by Jacobus, a notary active at Charlemagne's court between 787 and 792.[54] As Jacobus himself explains in these verses, he wrote them as a preface for a copy of the late antique poem of medical remedies by one Quintus Serenus, a copy that Charlemagne had ordered him to make and that apparently circulated widely across the realm.[55] Certainly, the large number of related extant versions of the poem, especially from the ninth century, and its appearance in several library catalogues and personal florilegia from that century, suggest that its popularity stemmed directly from Charlemagne's endorsement.[56] In his verses, Jacobus praises the health-giving powers of herbs, flowers, and trees and tells the reader that a wealth of information about the products of the earth, sea, sand, and air can be found in the following poem. He then links the curative potential of these earthly substances with the practice of medicine more generally and with Charlemagne's motives in soliciting a copy of Quintus Serenus's work. Addressing the audience directly, Jacobus indicates the king's desired effect on future readers: "By offering a pleasing draught to those languishing, you will be able to present a pious cure from the lord who reigns."[57] This is immediately followed by a reference to Charlemagne reigning by the "virtue of Christ," a stylistic decision that serves to obscure the precise identity of "the lord who reigns" and to suggest that the pleasing draught comes from both earthly king and heavenly Christ. Jacobus's verses thereby associate God's provision of earthly substances with "ancient" remedy books and royal support in alleviating suffering.[58]

Verses that emphasize the abundance of useful plants, particularly in the author's own vicinity, also appear in the *Lorscher Arzneibuch*, produced only years after Jacobus's poem, and in Walafrid Strabo's *On the Cultivation of Gardens*, composed in the 840s while Walafrid was abbot of Reichenau monastery.[59] In its praise for the properties of various flowers, plants, and herbs found in the monastic garden, Walafrid's poem is a work of thanksgiving to God for his largesse.[60] Although not an explicit endorsement of medical practice, *On the Cultivation of Gardens* borrowed from Quintus Serenus's work, and Walafrid could well have envisioned that it might serve as a type of herbal.[61] At the very least, he wished to alert his peers to the inconspicuous miracles of creation, like the rose's power to combat hidden toxins and the poppy's ability to inhibit a stomach ulcer.

In all of these ways, then, we see how the Lorsch apology articulated arguments grounded in scripture that were similar to those found in exegesis, other medical manuscripts, and poetry from the first four decades of the ninth century. The decision to focus on herbal remedies and natural substances as *things-to-be-used* was not simply a practical response but intersected with a broader political discourse characterizing the Carolingians as effective, useful leaders, in contrast to the *inutilitas* (uselessness) of their Merovingian predecessors.[62]

## Demarcating Medicine from Magic

If utility was considered in terms not simply of healing the body but also of advancing spiritual ends, then compilers had to contend with medical therapeutics that might have been considered efficacious but whose efficacy was guaranteed not by Christian faith but by superstition and sorcery. Not only did associations with paganism pervade medicine's past, but persisting intersections with illicit practices continued to trouble its status in ninth-century society. Accusations of "magic" had been exploited by hard-liners like Bishop Caesarius of Arles (d. 542) and Boniface the missionary (d. 754) in order to call out what they deemed incomplete conversion within Francia. Although this weighty accusation referenced an inherently unstable category, it served as a useful catchall for acts and beliefs that placed trust in powers separate or removed from those of the Trinity.[63]

Common medical treatments were vulnerable to condemnation for three main reasons. First, many of the remedies inherited from the Greco-Roman medical tradition included magical elements, such as incantations invoking the gods or seemingly superstitious instructions for preparing various medicines.[64] Second, some of the most popular (or at least prevalent) types of medical texts from the Carolingian period were various prognostic materials used to predict the length, severity, and crisis of an illness.[65] These bore a strong resemblance to the same divinatory practices proscribed as superstition in royal and canon law. Third, many of the cures recommended in recipe books assumed an understanding of the natural world in which certain substances were endowed with an unusual power (*virtus*) and might even be beseeched directly for help, as if they were independent agents.[66] Such confidence in mundane, material objects and humans' ability to manipulate them could be seen to detract from God's omnipotence over the created cosmos.[67]

Augustine's invectives in *On Christian Teaching* and *The City of God* carried a powerful warning about the coincidence between medical and magical practices. Although he condoned Hippocratic theories of disease causation against the explanations of astrologers, he forbade Christians from consulting prognostic texts that depended on the idea of lucky and unlucky days (including lists of so-called Egyptian Days on which bloodletting was forbidden), attributing such beliefs to demonic suggestion.[68] The bishop also counseled against herbs in amulets: "For it is one thing to say, 'If you drink that common herb, your belly will not hurt,' and another to say, 'If you suspend that herb from your neck, your stomach will not hurt.'"[69] The first action was acceptable medicine; the second was discredited magic. Yet, Augustine acknowledged a situation more complex than this simple binary. When a person fastened herbs externally on the body, without using incantations or engraved symbols, Augustine allowed that the herb might be efficacious through a "power of nature" (*vis naturae*) rather than through a magical binding. In the end, early medieval readers confronted an ambiguous directive from the authoritative Father—the "intention" behind herbal use was more important than whether the substance was found in a drink or amulet.[70]

Boundaries between medicine and magic were notoriously difficult to define and police. Although Hippocrates was lauded in histories of medicine as the inventor of a rational tradition, by no means did classical medicine embody a purely logical approach that gave way to folk superstitions at the dawn of the Middle Ages.[71] Instead, as historians trying to counter such stereotypes have observed, magical, medicinal, and miraculous approaches to mediating bodily sickness and health were all part of the ancient world and continued to be demarcated by perspective and circumstance rather than inherent character. Questions of discernment and categorization intensified in the midst of the late eighth- and early ninth-century reforming efforts.[72]

In the context of reforming councils held in eastern Francia in the early 740s, someone wrote down a list of proscribed pagan behaviors, which included the vague notations "On amulets and ligatures," "On incantations," and "On the brains of animals."[73] The fact that numerous recipes in early medieval collections recommended the use of charms, ligatures, and substances like animal brains and feces illustrates the precarious position in which Carolingian healers might have found themselves. The interpretive problems were manifold. How was one to distinguish a forbidden substance (like vulture brains) from the inherently powerful medicines of the earth? Which recipe instructions were superstitious and which were simply rational, given, for instance, that Bede had observed that earthly materials underwent transformations in accordance with the waxing and waning of the moon?[74] If twigs, stone shavings, and bits of bone might be carried around as holy relics, what demarcated Christian and magical amulets?[75]

The Carolingian dynasty had risen to power by cultivating alliances with church reformers like Boniface, who built his reputation on weeding out pagan customs and beliefs among both the general populace and the clergy in Bavaria, Francia, and Thuringia.[76] Charlemagne's violent military campaign against the pagan Saxons, which began in 772 and continued over three decades, fomented concern regarding the lurking presence of un-Christian practices within the Carolingian kingdom.[77] Reiterating denunciations against enchanters in Merovingian sermons and hagiography, Carolingian rulers evinced a fervent preoccupation with the persistence of magic and magicians among their subjects.[78] Capitularies issued by Charlemagne forbade the consultation of magicians, enchanters, weather wizards, soothsayers, diviners, or amulet makers, even drawing attention to the act of drinking an "unclean thing for the sake of medicine."[79] The Council of Paris in 829 devoted an entire chapter to how divine law would punish magicians, soothsayers, diviners, poisoners, enchanters, and dream interpreters. It likewise proscribed the use of love potions, amulets, and illusions that disturbed the stability of the mind.[80] Penitentials included penalties for those who had sinned by consulting magicians.[81] In his work *On the Magical Arts*, Hrabanus argued for both the demonic basis of these practices and their ultimate futility in a world controlled by God.[82] Yet, if some questioned the power of so-called magicians, others clearly believed in the real potency of magical rituals: two works from the middle of the century charged that evil sorcery lay at the root of troubled royal marriages and disturbances within the kingdom.[83]

While the sources imply that there was an alarming surge in suspicious, unlawful activities in the empire during the late eighth and early ninth centuries, there was likely little change on the ground.[84] Rather, a new emphasis on pastoral care of the common people prompted heightened attentiveness to practices that, while not necessarily new, were newly viewed as undermining monotheism. This was a concern at the local level as much as it reflected a centralizing agenda.[85] Because Carolingian legislation only proscribed illicit practices without positively defining *licit* medical procedures, those who sought to produce and promote medical literature had to develop their own strategies for situating Hippocratic medicine within the boundaries of orthodoxy.

Compilers of medical material resorted to various strategies as they addressed such questions. Sometimes translators excised pagan elements of texts, as occurred with the translation of Alexander of Tralles's Greek *Therapeutics* into Latin.[86] Sometimes copyists substituted Christian invocations for pagan ones, as may well have happened in a treatise on vulture medicine, loosely based on Pliny's *Natural History*, which instructed readers to repeat "Angel Adonai Abraham, on your account the word is completed" as they decapitated the vulture using a reed and then cut out various organs.[87] Other times, a strategy for Christianization may simply have rested on the inclusion of Christian elements alongside pagan traces. Thus, in an herbal compendium from the vicinity of Reims, one finds a remedy against pustules that instructs the user to petition Apollo: "Apollo the physician I entreat you to take away swellings and pains from the human body throughout all 365 days of the passing year."[88] Is it possible that the invocation to Apollo was defused by a Christian prayer a few folios earlier? This charm, to be used while applying medicines to a wound, left no doubt as to the practitioner's faith: "Just as our Lord Jesus Christ while hanging on the cross was pierced by a lance in his side and did not suffer pain or swelling or a fistula, thus also may you not suffer pain, swelling, or a fistula from injuries."[89]

Within a climate of uncertainty, compilers likewise asserted that what they copied was legitimate by visually proclaiming that it had divine approval. Particularly at the beginning and end of different medical texts, one often finds an invocation to God or Christ. These incipits and explicits served as declarations that, in copying these texts, the scribe performed a pious duty; they further suggested that divine assistance endorsed the medical codex as a whole. For example, in a later ninth-century manuscript that likely came to Saint-Gall from northern Italy, there are four supplications to God situated across the last few texts of the codex: "Here ends the book of medicine of Quintus Serenus. Thanks be to God. Amen. . . . In the name of Christ, here begin the teachings of Aristotle the chief doctor. . . . In the name of God, the chapters of this book begin. . . . In the name of God, here begins a selection from books of medicine."[90] These are all written in a distinctive red display script (canonical capitalis), different from the primary Caroline minuscule. They are found as framing devices around medical texts that bear some association with classical antiquity: Quintus Serenus was a late antique pagan whose medical poem begins with an appeal to Apollo; Aristotle was known as a pagan philosopher, and his authorship was attributed to a few medical texts that circulated in the early Middle Ages.[91] The two final invocations surround a list of head-to-toe cures, of a type that was likely recognized to be a classical inheritance given its resemblance to collections like *Pliny's Medicine*.

Though certainly not unique to medical manuscripts, invocations assumed a special significance when attached to texts that could possibly have been classified as sorcery or magic. Furthermore, these liturgical-like formulae often seem to have been located in proximity to those titles that, more than others, explicitly declared a pagan heritage, either through a recognizable name or a title that suggested a classical profession. One of the most decorated titles in a relatively unadorned late ninth-century Beneventan manuscript from Montecassino reads: "In the name of our Lord Jesus Christ, here begins the book of medicine focused on urines by Hermogenes the philosopher."[92] The same prefatory "in the name of Christ" is found in the incipit to a book of medicine attributed to Heliodorus (a Roman surgeon) and to one entitled "the medical art of the master Hippocrates," the first in a manuscript produced around 800 in southern France or northern Italy and the second in a contemporaneous manuscript possibly written at Saint-Gall.[93] In an early ninth-century codex from eastern Francia, "Amen" in a distinctive uncial script appears at the end of the *Prognostics of Democritus*.[94] Of course, such formulae were not exclusively used with texts attributed to pagan authors.[95] Thus, the Montecassino manuscript also includes a "Thanks be to God" at the end of a text on weights and measures by Isidore.[96]

In addition to textual Christian markers, some ninth-century manuscripts contain visual symbols of divine endorsement for the medical material copied within. Given the skill and planning involved, these decorative schemes (though few in number) signal a pronounced effort on the part of the compiler to proclaim the orthodoxy of the medical art. A striking example is a relatively small booklet from northern Italy (possibly the monastery of Bobbio), whose folds suggest usage by a traveling physician.[97] The original front cover of the *vademecum* features sketches of Christ, Mary, and monks.[98] The title running across the top of the first page reads, "In the name of Jesus Christ our Lord here begins the sacred art of medicine," the "I" being a braided cross running down the left side of the page, with a tang at the bottom and, at the crossbar, a medallion of a beardless Christ framed by a nimbus (see Figure 8).[99] The text below is a question-and-answer explanation of phlebotomy that opens with a decorated "Q" containing two figures holding a codex, almost certainly representing the *magister* and student participating in the didactic dialogue. Although the illumination seems hastily executed, it layers the rather mundane text with weighty theological associations. The letting of blood is set against Christ's sacrificial blood on the cross (emphasized by the red patches on his face); a relationship is established between the teacher-student pair and Christ (through their jointly encircled forms); and the so-named "sacred art" of human healing is framed within the "medicinal" grace of the Incarnation and Passion (with human healing represented by the technical skill of phlebotomy).[100]

Similar themes are at play in a medical manuscript produced around the turn of the ninth century at the scriptorium of Fleury.[101] Prefacing the start of the *Therapeutics* of the sixth-century Byzantine author Alexander of Tralles is a pair of arches with motifs common to Gospel book illuminations (see Figure 9).[102] Under the first arch sits Alexander, described as "the wise physician [who] published this little book of the art of medicine."[103] Under the second arch stands another braided cross with a tang, surrounded by the entreaty: "Holy cross save us because through you Christ will redeem us by his most holy blood."[104] The complementary archways again draw connections among recovery and resurrection, human sickness and sin, and divine blood and sacrifice—not to frame a liturgical or exegetical collection but a set of practical remedies for internal diseases, which included the use of amulets, incantations, and unusual substances (like wolf feces).[105]Alexander, encircled with a halo and holding what appears to be a cupping glass, is aligned with the "divine physician," his cures imbued with the grace of God's assistance. The utility of the material, manmade cross to salvific healing, as discussed by Beatrice Kitzinger, informs and emphasizes the utility of the human medical knowledge and manufactured remedies that follow.[106] This message is amplified by the incipit on the following page, which invokes Jesus Christ as a guarantor of Alexander's work.[107]

A final example comes from a medical compilation produced at Montecassino, where it introduces a late antique set of Latin texts on acute and chronic diseases.[108] The illumination is a decorated initial O, with a series of concentric circles, braids, and dots using red, green, yellow, and purple

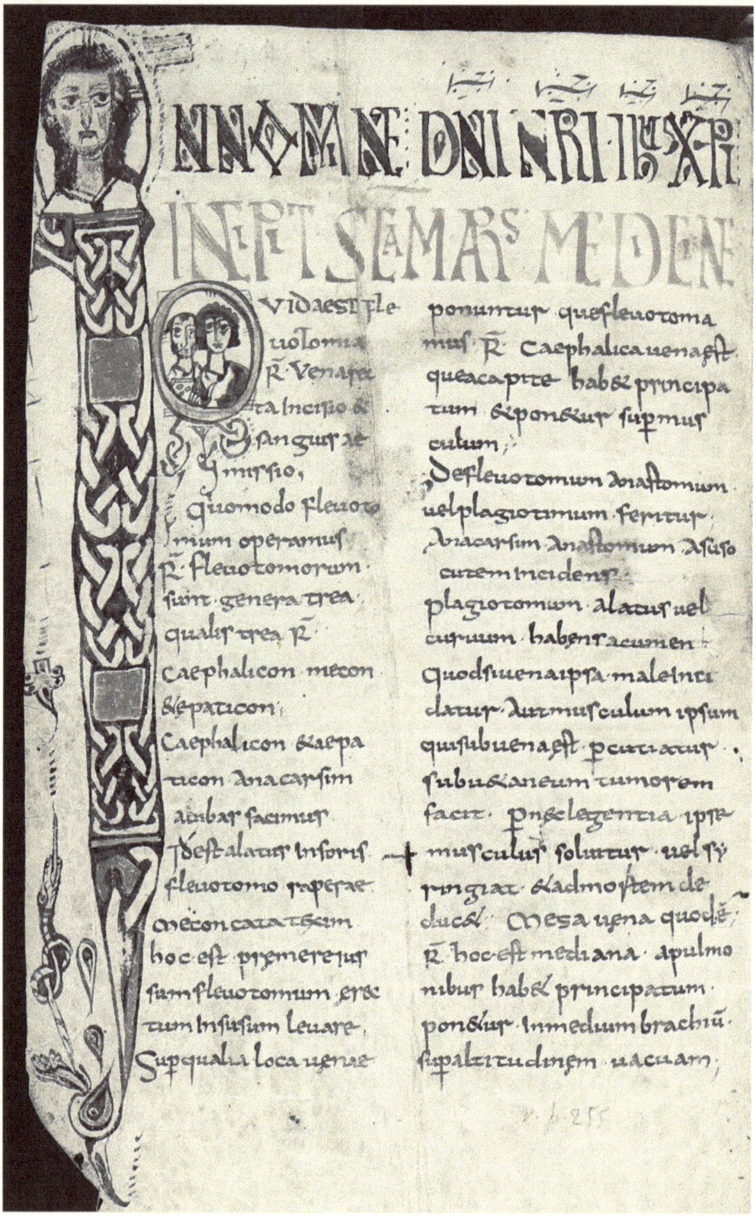

Figure 8. First page of a physician's *vademecum*, with a question-and-answer text on phlebotomy. St. Gallen, Stiftsbibliothek, Cod. Sang. 217, p. 252. By kind permission of the Stiftsbibliothek.

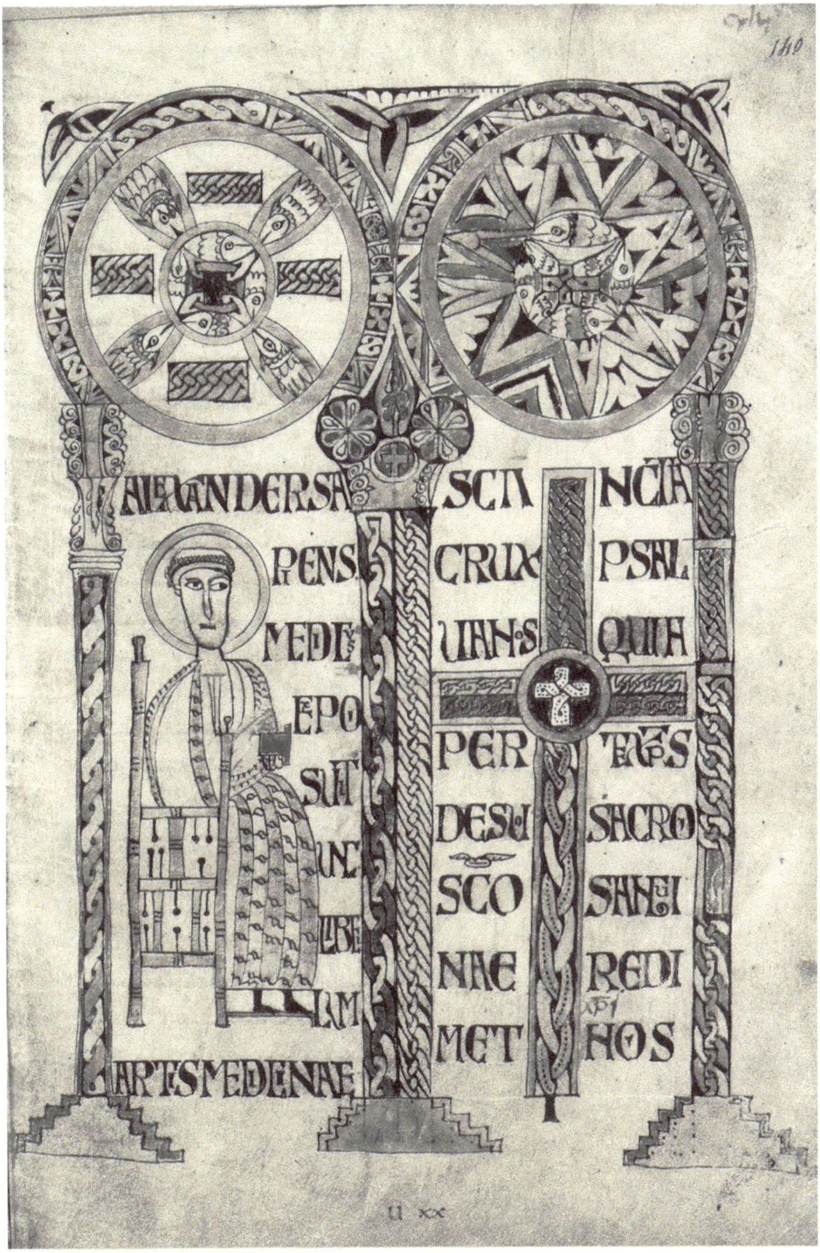


Figure 9. Author portrait of Alexander of Tralles as the frontispiece to the Latin *Therapeutics*. Paris, BnF lat. 9332, f. 140r. By kind permission of the Bibliothèque nationale.

ink. At the center is a right hand with the thumb and ring finger (also known as the *digitus medicinalis*) making the sign of a benediction.[109] Derived from Byzantine iconography, the same blessing gesture is given by the Christ in Majesty found in the Lorsch Gospels (ca. 810).[110] Similarly, an open-faced hand of God set against a diamond surrounded by several concentric circles prefaces the Gospel of John in the Codex Aureus produced for Charles the Bald in 870.[111] Thus, although the Montecassino manuscript is written in Beneventan script and dates from the early tenth century, the illumination shares motifs with ninth-century works from the heart of the Carolingian Empire, and its inclusion in a medical codex resembles strategies utilized in the Carolingian works discussed above.[112] Communicating God's endorsement of the text, the benediction conveys divine favor to the scribe's labor in copying medical knowledge, the reader's labor in studying the material, and the healer's labor in realizing the cures. The blessing is confirmed in the explicit of the paired treatise on chronic diseases, where the scribe has added "Thanks be to God" and filled in the space before the succeeding text with a large "Amen."[113]

These Christian symbols were visual signs of medicine's legitimacy that even an illiterate patient could comprehend.[114] In addition to sanctifying the text, they surely endowed the practitioner carrying the codex with religious authority (especially true in the case of the folded manuscript). Furthermore, images of Christ and the cross were instruments that could be activated within the "economy of healing," effecting thaumaturgic cures, endowing remedies with potency, warding off evil, and referencing cross-objects and physical gestures performed in visitations to the sick.[115] These illuminations were not practical in the sense of helping a reader identify a herb or execute a surgery, but they were far from ornamental. Though they do not surface in many extant manuscripts, they ought to be considered alongside apologetic introductions, liturgical incipits and explicits, prayers, and biblical proofs as but one technique for confirming medicine's status. While the Carolingians could turn to Augustine for verification that intention determined the orthodoxy of a therapeutic strategy, the discernment of intention was not necessarily easy, and because there was no canon of medical works, disagreement and contestation persisted when it came to drawing boundaries between "medicine" and "magic." Nevertheless, extant manuscripts point to a shared conviction that pagan aspects of the medical tradition could be neutralized. The devil was not, in this case, in the details but might be vanquished through strategies that transformed a medical codex into a Christian manual.

## Bodily Suffering and Medical Efficacy

Despite their confidence that medical texts could be purged of the interconnected dangers of magic and paganism, proponents of a Christian medical art still faced a problem that lay at the heart of human intervention in bodily health—the question of whether the pursuit of good health conduced to spiritual advancement. Medicine's claims to alleviate pain and infirmity potentially undermined a long-nurtured ascetic emphasis on the spiritual benefits of physical suffering, as discussed in Chapter 3. Again, the *Lorscher Arzneibuch*'s formulation of a cogent theological position on this matter offers strong evidence for the kind of counterarguments that some may have been employing to discredit human medicine.

The very first line of the Lorsch apology draws on a passage in Psalms, where a suffering King David, chastised by God for his iniquities, confesses his faith and begs God for assistance. While his enemies seek to malign and deceive him, David declares that he remains unmoved against them: "I, as if a deaf man, heard not [Ps 37:14]." Adopting these same words, the Lorsch author takes on the position of David, as a servant of God who faces criticism from wicked detractors and yet perseveres. Yet, there is another angle to this invocation of Psalm 37. David's suffering is described in vivid bodily language—God's arrows of wrath have pierced his flesh and caused sores that putrefy and weep. In the illustration of this psalm from the Utrecht Psalter (830s), David's body is covered in spots and arrows, tormented by small demons who grab at his clothes (see Figure 10). The message of the psalm is that God dispenses health, and spiritual repentance impels physical recovery. Just so, the apology indicates that the detractors "are accustomed to say: Why do we need to be cured by physicians, since we *cast our fears upon him who cares for us* [1 Pt 5:7]?"[116] Evidently, there were some people who argued that human medicine was worthless, and even impious, because true Christians should be cured by faith alone. Yet, the Lorsch author raises this viewpoint only to counter it; he alludes to the sickly, penitent David at the start of the apology but remains "deaf" to any suggestion that suffering should be simply endured rather than treated with medicines and comforts.

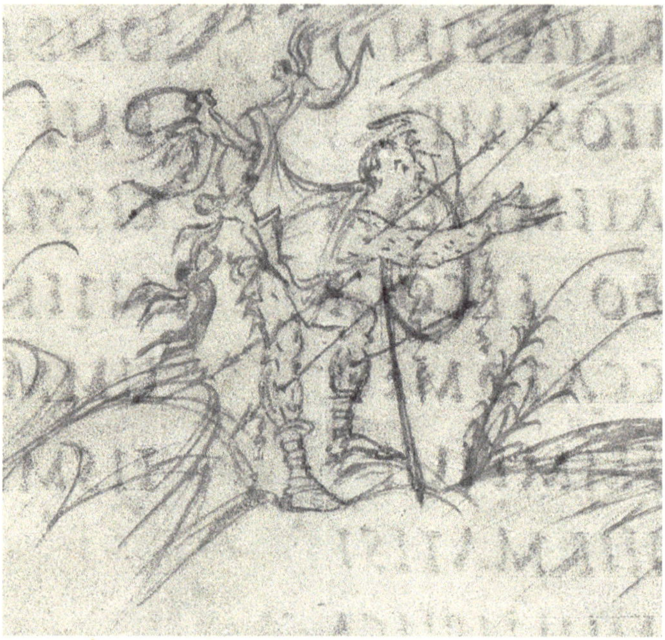

Figure 10. King David, pierced by the arrows of God's wrath and afflicted by putrefied sores, in the Utrecht Psalter (Ps 37). Utrecht, University Library, MS 32, f. 22r. By kind permission of the Universiteitsbibliotheek.

According to the apology, there are three reasons why people are struck by disease: they have sinned and are being punished; they are being tested by God; or they are suffering from a "malady of imbalance" (*ex intemperantia[e] passione*).[117] Following his source (Isidore's *Sentences*), the author declares at first that human medicine treats only diseases from intemperance; the other two must be cured by divine mercy. However, in an immediate qualification, he adds: "Nevertheless, even these [first two causes] sometimes are only cured with human aid."[118] In this shrewd rhetorical move, we see the apologist grappling with the weight of patristic authority yet creating license for his own agenda.

By turning to historical examples from scripture, the Lorsch author demonstrates the effectiveness of human medicine in treating each cause of illness (punishment, test, and natural imbalance). When the Apostle Paul sinned on account of his lack of faith, God blinded him as a *punishment* but then ordered the disciple Ananias to lay his hands on Paul's eyes, and the scales fell away (Acts 9:8–19). Tobit, whose blindness was a divine *test*, was cured only when fish gall was smeared on his eyes in accordance with the angel Raphael's instructions (Tb 11:10–14). Finally, when Timothy's stomach was weakened by sickness (an *imbalance*), Paul counseled him to "use a little wine for your stomach's sake and your frequent infirmities [1 Tim 5:23]." The Lorsch author frames *all three* cases as models of human medicine and human comfort (even crediting Tobit's cure to the medicine made from fish rather than the miraculous power of Raphael).[119] Blurring the distinction between divine miracle and human healing is central to the apologist's project. He concurs with his detractors that God absolutely *could* cure any disease through his command. But, he highlights, God dictated signs in scripture that clearly revealed his desire that human medicine be used. Hippocratic treatments, therefore, should be framed within the orbit of God's daily interventions in the temporal world, and medicinal substances conceived as gifts of divine creation.

If certain diseases were understood as a punishment or penance for sins committed, another theological uncertainty that the Lorsch author had to confront was not whether humans *could* be healed by earthly interventions but whether they *should* seek healing in the first place. The apology acknowledges that sickness can be beneficial because it "breaks the mind from its insensibility"—redirecting attention from temporal desires to eternal truths.[120] Furthermore, it points to individuals like Job who, despite leading a perfect life, was struck with a weeping sore as a trial of his faith. These holy exemplars are proof that "the Lord chastises him whom he loves," and that those who suffer in patience during the earthly life will merit eternal rewards in the next.[121] The apology does not ignore these examples. It cannot, because they represent a major stumbling block in any Christian attempt to defend the aims inherent to the art of medicine. They conjure to mind the ambiguity of illness and its equivocal link with internal sin, as examined in Chapter 3. It is thus at the heart of the apology, right in the middle of the text, that one finds the Lorsch author's answer to this central and urgent dilemma. The argument is subtle, relying on a delicate reframing of a quotation from Paul's letter to the Romans, but its conclusions resonate in the decision to produce the *Lorscher Arzneibuch* in the first place.

The author does not simply make a case for the orthodoxy of medicine but also presents an original and complex theological point about how Christians should care for the body. While Paul's original aim in Romans was to encourage a group of converts to cast off their old lives and dispense with their concerns over earthly matters, the Lorsch author significantly alters this message:

> Human medicine should not be rejected, but rather should be used in cases of suffering with thanksgiving, because no one ought to hate his/her own body for the reason that it was created, but neither should one relax the bridle on the body's delights for the reason that it easily falls into sin. Although Paul said, *make no provision for the body*, he immediately added *in its desires* [Rom 13:14]. For what he prohibited in desire, he conceded, without doubt, in necessity.[122]

As part of God's creation, the body cannot be inherently evil because everything God made is good. Thus, the body should be loved as God's work, but it should also be guarded because its weakness and desire for pleasure lead the individual into sin. In contrast to Paul, the Lorsch text does not argue that the body should be passed over to focus attention on the soul.[123] Instead, it acknowledges that the body should not be indulged with excessive care but casts medicine as a legitimate endeavor to protect a body in need and restore to it the health endowed by God at creation. By setting up a distinction between desire and need, the apology presents physical health as something good rather than threatening and human medicine as a response to need rather than desire. Although the author concedes that illness may be a tool employed by God, an experience that reminds sufferers of the transience of bodily delights and tests their faith, he returns to his refrain that *human medicine should not be opposed.*

A similar conception of health appears in two other Frankish manuscripts from the mid-ninth century, both of which contain a treatise that begins: "In all acts of curing the medicines of God ought to be employed, because divine power has deemed fit to bring back to life destroyed bodies (*revivificare corpora mortificata*)."[124] This opening declaration elides the distinction between God's future resurrection of dead, decaying bodies and his immediate, earthly care for the diseased and dying. The motive behind this is to emphasize that God's aims are consistent—if he will resurrect all bodies at the Second Coming, then he must have made some provision for those same bodies during their earthly life:

> And surely it cannot be that he himself did not foresee the pains that we suffer and types of infirmity? Because I believe that when he formed our bodies, then he also ordained various sicknesses to rule us. And for our sins he handed over himself and loved us to such an extent that he created all species of the world and beautiful things for human use.[125]

These lines read almost like a Christian creed. As in the *Lorscher Arzneibuch*, the text suggests that God always intended suffering to coexist with human endeavors to alleviate it. In this case, the text indicates that disease has existed since the *creation* of Adam and Eve, not since the Fall. The sacrifice of Jesus and his spiritual healing is then compared to the love God demonstrated for humanity by filling the earth with useful substances for physical cures—including, as the text goes on to elaborate, drugs, herbs, and trees providing medical ointments.

In the view of the Lorsch author, humans should *always* act to alleviate sickness and suffering. There is no guarantee, however, that human medicine will cure all illnesses because God ultimately has power over health and sickness, life and death. Thus, if an illness were precipitated by sin or as a divine trial, the apology acknowledges, God may decide not to grant a remedy through the work of the physician. "When one wants to become healthy in order to do good works, [only] then does one ask for a health-giving remedy."[126] God examines the patient's soul and, depending on what he sees, directs his grace toward the healing act and the power of earthly medicines.[127] The apologist walks a careful line between acknowledging that God may withhold a cure and encouraging his contemporaries to seek medical aid in all cases of suffering. He reiterates that the body itself is valuable and its health is something to be prized. Even if a sick person has failed to find a cure from a physician, "that person should not cease to pursue a cure for her body, but as much as possible she should endeavor to cherish it, not in order to fulfill its desires but in order to do good."[128]

## A Divinely Inspired Discipline

Authors like the apologist emphasized that the pursuit of cures was consistent with the ethical responsibilities of a faithful Christian. Such an orientation corresponded with an evolving understanding in the ninth century that medicine should be considered not simply a practical endeavor but a branch of learning that had the power to transform the one studying it. In this final section, we explore how medicine's inclusion within an educational program centered on the liberal arts allowed it to be recognized as a path toward divine wisdom.

In declaring that a "knowledge of cures" (*scientia curationum*) should be numbered among the gifts of the Holy Spirit, the Lorsch apology seeks to unify a biblical text with a liberal arts tradition that was popularized by Carolingian intellectuals.[129] To be sure, the Apostle Paul had enumerated the "grace of healing" (*gratia sanitatum*) as one of the nine gifts of the Holy Spirit (1 Cor 12:9), but by replacing Paul's terminology of grace with that of *scientia*, the apologist consciously references a definition of medicine he had cited earlier, which was itself drawn from Isidore's *On the Differences of Things*. "Medicine is the knowledge of cures (*scientia curationum*), which was discovered for the moderation and health of the body."[130] Thus, while Paul is said to call medicine a "gift" of the Holy Spirit, the Lorsch author makes clear that medicine is not performed solely through prayers or the laying on of hands. It is a set of practical treatments, discovered over the course of time, with demonstrated success at protecting and restoring the well-being of the body. Furthermore, it is a discipline of human expertise, a science acquired through education.

This Isidorian description of medicine sets the Lorsch apology within a clear textual community associated with the most prominent Carolingian intellectuals of the age. The same definition is found in schemata between Alcuin's *Dialogue on Rhetoric* and *On Dialectic*; in Hrabanus's *On the Natures of Things*; in the personal handbook of Walafrid; and in a letter from Ermenrich of Ellwangen to Abbot Grimald of Saint-Gall.[131] Many of these scholars shared strong personal and scholastic bonds—Ermenrich, for example, was taught by Hrabanus at Fulda and Walafrid at Reichenau, just as Walafrid himself had been the student of Hrabanus, and Hrabanus, the student of Alcuin at Tours. With the exception of Walafrid, in every case the definition of medicine falls within a discussion of the division of knowledge, one that the *Lorscher Arzneibuch* also cites. This larger framework, too, is Isidorian. *On the Differences of Things* presented a division of wisdom (*philosophia*) into three parts, each with its own subdivision: ethics, containing the four virtues; logic, containing dialectic and rhetoric; and natural philosophy (*physica*), containing arithmetic, geometry, astronomy, music as well as astrology, mechanics, and medicine.[132]

This more expansive list differed from the schema of the seven liberal arts that would become dominant at medieval universities—a development itself due, in large part, to Carolingian interest in an early fifth-century text by Martianus Capella, *On the Marriage of Philology and Mercury*. Martianus *excluded* medicine and architecture, for being too mundane, from the seven intellectual arts (grammar, rhetoric, dialectic, arithmetic, music, geometry, and astronomy).[133] Given the extensive circulation of Martianus's work in the ninth century, it would seem that medical learning faced the risk of being classified as a practical craft rather than a liberal discipline.[134] Yet, as Elspeth Whitney elucidates, the conception of the liberal arts remained relatively flexible throughout the Carolingian period, and for this reason early medieval scholars embraced Isidore's more expansive division of philosophy alongside Martianus's narrower classification.[135] As Faith Wallis and Florence Eliza Glaze observe, the successful incorporation of medicine within a well-recognized schema of wisdom was integral to the Carolingians' acceptance of this discipline and its preservation in monastic scriptoria.[136]

The Lorsch apologist himself candidly references an intellectual atmosphere of uncertainty regarding which ancient pagan disciplines could be Christianized. Of the seven subjects within Isidore's definition of *physica*, the text states, some can be harmonized with religion and some cannot; clearly, the aim is to prove that medicine ought to be.[137] We should see this maneuvering by the Lorsch text as one manifestation of what historians have described as the Christianization of the liberal arts, a gradual development spurred on, in large part, by Alcuin's writings.[138] In his *Dialogue on True Philosophy* (790s), Alcuin described the seven-pillared House of Wisdom from Proverbs as supported by the seven liberal arts, themselves equated with the seven gifts of the Holy Spirit; his argument was that the arts had sprung from divine wisdom and were a means to return to God.[139] In seeming imitation, the Lorsch apologist blended the gift of healing from the Holy Spirit with the Isidorian definition of *medicina*. Within a Carolingian framework of the liberal arts, it was possible, then, to consider classical medicine a discipline of divine knowledge.

Such a view of medicine's prestigious standing is unambiguously conveyed in a poem written by Alcuin for Charlemagne in 796. This poem, which vividly illustrates the operations of the court gathered around the king at Aachen, opens with an ode to the king and then proceeds to celebrate the work of the deacons, priests, and subdeacons within the kingdom. Immediately following these officers of the Church come the physicians:

The doctors hurry up at once, disciples of Hippocrates,
one taking blood from veins, another mixing herbs in a pot,
one brewing poultices, and another serving up potions.
And yet, doctors, tend to everyone without charge,
so that Christ may bless and guide your hands:
of all these things I approve, this is an order which I can praise.[140]

Here, Alcuin explicitly voices his endorsement for those who have studied the remedies of Hippocrates and are able to dispense them charitably. Given the hierarchical structure of the poem, it was certainly not by chance that Alcuin decided to insert his verses on physicians *before* his descriptions of other officers of the court, including members of the palace school, chancery, and scriptorium. This order was a sign of Alcuin's esteem for the medical art.

With similar motives, we can see the compilers of various manuscripts considering medicine's place within a Christianized scheme of ancient learning. One prominent way in which this manifests is in short histories of medicine scattered across larger compilations. These are fairly common and, as with the division of the arts, many are Isidorian at root. They reiterate what Isidore says in the *Etymologies* about the invention of medicine: Apollo discovered the art of medicine, his son Aesculapius expanded it (until he was killed by a lightning bolt and medicine was lost for five hundred years), and his descendent Hippocrates revived it at the time of Artaxerxes, king of the Persians.[141]

Such histories make frequent references to pagan gods, but Carolingian scholars were well accustomed to treating pagan divinities as historical persons.[142] It is in just this vein that a poem from the 780s describes medicine as the eighth liberal art, founded by the discoveries of a family (Apollo, Scolapius, and Hippocrates), and that a manuscript from the Loire valley presents large-scale author portraits of the same three ancient physicians (Apollo, Hippocrates, and Scolapius, the last of whom appears in a *Maiestas Domini* pose, enthroned on a flower-filled earthly orb).[143] Two additional portraits of Antonius Musa and Marcus Agrippa, the author and recipient of the first text in the codex, *On the Herb Betony*, face one another across the page in a clear staging of the historical circumstances under which the herbal was purportedly produced (see Figure 11).[144] Universal chronicles from the early Middle Ages reference the same famed pagan healers, setting their discoveries and writings alongside notable sacred events, such as the

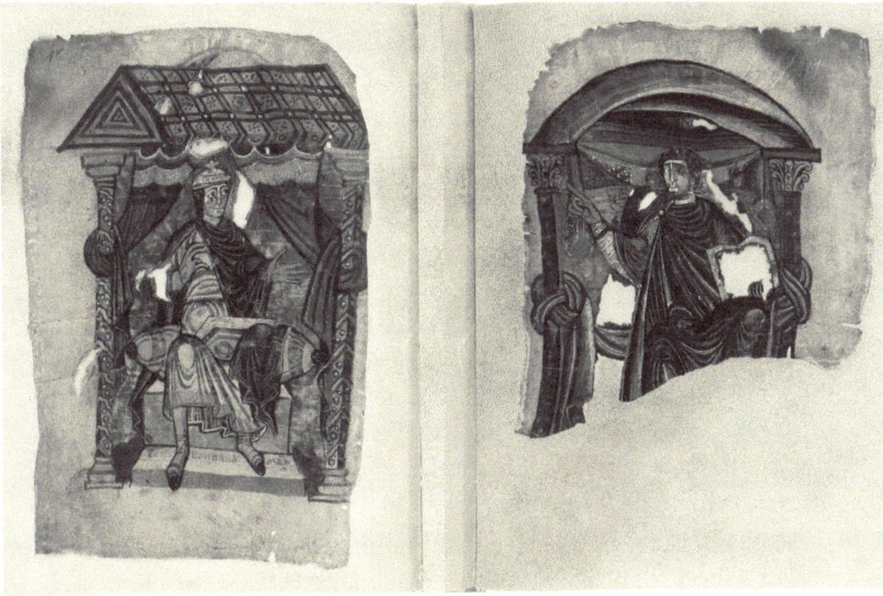

Figure 11. Marcus Agrippa and Antonius Musa, as patron and author from the preface to the *De herba vettonica*. Universitätsbibliothek Kassel, Landesbibliothek und Murhardsche Bibliothek der Stadt Kassel, 2° Ms. phys. et hist. nat. 10, ff. 1v–2r. CC BY-SA 4.0.

rebuilding of the city of Jerusalem.[145] These chronicles continued the late antique project of unifying all historical events into one teleological salvation story, such that even the pagan inventors of medicine could be seen as components of God's timeless plan for humanity.

A similar Christianizing impulse is evident in two histories (both, curiously, with Greek titles) that explicitly blend pagan stories of medicine's origins with biblical themes.[146] The *Epistola pepiodeotecon*, extant in an early ninth-century medical codex from Burgundy, locates the origins of medicine in humanity's decline from an ancient time of simplicity, peace, and health to an age of lust, envy, and violence, during which people began to require doctors because of the advance of ill health.[147] While the text seems to draw strongly on classical tropes of a golden age, it adapts its pagan sources by describing how "the highest creator, God," shortened human life, changed the temperate air, and ordered disease to spread across the generations. As in other narratives, Asclepius is named as the first inventor of herbal cures, but, in another Christianizing tweak, he is said to learn his cures from an angel.[148] Likewise, a medical manuscript from Saint-Denis presents a text entitled the *Epistola peri hereseon* (*Letter on the sects*), which, unlike other histories, does not simply repeat Isidore's origin story but carefully shapes it to Christian expectations. "After the flood, for 1500 years medicine lay hidden, right up to the time of King Artaxerxes of the Persians. Then Apollo, his son Scolapius, Asclepius the uncle of Hippocrates [and Hippocrates]—these four invented the art of medicine and the sects."[149] By inserting a remark about the flood in Genesis and leaving out mention of Asclepius's death by lightning bolt, the author has resituated medicine's origins in a biblical narrative of human history. References to "God's help" and "the will of the omnipotent God" at the beginning and end of the *Epistola* likewise emphasize that the Christian God inspired the development of medicine by pagans.[150]

Just as the *Epistola peri hereson* and the *Epistola pepiodeotecon* sought to Christianize the origins of medicine, so did a pseudonymous treatise ascribed to the Evangelist Luke strive to insert the distinguished Church Fathers into the historical development of the medical art. This text survives in only one witness and takes the form of a letter purportedly sent from Luke (evangelist *and* doctor) to all Christians and physicians; it prefaces the compilation of medical texts on generation and the soul discussed in Chapter 1.[151] In the brief letter, Luke openly acknowledges that Hippocratic medical works contain false pagan ideas, but he reassures his audience that this is not an intractable obstacle:

> It is well known that Hippocrates, a *medicus*, composed several works during the time of the pagans, and that, consequently, in these works, some things are obscure and others are heathen. . . . We who administer the cures of the art of medicine and are Christians and possess the books of Hippocrates give sanction to whatever [Hippocrates] said that was useful. But whatever he relayed either obscurely or insufficiently, we elucidate and rewrite, so that those reading [his works] may better understand. Whatever additional material we may insert there is from the books of Saint Isidore, Saint Augustine, Saint Gregory, and Luke the evangelist, because all these men dictated much about the art of medicine. [In these endeavors], we trust in the future help of our Lord Jesus Christ, that the work of our art may accomplish increasingly more, just as our books are corrected so as to become free from error by him who is an all-powerful *medicus*.[152]

As in the Lorsch apology, one finds here a justification of the utility of pagan knowledge and its ability to be converted to Christian ends. Relying on the authority conferred by Luke, the letter also emphasizes the precedent established by earlier holy and wise men who endorsed the art of medicine. With its focus on the unfolding of knowledge over time, the text offers a history of medicine framed within a Christian progress narrative. First, the origins of medicine are situated with Hippocrates in a time before the Incarnation, and the reader is provided with examples about the types of pagan beliefs to beware. Next, "Luke" treats Christian times, explaining how medical learning can endure by being regenerated, with the false components excised and the truthful ones augmented. Finally, the author anticipates God's oversight of medical learning into the future and the further perfection of the art.

With its emphasis on the procedures of textual editing, the correction of books, and the authority of the Latin Church Fathers, the epistle convincingly reflects the context of the Carolingian reforms.[153] The decision to insert it at the beginning of a set of texts concerning human development and anatomy aligns this manuscript closely with the *Lorscher Arzneibuch*, in that both authors prefaced their copying of older, Roman medical texts with an apology for the Christian legitimacy of this task. The lesson is indisputable—if Luke, who channeled the voice of God in writing the Gospel, sanctioned the continued practice of medicine, this art was always part of the divine plan for human society.

The function that classical education ought to play in the life of a Christian was hardly a new question in the ninth century; nevertheless, the years before Charlemagne's assumption of the imperial title represent a period during which the boundaries between pagan and Christian traditions were particularly contested.[154] The anonymous detractors mentioned in the apology may well have argued that pious Christians ought to shun medical learning because its development was inseparable from dangerous pagan beliefs. However, in line with contemporary claims for a Christian liberal arts program, the Lorsch author contends that, while the unbelievers compiled knowledge in pride, Christians can take what is "useful" in their writings, like discovering "gold from dung," and use it to glorify the goodness of divine creation.[155]

## Medicine, Demarginalized

In 2013, the *Lorscher Arzneibuch* was added to UNESCO's Memory of the World Register, in recognition of its "innovative, scientific approach to medicine."[156] Certainly, its survival allows us a unique lens onto Carolingian culture, but it would be a mistake to view it as an aberration within its time. The arguments that the Lorsch apologist presents for the legitimacy of medicine, while more theologically complex, are comparable to the arguments uncovered in similar ninth-century codices. Indeed, some of the arguments employed in the Lorsch apology resemble so closely interpretations advanced by Hrabanus and Hildemar of Civate, in their writings from the following decades, that one must wonder whether the *Lorscher Arzneibuch* or a copy of the apology circulated outside the monastery.[157] If these are not direct borrowings, they are, at the very least, textual parallels that link the production of the Lorsch codex to broader ninth-century scholarly discourses regarding bodily health.

In the late eighth century, not only did Jacobus offered a preemptive justification for Charlemagne's conservation of a classical medical poem, and only a few years later Alcuin composed a poem in which he, too, highlighted Christ's support for medical treatments. Such coincidences allow us to imagine the outlines of an intellectual debate among members of Charlemagne's court, within which emerged a forceful justification for medicine, one example of which was set down in writing in a codex produced at a royal abbey (Lorsch).[158] This debate encompassed the Christian appropriation of pagan learning, the boundaries of magic and legitimate practice, and the use of treatments in alleviating physical suffering. The fact that some kind of consensus emerged is suggested by the poem of an Irish scholar who settled in the Carolingian Empire shortly after Louis the Pious's death in 840. Little attempt is made to justify medical cures, and little fear is expressed regarding its pagan origins; rather, Sedulius Scottus promises to patients treatments "unknown to learned Greece," while praising *Medicina* as a Olympian goddess whose "breasts issue streams of healing nectar."[159] Compared to Jacobus and Alcuin, Sedulius appears more playful, assured in his use of classical allusions and confident that Carolingian healers have surpassed the wisdom of the ancients.

The Lorsch author, it would seem, was successful in answering the criticisms of his contemptuous detractors. Though medical cures and recipes would continue to be written into the marginal spaces of manuscripts, we can surely echo Sedulius's confidence that the medical discipline was no longer marginal to Carolingian culture but had been more firmly established as part of God's creative plan for Frankish society.

## CHAPTER 5

# A Ministry for the *Medicus*

On the Thursday before Easter in 817, the Emperor Louis the Pious was riding back to the palace when a rotten wooden portico collapsed on top of him and his companions. Although several of his companions fell to the ground with serious injuries, the *Royal Frankish Annals* reported that the emperor suffered only minor wounds to his chest, ear, and upper thigh, which were treated without delay. "Due to the presence of physicians, who applied [their] cures to him, he recovered extremely quickly—for [only] twenty days after this happened, he set out to Nijmegen to go hunting."[1] Unstable buildings continued to beset the royal family: several decades later, Louis the Pious's son, Louis the German, required more extensive care when the terrace he was standing on crumbled. Because he foolishly did not give immediate attention to his wounds, his physicians were forced to cut away his rotting flesh; while certainly painful, this skilled operation saved the life of the king.[2]

These are some of the rare cases in which ninth-century sources mention doctors and attribute a healthy recovery to their actions. Even though Louis the Pious was not gravely injured, the annalist made clear that no time was wasted in seeking expert care—the physical prowess of the emperor was no trivial matter in a warrior society.[3] Alcuin, too, highlighted the presence of Hippocratic attendants at court, describing them bustling about performing phlebotomies, preparing herbs and lotions, and offering healing drinks.[4] Yet, if doctors figure as heroes in these narratives, they appear in a more ambiguous light at other moments. According to his biographer Einhard, Charlemagne "trusted his own judgment more than the advice of his physicians, whom he almost loathed" because of their (unsolicited) recommendations concerning his diet.[5] In suggesting only that doctors might be figures of ridicule, the *Life of Charlemagne* set a light tone compared to the early ninth-century *Life of Saint Sturm*, which accused Charlemagne's personal physician,

Wintar, of poisoning the ailing abbot of Fulda.[6] Suffice it to say that the doctors at Carolingian courts were apparently the subjects of controversy as well as praise.

If the previous chapter analyzed the emergence of medicine as a Christian discipline, this chapter focuses specifically on those who put medical theory into practice. These individuals applied knowledge transmitted textually and orally about the workings of the human being to individual, volatile bodies, bodies that constantly hovered on the brink between life and death. This made the physician (*medicus*) an uneasy figure. His intervention in suffering situated him alongside holy saints whose miraculous relics healed all forms of bodily distress. Yet the *medicus* was no miracle worker. Hippocratic and Galenic tradition had emphasized that he was a rational investigator who relied on experience to understand the logic of the body. Christian pastoral literature, meanwhile, had long situated the physician of the body as a foil to the minister of the soul—the first embroiled in matter, the second involved in heavenly affairs. Accordingly, the physician's authority was severely limited because it dealt only with the mundane and temporal in nature. Hence, when Louis the German fell seriously ill in 869 and his physicians' treatments were ineffective, they could only despair for his life. Louis's piety offered a more powerful medicine: the king donated gifts to monasteries and the poor throughout his realm and "merited a cure from the Heavenly Doctor, to whom he commended himself and all his goods."[7] The *Annals of Fulda* acknowledge God as the true *medicus* and present human physicians as relatively weak individuals, with a precarious role in the divine order.

The difficulty in classifying the *medicus* as merely an investigator of nature is that this was only one discourse in Carolingian thought. Just like those ninth-century visionaries who traveled to the realm of the dead and carried back important information for the living, so was the human physician with his Hippocratic treatments positioned at a crucial juncture between this world and the next. His remedies could forestall the dissolution of soul and body or his poisons hasten death. From this perspective, if the *medicus*'s powers were to avoid being classed with the magician's as a challenge to the divine order, the ambiguity of his work needed to be reconstituted as a sign of his moral superiority and saintlike intercessory role. Just so, this chapter will demonstrate how Carolingian medical compilations challenged the binary in which the physician was contrasted to the doctor of souls and deemed to effect change only in the natural world. It will examine how a set of ideals regarding the physician's character, education, and motivations was presented as a means to promote his integrity and demonstrate that the authority he wielded was granted by God and was not an arrogation. Numerous developments, including a boom in the relic trade, the reform of rituals for anointing the sick, and renewed alarm about local magicians, intensified competition within the Frankish medical marketplace in the early ninth century. In this environment, delineating the role of the *medicus* became ever more essential. This chapter thus investigates the rhetorical tools through which the *medicus* was fashioned as an exemplary figure, with a distinct and valuable role within Christian society, and how such discourses, in turn, shaped assumptions regarding the care of the body in the Carolingian period.

## A Professional Identity?

Whereas high medieval Europe was populated by a variety of healers, including elite physicians (*phisici*) trained at universities, we know little with certainty about doctors in the early Middle Ages.[8] The terminology is straightforward but reveals nothing about status or background—*medicus* is the only term designating a medical practitioner in the Carolingian period.[9] Annals and biographies indicate that *medici* were part of a ruler's entourage but do not usually provide information beyond the fact that they were summoned in the case of grave illnesses and accidents.[10] Court physicians were not a new phenomenon but are attested for Merovingian, Ostrogothic, and Lombard rulers.[11] That they were a distinct group among Carolingian officeholders seems to be implied by the title "royal *medicus*" and Heiric of Auxerre's comment that "a crowd of physicians from the palace" (*turba medicorum e palatio*) treated a count's eye disease in 840.[12] That said, recourse to doctors was not restricted to the highest elite. The Salic, Alemannic, and Bavarian law codes indicate that *medici* might be called in the case of violent injuries to any free man or woman.[13]

Medical practice in the early Middle Ages has been cast as *Mönchsmedizin*, a term that carries derogatory implications about the decline of "scientific" practice when medicine moved within monasteries. Both Benedict's Rule (540s) and Cassiodorus's *Institutes* (560s) assumed that care of the sick would occur within the monastery, although the former refers only to the care of sick brothers, while the latter speaks of "those who seek refuge at holy places."[14] Cassiodorus notes that his monks should be familiar with late antique medical works, but the Benedictine Rule does not mention medical training, only a separate room for sick monks, the use of baths and meat, and compassionate attendants.[15] Nevertheless, ninth-century library catalogues from Benedictine houses indicate the ownership of medical books, and the production of many extant manuscripts has been assigned to such monasteries.[16] The Plan of Saint-Gall (an architectural schema for an ideal monastery, ca. 830) also suggests that health care was conceptualized as essential to Benedictine life. A corner of the monastic complex is devoted to medicine, including an herb garden; a separate chapel and cloister "for infirm brothers"; an infirmary with its own kitchen, dormitory, and bathhouse; a "house of physicians," with rooms for the critically ill, the storage of drugs, and a chief physician; and a space for bloodletting, receiving medicines (possibly laxatives), and eating (see Figure 18).[17] Other sources show monasteries procuring spices, honey, oil, herbs, sponges, mats, and leeches for the care of the sick.[18]

Although the full details of the plan may never have been realized, without doubt people recognized by society as doctors were located within the monastic domain; whether they were professed monks remains another question. Two individuals appear with the label *medicus* in the Reichenau confraternity book, but Alfons Zettler concludes that these were most likely laymen closely bound to the community.[19] Statutes for the monastery of Corbie explicitly indicate that the two *medici* serving the monastery should be laymen who, like the carpenters, masons, blacksmiths, and other craftsmen, possessed rooms within the monastic complex.[20] Despite this, there is strong evidence that at least some monks *did* hold the title of *medicus*: we find them as envoys, as abbots acclaimed for their medical learning, and even as practitioners on themselves (see Figure 2, where a monk performs cautery).[21]

Alongside monks, the secular clergy have also been cast as the primary representatives of Hippocratic medicine in the Carolingian age. Loren MacKinney argued that most young men entering a life in the Church were directed to study medicine.[22] The evidence for this is scant, but Achim Hack has pinpointed three royal charters that identify individuals as *clericus et medicus* or *presbiter et medicus*.[23] Similarly, Clare Pilsworth has found nineteen *medici* in charters from northern and central Italy, seven of whom are also identified as *clerici* and one as *presbiter*.[24] In terms of specific locations of training, John Contreni offers testimony that the cathedral school of Laon was a center of medical study, especially under Bishop Pardulus (848–856).[25] Episcopal seats like Reims, Chartres, and Hildesheim also seem to have been recognized as places with medical resources and scholars.[26]

In sum, the (albeit scattered) evidence suggests that the title *medicus* was one that could be held by laypersons, secular clergy, and monastics in the Carolingian Empire.[27] The term did not necessarily indicate a profession but rather a skill set that might be embraced simultaneously with other "careers." The one characteristic applicable to all individuals called *medici* is maleness—no woman is dubbed a *medica*, and female herbalists appear only as charlatans, foils to the legitimate male healer.[28] We can speculate about the existence of a range of local or informal healers (such as female birth attendants), but these do not appear in the written sources. Despite this strict gender divide, the general impression from the Carolingian period is that porous boundaries shaped the provision of medical care. Although prescriptive monastic sources state that medical care was only for the brothers, this was clearly not always the case in practice.[29] Einhard mentions a priest being carried to the same monastery where he had been educated in order to be treated by the *medici* there.[30] Similarly, a miracle collection relates a story of King Pippin ordering the lay abbot of Saint-Quentin to provide "the comforts of his *medici*" to an infirm man.[31] On the other hand, Ardo's *Life of Benedict of Aniane* and one of Lupus of Ferrières's letters speak of *medici* being summoned *to* the monastery to attend to the sick or wounded.[32] Sometimes, *medici* also seem to have traveled between different monasteries, according to the command of the abbot.[33] The best deduction, then, is that certain *medici* were mobile and likely treated patients in their homes, while others were concentrated at royal and episcopal residences, and others still ministered and trained in monasteries, whether as monks or as clerics.[34]

In the face of this elusive construction of a Carolingian medical "professional," one of the most fertile resources for investigating conceptions of the *medicus* remains the extant medical manuscripts themselves. Although these offer little information about the social realities of medical training, they are windows onto the ideological framework governing the practice of medicine and the moral dilemmas provoked by the work of the ambiguous *medicus*. It is to these manuscripts that we now turn.

## Education and Character of the *Medicus*

Although the scarcity of evidence from the early Middle Ages prevents us from reconstructing the training and background of an individual who was recognized as a *medicus*, the paradigms concerning this role, as expressed in the extant medical manuscripts, offer compelling clues as to how the physician wished to be perceived. To be sure, the obscure origin and transmission of these oft-called "deontological texts," and their similarity to certain Hippocratic and Galenic works, may lead one to question whether they reflect ninth-century thought at all.[35] Before dismissing them as simple reiterations, however, we might recall Robert Markus's comment that "the inherited literary tradition helps one to look for—and to find—things which have previously been allowed to remain blurred, in the shadows."[36] In this case, compilers of medical manuscripts were drawn to classical and late antique pronouncements about the physician because many themes accorded with contemporary ideals. In turn, these inherited ethical treatises (edited and refashioned as they were copied anew) sharpened beliefs about the proper conduct and education of a Christian healer, serving as a type of mirror for a ninth-century audience.[37]

Short pedagogical texts found in various renderings across different manuscripts argue that an extensive education was *de rigueur* for anyone wishing to assume the title of *medicus*.[38] Rather than a specific program of instruction, these emphasize a broad familiarity with different disciplines. "A *medicus* ought to be the type of person who is so exceedingly competent with literature that, while skimming through diverse numbers of books, he increases his thought and understanding and quickly discovers theory and skills. . . . And, above all, he should read the words of the philosophers."[39] One text explains that his education should include grammar, rhetoric, geometry, numbers, and astronomy, while another slightly differs in declaring that grammar, astronomy, arithmetic, geometry, and music are necessary subjects, but rhetoric is to be avoided for fear "that he become too loquacious."[40]

In general, these prescriptive synopses emphasize an idea also articulated by Isidore—that the study of medicine builds upon a foundation laid by the seven liberal arts.[41] The *Etymologies* states that the *medicus* must know grammar for understanding literature; rhetoric for defining true arguments; dialectic for rationally scrutinizing diseases and cures; arithmetic for calculating the rhythm of hours and days; geometry for appreciating the properties of regions; music for therapy; and astronomy for knowledge of the stars and seasons.[42] Not only did medical manuscripts include this section of Isidore's text, but compilers also evidently selected treatises with similar themes; the message they implicitly advanced was that medicine was taught by more than practical experience.[43] "Whoever has instruction and fear of God, with reading, talent, and reason is able to become an expert about the course of the time of life, the pulses of the veins, the stages of growth, the characters of men, birds, fish, herbs, trees, and rocks and everything that is made by craft and by hand."[44] Reading is said to be central to the practice of the *medicus*—a declaration that itself points to the production and use of the manuscripts within which these passages are found.[45] According to this view, *medici* were set apart from other craftsmen not only by their literacy but by their ability to relate their manual work to broader concepts about the cosmos that they encountered in texts.

Augustine's *On Christian Teaching* had categorized medicine as one of the mechanical arts, alongside agriculture and navigation.[46] While acknowledging that these "furnish a kind of service for God's labors (*ministerium quoddam exhibent operanti deo*)," Augustine claimed that Christian clergy should be familiar with these arts only in a superficial and cursory way, not so as to practice them but so that they might have the tools to interpret figures of speech in scripture.[47] The work does not disparage medicine, but it certainly distinguishes it from the elevated intellectual pursuits of the Christian scholar. Despite the importance of this text in Carolingian thought, however, attitudes toward medical learning did not follow the contours of Augustine's classifications.[48] Instead, compilers presented the art as an endeavor of intellectual reasoning, technical skill, and deeply rooted morality. Indeed, the *medicus* that emerges from ninth-century manuscripts resembles the preacher in *On Christian Teaching*, a figure who Augustine declares ought to read widely, speak eloquently, and model the Christian values he articulates.[49]

A treatise preserved in three ninth-century manuscripts, which directly addresses a student of medicine, underscores the need to cultivate intellectual expertise alongside the virtues of an upright character:

> I urge you, *medicus*, just as I, too, was urged by my teacher, read constantly and do not be lazy! Look after the ill whom you have received as patients and consider how to cure them. Pursue modesty, love chastity, guard the secrets of the home. If you learn anything in the homes of the infirm, be silent, and do not slander others.[50]

Rather than focusing on specific medical skills, this short text seeks to ensure that the student will be recognized as an honorable person.[51] It invokes a pedagogical genealogy in order to suggest that all *medici* adhere to high standards of behavior. Drawing on tenets of Hippocratic decorum found in the Oath, the passage highlights the intimacy of medical care and the corresponding need for discretion and sexual purity. But it also speaks more generally of virtues such as studiousness, diligence, charity, and compassion. Similarly, other didactic texts, including one that is even entitled *What Type of Person a Medicus Ought to Be*, mandate a long list of qualities—the physician must be amiable, patient, gentle, chaste, sober, clement, detached, modest, reliable, vigilant, pious, competent, and agreeable in conversation.[52] Unfit are those who are proud, intoxicated, lazy, fearful, angry, squeamish, lustful, vulgar, deceptive, or timid.[53] While primarily emphasizing the internal disposition of the doctor, these texts also indicate the importance of making virtue visible to others by means of outward signs such as walking in a dignified manner and patiently dealing with fractious patients. For "gravitas signifies many things about the soul," one treatise reminds its readers.[54]

These writings do not assume that it is training or education that instills righteousness; rather, the aspiring student must first have his character tested (*probare*) to determine if he is worthy of continuing.[55] "Just as the whole earth was not made optimal for the receiving of seed but only that part which after it has received the seed makes it fruitful—likewise neither is every [person] on earth made fit to receive teaching but only one who has a good will and is able to sustain himself steadfastly."[56] In eloquent language such as this, medical practice is established as a restricted field, with those admitted to it deserving of the trust of society. The message is clearly that not everyone is suited to the study of this elevated art: "Truly, medicine has passed through many but found few who are wise."[57]

Without doubt, these reflections on the *medicus* should be considered prescriptive, not descriptive. The question of what influenced these ideals is more difficult to pinpoint. Were these texts viewed as vestiges of a classical Roman heritage that seemed even more important to preserve in the imperial climate after 800? MacKinney has suggested that these treatises prove Hippocratic ethics continued in an "unbroken line" from classical times to Salernitan medicine as a result of a (tenuous but persistent) secularity when medieval monks dealt with practical matters like health.[58] The previous chapter has sought to dispel the assumption that "medical culture" exists in proportion to secularization. And, in any case, can we be certain that these prescriptions were not shaped by Christian values? Certainly, some of the statements in these texts would have been *read* as innately Christian: "For humility is always learning, always accruing [knowledge], disregarding nothing and offending no one."[59] If, around 400, Jerome held up the Hippocratic doctor as a benchmark against which the clergy could demonstrate their superiority, around 800, the assumption was that caretakers of the body would model their comportment on that expected of caretakers of the soul.[60]

I want to suggest that the appearance of these texts in ninth-century medical manuscripts owes much to a culture of defining roles and responsibilities, a culture that dominated church councils, palace affairs, and elite writings early in the ninth century, particularly in the years between 813 and 833. Reforming councils called by Charlemagne in 813 and by Louis in 816 and 829 encouraged processes of self-reflection by which different orders within society identified their own offices and obligations and where they had fallen short, devoting special attention to the *ministerium* (duty) of bishops and kings.[61] Sifting through diverse traditions, these elites did not simply repeat old rules about monks, canons, nuns, abbots, priests, and prelates but shaped new assumptions about social power and moral authority. Their approach to the relationship between duties and morality has many parallels with the delineation of the physician in medical codices. The lists of qualities demanded of a *medicus*-in-training even share similar terms to those used to set expectations for various ecclesiastical personnel: mandates from the Council of Frankfurt (794), for example, proclaim that the cellarer within a monastery ought not to be a greedy person but "a wise man of mature conduct, moderate, not a glutton, or arrogant, agitated, unjust, sluggish, or wasteful, but a God-fearing man."[62]

As one means to secure the success of this definitional project, Charlemagne seized on the growing ubiquity of oath-taking across the early Middle Ages, turning the oath of loyalty into a type of sacrament, a double-fold promise of faith (*fides*) toward the emperor and toward God.[63] In this context, how should we identify references to the swearing of an oath by medical students? In truth, there are only sporadic allusions to the Hippocratic Oath in ninth-century manuscripts and no complete copies of the original text.[64] But when the treatise *On Giving the Oath* (*De sacramento dando*) declares that "he ought to swear who wishes to begin [to learn] the medical art and the science of nature," we can nevertheless see parallels with Carolingian assumptions that oaths could regulate Christian behavior in the service of the proper functioning of society.[65] The very idea of a *medicus* whose responsibilities to care for the body were secured by "the sacrament of an oath" (*per sacramentum iuramenti*) might have allayed anxieties about this figure's power over life and death, whether or not there was a consistent ritual of oath-taking. If excerpts of the Hippocratic Oath seemed significant to ninth-century compilers, this was because they already accepted that oaths were not simply promises of political loyalty but were pledges to uphold ethical standards in a demonstration of religious faith.[66]

## Competing for Patients

Although the collected texts within medical manuscripts mostly portray the *medicus* as a respected figure, contemporary sources like the *Life of St. Sturm* suggest that taking up this role could attract danger. Indeed, the very insistence on the virtuousness of the doctor belies a context in which practitioners of medicine occupied contested ground. In their repeated characterizations of the healer of the body as highly educated and deeply virtuous, medical manuscripts were performative texts, intended to shape the reality of ninth-century society. In the words of Robert French, these manuscripts told a "Good Story" about the learned, righteous expertise of the *medicus* to convince contemporaries of the authority vested in this role.[67] While French and others have revealed the discursive, legal, and institutional processes by which university-trained physicians of the thirteenth and fourteenth centuries sought to establish a hierarchy of healers that affirmed their own superiority, the negotiations of the ninth century focused more on contrasts than hierarchies.[68] It was not a question of categorizing healers according to the subdivisions of medical practice (diet, pharmacy, surgery) but a problem of legitimacy or illegitimacy in the very nature of human intervention on the body.[69] As we saw in Chapter 4, prescriptive texts issued by Carolingian rulers and pastoral leaders stridently forbade any consultation with those involved in superstitious dealings and any act associated with demonic powers. The sick were not to turn to magicians, charmers, or soothsayers in times of suffering but rather to depend on the orthodox learning of a virtuous *medicus*.[70] Yet, it was not simply accusations of magic with which early medieval doctors had to contend; it was also enduring stereotypes regarding the types of people who entered the profession.

Hippocratic medicine had long suffered negative associations in the Latin-speaking provinces of the Roman Empire, in large part because many physicians there were originally of low or servile status.[71] While the situation changed over the course of Late Antiquity, certain associations probably persisted into the early Middle Ages, particularly those that tarred the physician as immoral, greedy, and incapable.[72] Perhaps the most vituperative critique derived from Pliny the Elder's *Natural History* (ca. 77 C.E.), wherein he excoriated physicians for their ignorance, avarice, and lack of accountability, accusing them of perpetrating frauds and criminally experimenting on their weak and susceptible patients.[73] The *Natural History* was well known to the Carolingians, and a toned-down version of Pliny's original denunciation also circulated as the preface to *Pliny's Medicine* (a heavily revised version from the fourth century).[74] This preface offered a justification for the remedy collection that followed, as "Pliny" explains that he composed the work so that those traveling need not have recourse to unfamiliar, corrupt healers, who sell "useless remedies at enormous prices," turn short-term illnesses into long afflictions for the sake of profit, and accept incurable cases "on account of greed."[75]

Just as *Pliny's Medicine* raised the specter of caretakers of the body who were extortionists, so did other stereotypes of the physician suggest that he might be a duplicitous character because of his "potions." The mystery surrounding the power of concocted drinks could easily incite convictions of both poisoning and magic, as indicated in the *Life of St. Sturm*.[76] When Charles the Bald died of a fever in 877, the *Annals of Saint-Bertin* accused his royal physician, a Jew named Zedechias, of poisoning him with a deceitful draught.[77] As we see here, Jewish involvement in healing could be wielded as a rhetorical device, to taint perceptions of the *medicus* and raise suspicions about the medical art in general. Fears surrounding a nonbeliever treating a Christian body had potency, even if there were few Jewish doctors in early medieval Francia.[78] When a cure was unsuccessful, a healer's Jewishness became an obvious target and could fuse with other denunciations.[79] The easy slippage among various negative characterizations is seen most clearly in Regino of Prüm's early tenth-century chronicle: Charles the Bald is described as misplacing his trust in "a certain Jew" who delivered to him "a drink of death" and tricked many with his "magical illusions and incantations."[80]

In cases where physicians were not accused of deliberate harm, one of the most prominent accusations they faced was that they were simply ineffective. The Gospel of Mark (5:25–29) described how a bleeding woman suffered the useless treatments of doctors for twelve years before being healed instantaneously by Jesus. In this model, medieval hagiography often contrasted the futile human doctor to the effective saintly "physician."[81] In his *Miracles of Saint Martin*, Bishop Gregory of Tours (d. 594) frequently noted the number of years that disabled individuals suffered before finally being cured at the tomb of Martin, and Einhard's account of his saints included several references to the "ignorance of physicians" and their "useless" remedies.[82] Valerie Flint has proposed a reading of hagiography that highlights the series of juxtapositions among the saint, doctor, and magician.[83] In order to bolster the saint's *supernatural* cures, the hagiographer often made the doctor into the "fall-guy" for the saint by indicating the failure of his *natural* remedies. At the same time, however, the *medicus* might appear as a Christian ally to the saint, with both standing against the demonically driven enchanter. Flint contends that the attention hagiography devoted to denigrating the *medicus* and vilifying the magician suggests a reality in which both figures commanded significant social standing, an argument that enables us to see past the topoi within hagiography to the contested positions various healers occupied within early medieval society.

In a similar fashion, we can analyze the presentation of the *medicus* in medical compilations as indicative of broader tensions regarding cures for sickness within the changing landscape of healing propelled by the Carolingian *correctio*. Descriptions of the physician and his role, copied and edited anew in the ninth century, were implicit responses to longstanding stereotypes but also attempts to propagate a set of contrasts and comparisons that worked to the advantage of practitioners of human medicine in the Carolingian medical marketplace.[84] As manifestations of those who sought to undermine the foundations of Christian society, Jews, poisoners, extortionists, and magicians were frauds whom the *medicus* had to oppose if his activities were to be sanctioned by ecclesiastical authorities. Yet, concurrently, he jostled for attention with healing methods that were under the purview of those same authorities and were being endorsed with mounting vigor.

"By 826, the saints were rushing north to rescue the kingdom of Louis the Pious," as Paul Dutton observes.[85] According to contemporaries, large crowds of the ill and disabled flocked to be healed by the relics.[86] In fact, the translation (relocation) of corporeal relics from Rome to sites north of the Alps was not unprecedented in the 820s but had taken place in the decades after the Carolingian dynasty first came to power. Yet, because the traffic in Roman saints ceased around 780, when it was initiated again by Carolingian elites like Hilduin of Saint-Denis and Einhard, it sparked a new wave of translations that lasted until the 850s.[87] In combination with Charlemagne's repeated order (in 801 and 813) that all altars contain relics, these developments resulted in the multiplication of sites of "heavenly medicine" across the Carolingian realm.[88] The influx of relics sparked new lines of competition among healers, not only between doctors and saints but also among the saints themselves. In the *Translation of Saints Marcellinus and Peter*, for instance, criticisms of other relics outnumber criticisms of useless physicians, and with understated smugness, Einhard emphasizes repeatedly that his martyrs are due all the credit for miracles that occurred when they visited the resting places of other relics.[89] The multiple rivalries in Einhard's text point to the manner in which allies and competitors were continually being reconfigured in response to a dynamic social reality of healing possibilities.

Entangled in these same developments was the Christian rite of unction for the sick, which Carolingian ecclesiastics increasingly began to promote shortly after 800, as Frederick Paxton has revealed.[90] Relying on the Epistle of James (5:14–15), Bishop Gerbald of Liège ordered the priests in his diocese to anoint the sick with holy oil and diligently pray over them.[91] Just over ten years later, the 813 Council of Chalon-sur-Saône decreed that "according to the teaching of the blessed Apostle James, with which the doctrines of the Fathers also agree, the infirm ought to be anointed by priests with oil that is blessed by bishops. . . . And this type of medicine should be given no little attention because it cures the weaknesses of soul and body."[92] Bishop Jonas of Orléans, too, sought to amend popular behavior, criticizing the sick for seeking remedies from male and female diviners rather than from priests who could administer the unction of sanctified oil.[93] Roman sacramentaries included no rite for the unction of the sick, only a rite for blessing the oil. However, Benedict of Aniane's composition of a reform ritual for Frankish priests to follow in carrying out holy unction (completed between 815 and 821) spurred on the availability of this ecclesiastical "medicine."[94] Like the cures of the relics, the ninth-century rite of sacred anointing promised to remedy the suffering of the body as well as the ills of the soul.[95]

In light of this greater diversity of healing options, we can more precisely situate the ninth-century didactic descriptions of the *medicus* within specific dynamics emerging from the Carolingian rise to power. Texts outlining the *medicus*'s learning and character responded to long-standing negative tropes by instead casting physicians as shining models of Christian virtue. Against accusations of greed, writings in praise of the physician frequently emphasized his charitable endeavors—take, for instance, Alcuin's admiration for how the Hippocratic practitioners at court "tend to everyone without charge" and the Lorsch apologist's emphasis that heavenly, rather than earthly, rewards are the physician's compensation for services.[96] Finally, attempts to fashion the *medicus* as another type of miracle worker reflected a climate in which avenues for divine healing had multiplied. The rest of this chapter takes up this final agenda, examining various formulations of the physician's status and responsibilities in order to demonstrate the ways in which such healers were cast as eminent, even sanctified, members of Carolingian society. To sanctify the *medicus* was not to denigrate the saint or to pit rational medicine against religious authority—on the contrary, the same monastery or cathedral might be the site at which one could receive a cure from relics, holy unction, or trained physicians.[97] However, this move did mark an important shift in the history of the *medicus*'s ministry.

## Christ as the Model *Medicus*

In the Synoptic Gospels, Jesus declares to the doubtful Pharisees that he communes with sinners because "it is not the healthy who need a doctor, but the sick."[98] His ability to cure human sin invisibly is showcased in his miraculous healing of disabled and diseased bodies, as he informs those gathered to hear him preach.[99] Drawing on this biblical theme, as well as a long Greek tradition of comparing the medical care of the body with the philosophical care of the soul, Christian apologists from the second century on popularized the metaphor of "Christ the Physician."[100] While this comparison reflected the thriving medical culture of Late Antiquity, it did not necessarily encourage positive attitudes toward Greco-Roman physicians. Instead, as this section demonstrates, it was only with the reappropriation of the metaphor in medical writings, and its application to human *medici*, that physical healing was aligned with divine power in ways that affirmed the care of the body.

Among some of the earliest Christian theologians, metaphors emphasizing Jesus's therapeutic skill pitted him against Asclepius, the most prominent Greco-Roman god of healing and a patron of physicians, invoked by name in the Hippocratic Oath.[101] Like Jesus, Asclepius cured the incurable and raised the dead. Thus, in an effort to undermine this pagan authority, apologists such as Tertullian and Origen argued for Christ's status as the Supreme Physician, the only god who could treat all afflictions of human bodies and souls.[102] Into the fifth century, even after Christianity became the official imperial religion, the pagan cult of Asclepius remained such a threat that Augustine heaped particular scorn upon Asclepius's "supposed" powers throughout his *City of God*.[103] Lambasting those who trusted in the false pagan god as the divine physician (*medicus deus*), Augustine also criticized Christians who turned to human doctors in their need, cataloguing a multitude of testimonials juxtaposing the miraculous cures of the saints against the ineptitude and gruesome torments of the medical profession.[104] In foundational Christian texts such as the *City of God*, then, the metaphor *Christus medicus* came to symbolize the preposterousness of bestowing the title "physician" on any figure who did not channel the unparalleled healing power of the omnipotent God.

Of all Latin theologians in Late Antiquity, Augustine turned most frequently to the concept of the Divine Physician in elucidating the salvific work of God and showing how Christ's omnipotent grace cured human frailty.[105] But he was not alone. Jerome, too, referred to Christ as the true physician (*verus medicus*), the only physician (*solus medicus*), and like a spiritual Hippocrates (*quasi spiritualis Hippocrates*), and his writings are replete with concepts drawn from surgery, pharmacy, and dietetic medicine.[106] Further, in his foundational work on the duties of bishops, the *Pastoral Rule*, one of Gregory the Great's key conceptual frameworks was the model that physicians of the body offered for spiritual leaders, whom he described as doctors of the soul.[107] Outlining the techniques to be employed by the developing Church ministry, Gregory praised physicians of the body for their discernment and ability to adapt treatments to the unique condition of every individual: "These are the [treatments] that a caretaker of souls ought to preserve in the diversity of his preaching, so that he may apply the appropriate remedy to the wounds of each person with anxious attention."[108] Gregory's pastoral directives proved extremely influential with Carolingian scholars, and his paradigm of the care of the soul as a form of personalized medical treatment permeated the language of ecclesiastical councils convened in 813, 816, and 836.[109]

Gregory's contemporary, Benedict of Nursia, likewise inspired a strong tradition of medical comparisons in ninth-century discourse. The Benedictine Rule described the ideal abbot as a "wise physician" (*sapiens medicus*), who cared for the "sickly souls" of his flock with his diverse range of "poultices," "ointments," and "medicines." Yet, just as a doctor might have to employ drastic treatments in dire cases, the abbot had to recognize when a brother could not be healed and apply the "cauterization of excommunication" and the "knife of amputation," evicting a monk from the monastery lest contagion spread to the rest of the cloistered body.[110] Over several decades,

Benedict's Rule was adopted as the singular standard for all monasteries in the Carolingian realm, and its dictates shaped ninth-century theories of ecclesiastical (and royal) ministry.[111] Just so, the bishops involved in the rebellion against Louis the Pious in 833 explained their actions as a Benedictine duty, whereby they were "spiritual doctors" responsible for correcting the emperor's unhealthy condition.[112]

In precisely this way, the long lineage of the *Christus medicus* metaphor, in its wide variety of forms, infused Carolingian conceptions of divine and pastoral governance within the *ecclesia*. Small books of devotional prayers, for example, frequently referred to the Trinity as "my most powerful physician" (*medicus meus potentissimus*), and Alcuin's penitential works likewise described God as a *medicus* who could heal any illness without effort or delay.[113]

Although the recurrence of these metaphors suggests some familiarity with medical procedures, this figurative language did not necessarily validate the practitioners of Hippocratic therapeutics. The comparisons presumed an analogy between the care of the body and of the soul, but the message in pastoral writings was *consistently* that caretakers of the flesh were inferior to those who treated the spiritual. Jerome, for instance, described the Evangelist Luke as someone "who was turned from a doctor of bodies to a doctor of souls (*medico corporum in medicum est uersus animarum*), in the same way that the apostles, from being fishers of fish, were made into the fishers of men."[114] In doing so, this Father appealed to a dualistic relationship between *medici* and clergy, in which the latter surpassed the former by nature. Similarly, the 813 Council of Chalons-sur-Saône, noting that physicians took no regard for a patient's station in applying harsh cures like cautery, decreed "how much more should this be observed by those who are not *medici* of the body but of the soul."[115] Hrabanus Maurus, too, propagated this hierarchical assessment: "Just as corporeal [doctors] cure the sicknesses of bodies through herbal medicines, so do the spiritual heal the infirmities of souls through the remedy of divine precepts. Both ought to be held with honor, but the spiritual ought to be preferred, since their reverence is greater to the degree that their works are found to be longer lasting and more salubrious."[116]

The very fact that a certain binary thinking underpinned the *Christus medicus* metaphor makes it all the more significant that it appeared in a new genre in the ninth century—medical treatises. This new context for the metaphor utterly transformed how it was to be read. A text found in several early medieval manuscripts ends with the exclamation: "May the grace of God be with you and in the use of medicine and may health (*salus*) come to your patients from God, who alone is a *medicus*."[117] This phrasing undermines any distinction between physical health and spiritual salvation with its invocation of divine grace and its use of the multivalent word *salus*. If the human physician is cast as a tool of divine grace, the text insists that the reader recognize God as the only healer, the one who ultimately bestows physical health when medical remedies are utilized on the body. Yet, here, the relationship between *medicus* and God advances the human practitioner—he is established as an agent of the divine, and his work is empowered by divine oversight.

Likewise, the pseudonymous letter from Luke (discussed in Chapter 4) describes Christ in the well-worn patristic tradition as an "all-powerful physician" (*omnipotens medicus*).[118] And a dictum associated with Luke's name reads as follows: "Luke says, where the Lord works, there the *medicus* is praised. Hippocrates also said: however much the Lord permits, this much the *medicus* accomplishes."[119] Here, too, the physician's influence over the body's state is shown to be limited by the hidden will of God. But, again, the appearance of this statement in a manuscript of Hippocratic teachings and treatments does not undermine the physician's power but rather bolsters it.[120] Even the famous Hippocrates confirms the Christian God's role as foundation and facilitator of every successful poultice, herbal cure, or bloodletting procedure!

I conclude with an example from the *Lorscher Arzneibuch*. In order to find biblical support for human medicine, the apologist asserts that God deserves to be called a physician because he healed the world from the weakness of unfaithfulness by the medicine of the Incarnation and the sacrament of baptism. Citing the Synoptic tradition comparing Jesus to a physician, the apologist concludes that the Lord acted according to "medical practice" (*medicinalis mos*) in how he converted the bitterness of the Old Testament to a sweet healing tonic.[121] We see how the original meaning of the God-as-physician metaphor has been inverted in this Carolingian text. Rather than proving the superiority of the Christian God to all pagan and human healers, the comparison advances the legitimacy and authority of human *medici* trained in a discipline developed by pagan experts. The above examples from ninth-century medical manuscripts stem from a long Christian tradition; they depend upon concepts developed in Augustine's sermons and phrases scattered throughout Jerome's scholarship. However, they presume a different kind of argument—rather than using the visible care of the body to explain the invisible care of the soul, they present those who heal the body as crucial components of God's salvific operations. The analogy now credits the *medicus* and no longer points to his comparative inadequacy.

## The Doctor and the Saint

Appropriating the *Christus medicus* metaphor was one way in which medical texts circulating in the ninth century repositioned the physician as an associate, rather than antithesis, of those with a specific *ministerium* in the care of Christian souls. Yet, if the clergy claimed titles as "doctors" in a spiritual sense, the saints who populated the Carolingian realm competed with *medici* by offering physical healing together with spiritual cleansing. Thus, if human *medici* were to hold their own, they had to grapple with both the natural and supernatural worlds. Focusing on two particular manuscripts, produced around 800 and 850, this final section argues that the ways compilers gathered and presented materials created manuals of medical instruction that resembled the mirrors (*specula*) for lay noblemen discussed in Chapter 2. Just as those manuals were didactic guides that reflected new assumptions about the laity, so were these medical manuscripts intended to educate the *medicus* and signify his position. That position rested not only on the rational management of nature but also on an intervention in the invisible and miraculous layers of the cosmos.

A manuscript likely compiled in Burgundy stands as one of the earliest extant Carolingian medical collections and is a rare example of medical treatises being combined with hagiographical material in a single codex. The codex was put together in stages, yet over a relatively short time, such that it probably existed in its current state by the early ninth century.[122] An original unit of medical treatises—consisting of texts on anatomy, urines, fevers, humors, bloodletting, herbs, weights and measures, and remedies and antidotes (attributed to authorities like Hippocrates, Galen, Vindicianus, and Soranus)—was expanded by insertions at the beginning of the codex and in between certain quires. The most significant addition was the two texts that now preface the medical collection, the *Passion of Saints Cosmas and Damian, Physicians* and the sole witness to a moralizing history of medicine titled the *Epistola pepiodeotecon*. Examining the lessons imparted by the scribe's layered construction of this manuscript reveals an argument about interconnected systems of healing in the Carolingian world.

The very title of the *Passion* declares that Cosmas and Damian exemplify the roles of both saint and physician.[123] The two brothers, we are told, were raised in the Christian faith by their mother and persecuted in Syria during the reign of the Emperor Diocletian. Most of the text vividly describes the brothers' torments and death, but the beginning explains that they were taught "by the revelation of the Holy Spirit much knowledge of the art of medicine, and they cured [people] according to divine scripture."[124] The examples of the brothers' deeds focus not on their technical skills but on their spiritual power; like Christ, they cure the blind, expel demons, and restore an invalid woman who has spent all her money on doctors. Faith, not herbs, animates the brothers' remedies. And yet, the passion does not state that Cosmas and Damian received "the grace of healing" (as in 1 Cor 12:9) but learned knowledge (*scientia*) from the Holy Spirit. Furthermore, as compared to other ninth-century hagiographical accounts of doctor-saints, this text presents no stark contrast between those who offer miracle cures and those who, "enslaved to earthly teachings," offer only Hippocratic treatments.[125] Rather, Cosmas and Damian perfectly embody the harmony that ought to exist between Christian faith and human medicine. This is evident in the promise written immediately under the title: "Whoever is sick and has this passion read over her, the Lord will have mercy on her."[126] The text even ends with an antiphon, which indicates a possible liturgical use for the manuscript or, more likely, a chant to be uttered either by sick patients in monasteries or by clergy visiting the sick in their homes (where the passion may have been used alongside ritual anointing). Either way, the message is undeniably that this history of the brothers' suffering is another remedy—among the many others found in the pages of the manuscript—for purging pain from an ill body.

The *Epistola* that follows the *Passion* is difficult to categorize.[127] It begins as a history of medicine, drawing heavily on pagan narratives of a golden age, but morphs into a sermon-like text on the character of the *medicus*, with a long Christian discourse on the omnipotence of God. We already encountered the opening, which outlines how disease first disrupted the idyllic health of the ancients, in Chapter 4. The section on the *medicus* starts by emphasizing that "perfect physicians" (*medici perfecti*) must have experience, learned knowledge of Hippocratic texts, and fear of God. With the ancients, medicine was considered miraculous, but as a result of moral corruption, it deteriorated and was scorned. Here, the authorial voice intensifies with agitation, asking the reader why the art of medicine should be dismissed because of the weakness of certain human practitioners and denouncing those patients who do not seek out a virtuous physician:

> Oh you wise one, why do you slander wisdom if human fragility errs? . . . Oh you sick person, who entrusts yourself to the foulness and evil of another, you will not be able to make a petition pleasing to the Lord on your own. And your [chosen] advocate the [false] *medicus*, who is full of foulness, is not heard.[128]

Humanity is prone to vices that undermine the pursuit of wisdom—hence the physician must "manifestly guard himself" in order to be an effective healer. The text insists that those who are proud, greedy, or blasphemous are not able to exercise the art, and thus "their patients are flagrantly and quickly brought near to death."[129] Indeed, a bold heading in the middle of the page highlights a list of qualities that closely resemble the characteristics in the didactic texts discussed above: "The Life of the Medicus: chastity, faith, and sobriety cause the wise to remain in wisdom."[130]

In an apologetic fashion, the *Epistola* chastises those who believe that medical skill or success can exist separately from proper Christian devotion. A physician mired in sin, or one with a false conscience, is unable to invoke God's necessary aid for his patient.[131] Consequently, "it is better to live with an ignorant but holy [*medicus*] and to bear with his little art, however unskilled it is, than to consult with a perfect one full of every iniquity and immorality."[132] The message of the text is certainly not that medical care is unwarranted or illegitimate, but that it is useless to turn to a physician who is not also an intercessor with the divine judge. The Lord acts as a mediator in three possible ways, the author explains: he shows mercy to the holy *medicus*; he holds his pure art back from an impure *medicus*; or he renders judgment on the sick person. As the text expounds at length, God alone has free will and dominion over all of creation; he alone has authority over the life of the body and soul. "You"—the text once again inquires of its reader—"what care do you show to the body, which you are able to see; surely you are not able to master cures for the soul, which you cannot see?"[133] Humans have limited agency over their health, even the physical, visible aspects of it. The author promises that the following pages will explain the condition of the fragile and fearful earthly body, inherited from the first man (Adam), and what happens to it on account of an abundance of phlegm, humor, bile, and blood. The medical texts set after the *Epistola* proceed to do precisely that.

In deciding to preface a collection of medical texts with the *Passion* and the *Epistola pepiodeotecon*, the Carolingian compiler created a manuscript that functioned as a healing device on multiple levels. First was the miraculous level, in which simply reading about Saints Cosmas and Damian could effect a cure in a listening patient. Second was the moral level, in which learning about the history of medicine taught a patient how to properly care for the body and seek a virtuous facilitator of health. Third was the medicinal or physical level, in which the treatments and herbal cures outlined in the core of the codex promised to return the body to a state of nonsuffering. That these layers could work independently or simultaneously would surely have been understood implicitly by a Carolingian audience accustomed to interpreting the manifold levels of scripture.

The passion of Cosmas and Damian served not only as a type of liturgical "charm" but also provided a model for the physician who might utilize the manuscript.[134] As the *Epistola* offered cautionary advice to those studying Hippocratic cures, reminding them that knowledge of plants and anatomy was only effective if a doctor begged the assistance of God, so did the saints embody the paradigm of a Christian healer. The *medicus* was supposed to conceive of his treatments not in opposition to the healings provided by the saints but rather as another type of miraculous intervention. Just like Cosmas and Damian, in fact, the Hippocratic practitioner might be able to provide "a remedy for demons," not, in this case, by undertaking an exorcism but by mixing a cure with hog's fennel and jet stone.[135]

This image of the *medicus* exhibits strong similarities to ideas found in the contemporaneous *Lorscher Arzneibuch*. At the end of the Lorsch apology is a set of verses praising the pharmaceutical offerings of local fields and mountains, drawn from a poem by Isidore of Seville about his library.[136] It was unusual to excerpt the medical verses rather than those about the Church Fathers, though one other Carolingian medical manuscript likewise included a few of these lines (albeit in a different order).[137] Completely atypical was the compiler's decision to draw stark attention to the title of these verses, by highlighting it in the middle of the page in a canonical capitalis script: "Cosmas Damianus Ippocratis Galienus" (see Figure 12).[138] This was a statement that these four names belonged together in the estimation of the scribe. For a Carolingian book of medical recipes to consciously equate the status of two popular saints with that of two famous physicians of the pagan past was a message about how contemporary *medici* could be seen to embrace both traditions simultaneously.

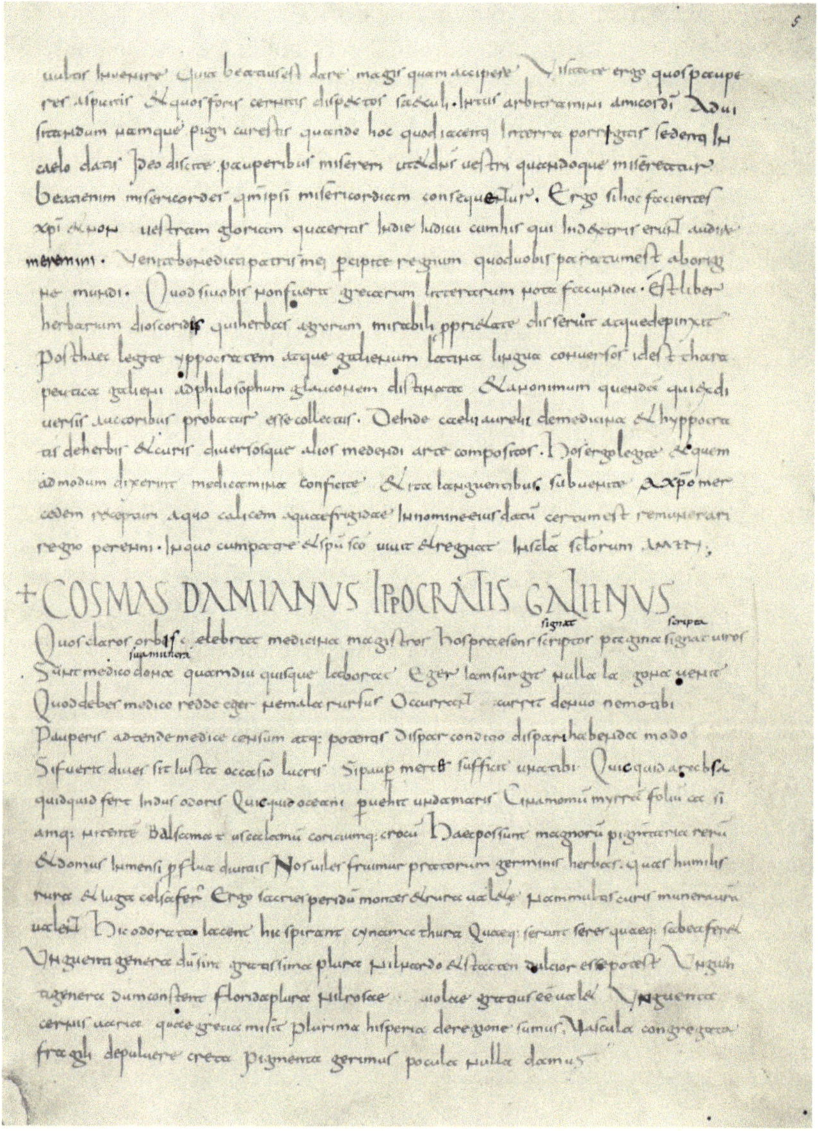


Figure 12. Medical verses from Isidore of Seville's poem on his library, as excerpted in the *Lorscher Arzneibuch*. Staatsbibliothek Bamberg, Msc. med. 1, f. 5r. Photo: Gerald Raab. CC BY–SA 4.0.

The cult of Cosmas and Damian was already well known in Carolingian lands by the ninth century. A claim circulated in Gregory of Tours's *Histories* that their relics lay near to Saint Martin at his church in Tours.[139] The sacramentary that Charlemagne received from Pope Hadrian around 790 included a mass for them on September 27, and several manuscript witnesses to their passion survive from the ninth century.[140] The saints' popularity spread from Rome, where their feast day was long established and several churches featured depictions of the saints.[141] A stunning apse mosaic of the two brothers, holding red surgeon's boxes and being presented to Christ, can still be seen in a basilica in the Roman forum that Pope Felix IV (526–530) dedicated to them (see Figure 13).[142] As part of their strong cultic presence in the Mediterranean, Cosmas and Damian were associated with various forms of healing—incubation may have taken place in Roman sites bearing their images, *xenodochia* (hospitals) connected with their names provided care to travelers and the infirm, and oil used in the ritual anointing of the sick was blessed on their feast day in the Visigothic Church.[143] Yet, in Francia, Gregory of Tours's *Glory of the Martyrs* (the earliest passion to circulate) suggested a more limited correlation between these saints and healing activities. It makes clear that Cosmas and Damian only employed human science *before* their conversion; after they became Christians the saints cured illnesses "solely by the merit of their powers (*virtutum*) and by the intervention of prayers."[144] It was precisely this kind of dichotomy between pagan and Christian healing that the Burgundian manuscript sought to overturn with its argument that the saints were suitable models for those enacting the Hippocratic remedies in the rest of the codex.

* * *

Our second example of a Carolingian effort to present the *medicus* and the saint on the same continuum of divine intervention comes from a manuscript produced around 850 at the monastery of Saint-Denis near Paris.[145] Consisting entirely of various medical materials, the codex is clearly demarcated into different sections, the second of which contains a series of short introductory texts; these range widely over different subjects but almost all of them are titled as *epistolae*. Not only did the scribe purposefully group these texts together, but he also drew the reader's attention to the fact that he had done so by labeling the section *Book of Letters* in a prominent red capitalis quadrata

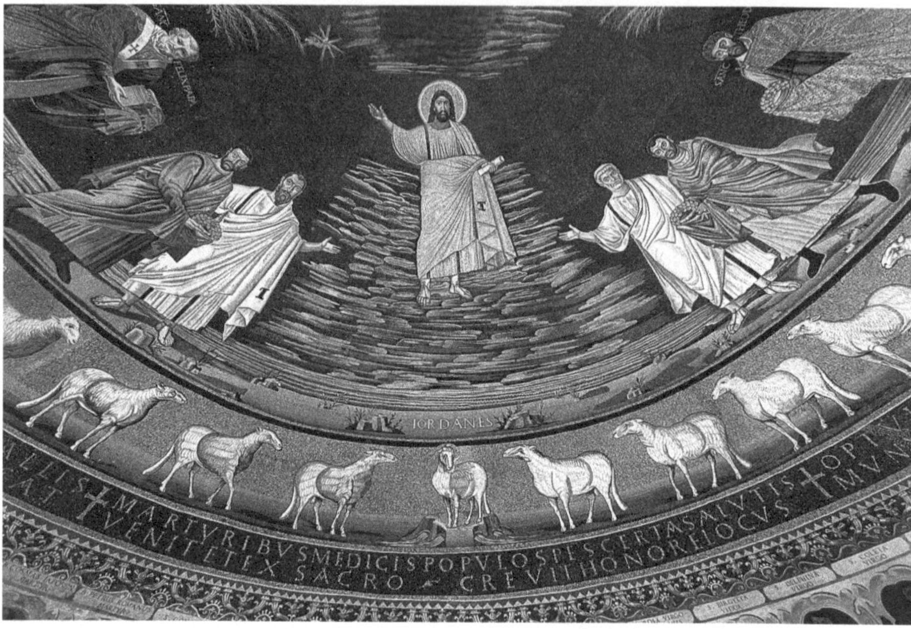


Figure 13. Saints Cosmas and Damian being presented to Christ by Peter and Paul, with Pope Felix IV and Saint Theodore standing at the sides. Apse mosaic, Basilica dei Santi Cosma e Damiano, Rome, early sixth century. Scala/Luciano Romano/Art Resource, NY.

script.[146] While the origins of many of these letters remain obscure, we can see vividly how the texts selected for inclusion, and their ordering, reveal the agenda of the ninth-century "author"—presenting the *medicus* as an intercessor whose work is by no means restricted to the physical and visible world but also concentrates on the healing of the soul. Like the Burgundian manuscript, then, this collection evinces a concerted attempt to claim for the *medicus* the realm of the spiritual as well as the natural.

A letter preserved only in this collection and one other mid-ninth-century manuscript outlines the dual responsibilities of the Christian *medicus*. It offers a brief rationale for God's dispensation of the art of medicine (touched on in Chapter 4), linking Christ's sacrifice for human sins with God's foresight of the sicknesses that would plague humans and praising God for his provision of food, drink, drugs (*pigmenta*), herbs, and trees to be used in various medications. Interspersed with this justification of herbal cures for destroyed bodies (*corpora mortificata*) is an explanation of the physician's purpose:

> It is a worthy declaration to call such a person a *medicus* who is responsible for the health (*sanitates*) of the soul and the health (*salubritates*) of the body—by which means let us not ask of him who fashioned the soul and the body by his order. . . . Thus, he constituted workers (*operatores*) whom he taught by his grace so that they might dedicate themselves to spiritual services. With diligence, may they cure bodies and restore souls. But there are many who do [not] seem devoted to their pursuits: they seek help for the body and damage the soul with their neglect. Whoever, instead, devotes himself to saving the soul and the body will deserve to receive perfect health (*pristinam sanitatem*) and freedom from his sin, made immortal by the omnipotent God.[147]

This passage unambiguously establishes human physicians as practitioners of spiritual healthcare. Indeed, the text equates the responsibilities of the physician in protecting the well-being of his patients with the love that God demonstrated toward humanity in his original fashioning of Adam and Eve. God is the creator of the body and soul, but the *medicus*, here, becomes the divine protector of these entities during their temporal life.[148] The implicit argument is that the health of body and soul are symbiotic; the body cannot be treated effectively without consideration of the soul.

In its framing of the domain of medicine, this letter suggests parallels between the remit that the *medicus* possessed and the type of intervention that ecclesiastical rituals of anointing were intended to achieve. Such rituals were reformed and rewritten by Benedict of Aniane in the second decade of the ninth century and involved a bishop or priest visiting the home of the sick person, anointing him/her with holy oil on various body parts, and chanting a number of prayers, antiphons, and hymns beseeching God to remove pain and expel any unclean spirits from the interior of the body.[149] According to Paxton, Benedict's reform rite returned attention to the physical therapy provided by anointing rather than designating it primarily as a rite for spiritual purification (as in the Irish tradition).[150] The clergy entreated God to "heal the diseases of soul and body," so that the infirm one could be "restored to pristine health" (*pristina sanitas*).[151] There are clear correspondences between Benedict's ritual and the Saint-Denis letter, especially when it comes to the language of health. The liturgy of the sacrament turned to medical metaphors in its appeals to divine assistance, addressing "Christ the true *medicus* of human health" and "Lord God, you who are the true health and medicine."[152] As we have already seen, these metaphors also surface in ninth-century collections of Hippocratic medicine, and the Saint-Denis codex is a good example: it emphasized the *medicus* as channeling God's mercy (like the priest) by describing a set of therapies as intended "for curing vexations of bodies with the grace of God" using remedies revealed "from then, now, and right up into eternity with God's help."[153]

The Saint-Denis *Book of Letters* is permeated by a desire to make abundantly clear that caretakers of the body are not tarnished by the corruptibility of the earthly flesh but elevated by their role in preserving God's creation. In an epistle on those beginning their training as students, medicine is twice referred to as a "sacred art" (*sacra ars*).[154] The rhetorical question "What is a *medicus*?" asked in a treatise entitled *A Letter of Arsenius to Nepotianus*, generates a long list of affirmative qualities.[155] "Arsenius" answers that the *medicus* is "a gentle helper, vivifying the body, curbing pains, drying out the humors, he encourages diets and puts fevers to flight."[156] He is defined as a "laborer for health" (*operarius sanitatis*), in language mimicking that found for God's workers in the letter above. An appealing metaphor is employed to depict the less tangible effects of the physician's work: "Just as a lamp, which illuminates the house, allows everyone to see by preventing the encroaching darkness, thus also does the cheerful ingenuity of the physician convert all sorrows into joy, comfort all parts of the sick person, and revive the soul."[157] Here, again, especially when this text is read against the others in the *Book of Letters*, does the caretaker of the body become the protector of both visible and invisible components of the individual, managing the health of the soul alongside the body.[158]

The point is further elaborated when the *Letter of Arsenius* declares that, as part of his operations, the *medicus* is always "demonstrating present things, announcing future things, making evident eternal things."[159] This line plays off Isidore's statement (also found in the Hippocratic *Prognostics*) that "a physician should recognize the past, know the present, and foresee the future."[160] Crucial to the prognostication that Isidore describes is the physician's ability to draw rational connections among phenomena perceived in the past, the current state of the patient, and the likely outcome of the disease. As Cassiodorus acknowledged, to an ignorant person this might seem equivalent to prophecy, but it was, in truth, merely an act of logic.[161] Yet, the *Letter of Arsenius* did not ascribe simply the power of interpreting the future to the physician but claimed that his work revealed eternal truths. This explicitly defined the *medicus* as an intercessor between earth and heaven, as one who could expose the true meaning of seemingly random events. Just like the saint, he had access to the divine realm; he relied not only on reasonable conjecture but also on supernatural insight.

Given the numerous denunciations of divination in capitularies from the period, it might seem dangerous to associate the *medicus* with the practice of predicting the future. However, this danger was dispelled by the emphasis on the physician as a conduit of divine grace, as indicated at several points in the Saint-Denis *Book of Letters*. Just as saints might "see" deeds taking place far from them and be able to predict the course of future events (including their own deaths), so was the physician capable of comprehending the invisible—the life of the interior, hidden body and the cosmic patterns of God's creation.[162] The very exceptionality of the physician's abilities posed a theological dilemma that the authors of hagiography had likewise confronted. While praising the miracles of saints, authors had to tread a careful line between attributing deeds to the saints' own agency and acknowledging that power merely flowed through them from God. Thus, Alcuin, in his *Life of St. Willibrord*, underscored that God, not the saint, was the true healer: "Just as he deigned visibly to heal their bodily diseases, so also through the intercession of the saint on our behalf . . . he will continue daily to cure the hidden disorders of our souls."[163]

In similar fashion, medical writings from the ninth century asserted that a successful treatment should not be credited solely to the *medicus*'s training, ingenuity, or wisdom. A cure was the result of both the visible, rational application of appropriate medicines and the invisible, mysterious working of God's will. Appealing to the language of hagiography, the *Lorscher Arzneibuch* characterized the *medicus*'s healing acts as miracles (*mirabilia*) through which God desired to be honored.[164] With strong parallels to the themes found in the *Epistola pepiodeotecon*, the apology delineated three players in any healing encounter: the patient, the *medicus*, and the Divine Physician:

> When someone is ill, she should ask the *medicus* with deference for a suitable medicine for her illness, and she should beg God with humility for an effective remedy for her disease. For when she wants to become healthy in order to do good works, *then* does she ask for a health-giving remedy. On the contrary, when she seeks to become

> healthy for another reason, she negates the effect of her prayers, with the consequence that she fails to obtain health.[165]

This passage highlights the importance of the patient's inward orientation in effecting a cure; the patient asks for health "with reverence" toward the *medicus* and "with humility" toward God.[166] God examines the patient's soul and, depending on what he sees, directs his grace toward the *medicus*'s actions. Here, the physician's visit begins to look remarkably similar to an invalid's faithful pilgrimage to a holy relic with a pure heart and hopes of divine intervention.

With these examples from the Burgundian and Saint-Denis medical codices before us, we can offer an amendment to Flint's conceptualization of the competitive landscape of early medieval healers. In contrast to her finding that hagiographical texts distinguished between the saint and the *medicus* by assigning to the former a purview over the supernatural realm and to the latter a purview over the natural world, ninth-century medical collections evince a conscious agenda to establish the Hippocratic healer alongside the saint.[167] If new relic cults and rituals of clerical anointing threatened to disenfranchise medicine, certain compilers responded not by trying to further distance medical care from rituals and repositories of the sacred but by aligning the *medicus* with such holy intercessors.[168]

## Doctors Without Borders

Many scholars have argued that the ninth-century elite evinced a particular concern with establishing the notion of a *ministerium*, or office, for different groups within society.[169] That is, a significant portion of the outpouring of literary activity in the early ninth century consisted of treatises, handbooks, and exegesis that sought to delineate the activities and duties essential to certain roles within society, especially kings, bishops, abbots, monks, and canons. As we saw in Chapter 2, there is evidence that the laity, anxious to secure its own *ministerium*, requested handbooks that would outline a manner of living capable of sanctifying the duties of a lay noble. In this context of categorizing and demarcating responsibilities, it is not surprising to discover that the definition of a *medicus* was also something that provoked literary endeavors. If the body was to be respected as an integral component in the divine order of society—as a sign of God's goodness and also as a means by which he might test his faithful—the caretakers of those bodies needed to reflect the values and principles of the Carolingian *correctio*.

This chapter has shown that there was continuing uncertainty about the *medicus*'s role into the ninth century, uncertainty that Carolingian intellectuals answered by compiling, arranging, and editing texts so as to create an authoritative record of how the *medicus* ought to be—as a moral attendant, an educated person, a mediator of time, nature, and the body, and, most importantly, a cosmic link between God and human society. Not all ninth-century answers to these problems were the same; nevertheless, I have charted connections across the extant sources in order to highlight efforts to formulate a privileged *ministerium* (so to speak) for the *medicus*. The urgency behind this task reflected not simply a growing competition among Carolingian healers, with the rise of saintly translations and a reforming zeal surrounding holy unction, but also the theological complexity of the material, created body. The body's status as container for the soul made its internal mysteries all the more fraught. Thus, the *medicus* needed to be an expert at accessing the invisible truth of creation and interceding with the one true Physician.[170]

# PART III

## Medical Order and Disorder for Self and Society

CHAPTER 6

# A Necessary and Timely Intervention

In the spring of 837, an unusual comet sped across the night sky of the Carolingian realm, striking many with apprehension about what it foretold.[1] This omen prompted Louis the Pious to consult an expert in astronomy, or so we learn from an anonymous life of the emperor composed shortly after his death by none other than the expert himself, now known simply as the Astronomer. Although the Astronomer says that he hesitated in offering one definitive interpretation of the comet, Louis acknowledged that such a sign was known to presage the death of a prince.[2] And, indeed, Louis died only a few years later, when, as the biographer elucidates, the emperor's normal physiological fluctuations were disturbed by political disorder within his own family.

The Astronomer included considerable detail as to what he deemed to be the precipitating cause of death—Louis "was already burdened with old age, and his lungs were weighed down with an abundance of phlegm (beyond the customary increase in the winter), and his chest was shaking [with coughing]," when he received the news that his son Louis the German was in revolt against him. Although an exceptionally mild man, the emperor "was so afflicted with bitterness (*amaritudine*)" that, as the text states, "the phlegm grew and hardened into an abscess, and a deadly ulcer congealed in his inner organs."[3]

The Astronomer's interpretation of this sequence of events (comet, rebellion, physical collapse) reveals his expertise in both the movements of the heavens and the workings of the inner body. Compared to other Carolingian biographers, this author displays considerable interest in the pathology of the protagonist's final illness. He seems familiar with humoral models of seasonal change, the dangers of excess phlegm, and substances that do not evacuate the body but stagnate and fester. And he suggests that the "bitterness" Louis experienced was a movement of the soul that also had a physical effect, coagulating and hardening the phlegm settling into his lungs.

The Astronomer's report has long attracted interest for what it reveals about Louis, the possible identity of his biographer, and the revival of Roman astronomy in the ninth century. Much less attention has been shown to its account of physiological processes.[4] Yet it should not surprise us to discover an apparent affinity between astronomical knowledge and Hippocratic medicine; these two fields of thought moved in similar circles in the ninth century.[5] They were both caught up in Carolingian concerns regarding the calculation of time and the underlying patterns governing the material cosmos. Certain types of medical material were often copied alongside collections focused on the calendar, and medical manuscripts, in turn, reflected a strong emphasis on the division of the seasons, months, days, and lunar cycles.

This chapter analyzes some of the most popular medical treatises of the early Middle Ages against contemporaneous understandings of the material universe, time, and divine order. It reveals, above all, a conviction that the body's nature was equally poised between the regular fluctuations in elemental cosmic structures and the unpredictable events that interrupted these cycles with their display of divine omnipotence. Comets like the one of 837 were recognized to be anomalous *because of* a belief in the consistency of the heavens. So, too, medical writings had to develop an approach that balanced instruction regarding the rules of bodily flux with an acknowledgment that rules were ultimately contingent on God's hidden judgment, which intervened in human affairs ceaselessly, if mysteriously. In investigating the answers that medical compilations offered to fundamental questions about order and disorder, this chapter challenges, from an oblique angle, the persistent characterization of early medieval medicine as atheoretical.[6]

To be sure, the Carolingians approached medical learning as knowledge that was, above all, meant to be applied. However, the theoretical framework of ninth-century thought on the body becomes clearer once we accord due attention to the intersections between medical and spiritual literature. Across various genres, then, this chapter pursues a new emphasis on the rational, divine order imbuing the temporal, material world. Concurrently, it explores a Carolingian enthusiasm for medical concepts and techniques by which the rational soul, having perceived this order, could regulate the body's instability and ensure its congruence with broader social and cosmic patterns.

Although very few ninth-century texts contain a theoretical apparatus resembling that in contemporary Arabic Galenism, we feed Galen's already oversized ego if we subscribe unreservedly to the belief that without his systematizing impulse medical learning lacked theory.[7] Rather than posing the problem as a search for Galenic theory, it is more useful to locate patterns of thought that seem to have structured a diverse array of approaches to healthcare. This chapter demonstrates that medicine as applied knowledge was indeed enmeshed in a theoretical scaffold, whose scale is possible to comprehend only when we expand our gaze beyond the healing arts, to a wider set of theological and philosophical concerns that preoccupied Carolingian thinkers.

## Popular Medical Texts and Theory

Let us start by considering the contents of a *liber medicinalis* (book of medicine). What types of treatises did compilers favor when they gathered and edited material on the care of the body? What were the concepts that Carolingian scholars encountered when consulting medical manuscripts? Here, I focus on two of the most common medical texts of the ninth century. While these (unlike, say, the Lorsch apology) are not products of Carolingian authorship, their frequent copying attests to a belief that they relayed useful and trustworthy information. There was certainly no definitive model of how the body functioned across the Carolingian realm, and even within a single manuscript, various (and sometimes conflicting) ideas might be presented. That said, the following treatises claimed to offer a comprehensive explanation of bodily processes, and, accordingly, Carolingian practitioners may well have assumed that they summarized all the medical theory necessary to learn.

The most popular medical treatise in the ninth century was the *Letter to King Antiochus*, purportedly written by Hippocrates for an ancient Seleucid ruler.[8] The text thus presented itself as a witness to ancient knowledge, especially since Carolingian readers encountered Antiochus IV (Epiphanes) in 1 and 2 Maccabees.[9] The first extant copies of the letter are in manuscripts from the end of the eighth century,[10] but it originated from a (probably) spurious Greek text composed in Late Antiquity, which was then edited, interpolated, and retranslated many times over the intervening centuries.[11] Carolingian scholars may have been particularly interested in the *Letter* because parts of it appear in *On the Reckoning of Time*, one of Bede's most popular works on the Continent in the ninth century.[12]

In the preface, "Hippocrates" promises the learned Antiochus that he will explain how sicknesses occur, the signs by which they are known, and how they may be cured.[13] He begins by describing how the human body can be divided into four parts—head, chest, belly, and bladder—each of which can exhibit specific signs of an internal sickness. A relatively long list of these signs is then provided for the different corporeal "areas" (the bladder being the only part that corresponds to an organ). The head, for example, communicates sickness through the following symptoms: lack of smell, clouded vision, frequent throbbing of the temples, ringing in the ears, weeping of the eyes in the morning, and heaviness around the eyebrows.[14] Illness in the belly, meanwhile, brings forth nausea, shaking in the whole body, mild fevers, a problem with the spleen, and numbness of the calves.[15] The implicit argument is that all symptoms relate to a problem in one of the four key areas of the body, and once one has identified the area, one can apply the appropriate remedy. Each of the four zones demands its own particular remedy, although, for the most part, the courses of treatment differ solely in terms of the mixture of herbs to be used. All four call for fasting or abstinence before taking the assigned medication (usually a drink), the purpose of which is to purge the body (by draining liquids, vomiting, or defecating).

As "Hippocrates" moves through each of the four parts, he first lists the signs, then instructions on the cure, and finally an emphatic warning about the consequences of ignoring these instructions. For instance, if someone suffers a condition (*causa*) in the chest and does not treat it, "these things happen to those neglecting such [signs]: pain in the lungs, black bile, mild fevers, pain in the spleen, lethargy, complaints in the liver, frequent hiccups, and insomnia."[16] The message is that each root cause can sprout many more conditions (often increasing in severity) if one overlooks a problem arising within the body.

The conception, diagnosis, and treatment of illnesses outlined in the *Letter to Antiochus* is exceedingly simplistic. The text assumes no understanding of complex internal processes and, indeed, even suggests that such knowledge is not necessary. Given that Carolingian medical manuscripts typically contained long lists of head-to-toe illnesses divided according to the members, senses, organs, or features of the body, readers of medical texts were naturally aware that bodies consisted of more than a head, chest, belly, and bladder.[17] At the same time, these lists of head-to-toe conditions were simply more specific than the *Letter to Antiochus*; they did not offer a fundamentally different approach to disease. An entry in a remedy collection like the *Tereoperica* (discussed in Chapter 3) typically begins with a definition of the complaint—headache, for instance, "is a pain in the head which lasts a long time (that is, it is not recent but long-standing) and is always invisible, sometimes getting worse and sometimes diminishing." It then lists the "signs" of this condition (in this case, pulsing temples, ringing in the ears, a heavy head, and sore neck muscles) and, finally, one or more cures to resolve the problem.[18]

The focus on discrete treatments in texts like the *Tereoperica* has encouraged the perspective that the Carolingians were not especially concerned with investigating the body as a unified system, while the simplicity of texts like the *Letter to Antiochus* has been read as indicating a widespread lack of interest in theoretical approaches to medicine. The assumption has been that medicine was low in a hierarchy of intellectual priorities, and thus the basic practicalities were preserved but little else. Before taking the view that few resources were directed toward caring for the body, however, it might be helpful to compare the patterns of thought within these texts to those in the treatise on self-care that Alcuin composed for Wido. In Alcuin's account of the *vitia* that can attack the soul, there is a clear conceptual resonance to medical texts like that we have just examined. Here, for example, he describes to Wido the nature of greed (all seven chapters on the other vices follow the same format):

> Greed is the excessive desire of acquiring, having, or hoarding riches, which is an insatiable pestilence. . . . The shoots of this are envy, deceptions, robberies, homicides, lies, perjuries, plundering, violence, disquiet, unjust judgments, contempt of the truth, forgetfulness of future blessedness, and hardening of the heart. It occurs in opposition to mercy. . . . It is conquered through fear of God and through brotherly charity.[19]

As in the *Tereoperica*, Alcuin begins by briefly defining the vice, then lists the signs by which it is recognized, and finally offers various remedies for overcoming it. As in the *Letter to Antiochus*, the root of ill health within the individual is diagnosed through symptoms that are simultaneously the effects of a hidden, untreated *causa* within the soul. None of these texts focuses on the development of disease; rather, they prioritize categorizing conditions and their remedies.[20] In this sense, the practical emphasis of texts like the *Tereoperica* is comparable to pastoral works like the penitentials, which also divided sins into a schema of categories and subcategories and set the discrete sin alongside its "medicine" in long, simple lists.[21]

In the second half of the *Letter to Antiochus*, the author *does* address how sicknesses occur but draws few connections between this and the first half, on the four parts of the body. The only point of linkage between the two sections is the number four: there are four zones in the body and, we are informed, there are four causes of sickness related to the four times of the year. "Hippocrates" gives exact dates for dividing the year into seasons, with each season said to give rise to an increase in one of the four humors (phlegm in winter, blood in spring, yellow bile in summer, and black bile in fall).[22] Each particular humor, as it grows in the body, allegedly provokes specific issues, including fevers, catarrh, coughing, and stomach discharge. One can counter these effects by focusing on regimens of food and drink, physical exertion, fasting, and sexual activity (or its renunciation). In summer, for instance, when yellow bile (*colera rubea*) increases, "you ought to eat cold foods, very sweet and pleasant and nice smelling, which are easily digested; you ought to drink cold and watery things, and you should not have sex at all."[23] The theory behind the foods recommended rests on the notion of contraries—cold foods in summer and warm foods in winter—but no specific rationale is provided for the different routines.[24] Nor is an explanation offered for how the conditions provoked by the humors relate to the sicknesses that take root in the four parts of the body and produce the aforementioned signs.

The *Letter to Antiochus* presents itself as the most condensed advice possible for ensuring the health of the individual. It covers all actions necessary in both a prophylactic and a reactive sense, as it elucidates the almost imperceptible changes experienced by the body over the course of the year and the signs that are most helpful for assessing the individual's internal condition. Whatever doubts we may have about the usefulness of such a short and somewhat disjointed treatise, it was remarkably popular with the Carolingian elite. It is found in a manuscript compilation put together by Walafrid Strabo and another associated with Grimald, abbot of Saint-Gall and archchaplain to Louis the German.[25]

Several of the ideas expressed in the *Letter to Antiochus* overlap with themes present in a second popular medical treatise, again presented in the form of a letter. This *Letter to Pentadius* is preserved in multiple Carolingian medical compilations, where it is typically attributed to the fourth-century North African physician Vindicianus (though it possibly derives from a later translation of a pseudonymous Greek text).[26] Although a relatively short treatise, it likewise claims to be a comprehensive explanation of the "whole world" and the "nature and ordering of every single body."[27] This "nature," the reader quickly learns, is grounded in the four humors (blood, phlegm, black bile, and yellow bile), the building blocks of the flesh. It is worth exploring this text in detail, because while the ninth century is often slotted into a broad (and undifferentiated) period in which "humoral theory" predominated, little attention has been paid to what humoral medicine actually encompassed at this time. By considering the text's major emphases, we gain a tantalizing sense of the particular strains of humoral thought known to the Carolingians, and also the limits and specificities that rendered them different from similar approaches in other periods.

Vindicianus begins by declaring that all the humors "rule in their places," that is, in a different organ of the body (although, in fact, he names five organs and suggests some humors rule multiple organs).[28] Each also exits the body through its own special "breathing hole," whether the nose, ears, eyes, or mouth.[29] While the connection between the elemental level of the humors and the functional level of bodily systems is not entirely clear, the articulation of the body in the *Letter to Pentadius* unites fluids, anatomy, and the senses through loose associations.

These bodily structures are then situated in a broader framework through linkages with an individual's temporal experience. On the lowest level, there is a quotidian exchange of humors over the course of a human day, with each humor dominating the body for six hours. Next, as in the *Letter to Antiochus*, each humor is said to rotate in an annual cycle over the course of the four seasons. Lastly, Vindicianus articulates a lifetime transformation, which begins and ends with phlegm but cycles through the other three humors over the four stages of childhood, youth, adulthood, and old age. The various humors impart to the individual distinct qualities, whereby they make themselves manifest to external detection. Vindicianus notes the type of pulse (weak or strong, quick or equal, for example) that a humor conveys when it is ruling the body. He also records the unique *virtus* of each substance—yellow bile, for instance, is "bitter, vigorous, fiery, and dry," while phlegm is "cold, salty, and wet."[30] These combinations of qualities, in turn, impart certain physical and personality traits—thus, yellow bile makes a person angry, talented, sharp, light and thin, voracious in appetite, and quick in digestion, but phlegm makes him/her physically robust, alert, thoughtful, prematurely gray, and rather timorous.[31]

Central to the *Letter to Pentadius* is the conviction that the humors underpin everything related to bodily function and might even affect moral and intellectual traits.[32] Yet, the text avoids suggesting biological "types" by emphasizing the constant flux of the body's interior state. Furthermore, although age provides the basis of a taxonomy, gender is not treated as a noteworthy category. Compared to a later medieval emphasis on men's humoral composition as dry and hot, and women's as wet and cold, nothing here indicates that males and females are constituted differently.[33] The object of acquiring knowledge of all these permutations and their distinguishing signs is *not* primarily to categorize people according to complexion (as would be the case several centuries later) but rather to diagnose "from which humor the sickness is born."[34]

Sickness, Vindicianus explains, occurs when one humor grows beyond moderation and balance.[35] To some degree, then, sickness is inevitable, given that the humors are always alternating in ascendency. And yet, the text implies, knowledge of the cyclical nature of the humors should allow a physician to apply substances with contrary qualities accordingly, and thereby diminish or restrain excess and its accompanying illness. When each humor observes its appropriate measure and place in the body, health is maintained. But when one seeks to dominate outside of when it is proper for it to dominate, the body's order is disrupted. The individual's inherent fragility is an essential aspect of this conception of physiology, since, as the text emphasizes, the things that sustain the body also endanger it.

## The Body Within Cosmic Patterns

Uniting the *Letter to Antiochus* and the *Letter to Pentadius* is an orientation on the number four. These texts implicitly assumed that the four humors, though hidden, could be ascertained rationally for the very reason that they corresponded to observable phenomena—namely, the four seasons of the year. Although many of these layered associations can be found as early as the fifth century B.C.E. in the Hippocratic treatise *On the Nature of Man*, it was only in the centuries after Galen that the theory of the four humors was systematically expounded and became a cornerstone of late antique medicine. Galen himself advanced a fourfold humoral framework by highlighting the importance of *On the Nature of Man*.[36] Yet, as Jacques Jouanna has detailed, it was writings that postdate Galen that first methodically developed a theory of the four associated humors, elements, and temperaments.[37] Against those who would date the *Letter to Pentadius* to fourth-century North Africa, Jouanna argues for a significantly later date, with the original Greek text likely composed in sixth-century Alexandria.[38]

If theories of the four humors and temperaments were rooted in the late antique Greek-speaking East, Latin translations of these texts were reproduced and diffused because of Carolingian interest in this schema. Consequently, a basic theoretical framework that highlighted fourfold divisions represented a continuum across contemporaneous Carolingian, Byzantine, and Abbasid societies. If we turn to the *Book of Letters* in the medical codex from Saint-Denis (ff. 12r–41v) that we examined in Chapter 5, it is clear that one of the compiler's principal objectives was to present a consensus on the quadripartite logic of the body. In a text on the stomach (f. 15v), we hear repeatedly about the fourfold elements of the body, as well as the four-stage process of digestion. In a text on the division of time (f. 17r), we are told that the body is divided into four parts; one folio later, another letter (f. 18r) similarly states that the Latins divide the year into four. The following text (f. 18v) is entitled *Letter of Hippocrates on the Four Humors*; two folios later (f. 20v), a text opens by proclaiming that all sicknesses stem from four humors. A question-and-answer treatise (f. 28v) finds that sicknesses have four distinct phases and confirms (f. 29r) that there are four humors in humans; another question-and-answer text (f. 39r) further states that there are four humors and four elements. A treatise that includes many references to quadripartite divisions (f. 39v) uses a display script to highlight the phrase "There are Four Winds." And, finally, the last letter in the collection (f. 41r) is entitled *A Letter of Hippocrates to Antiochus and Anthony on the Four Members.*[39] Though this catalogue is not exhaustive, it demonstrates how the monotonous repetition of the same information created the impression of unanimity among "the ancient" medical authorities and of absolute harmony in the material world.

A treatise in a medical manuscript produced in eastern Francia in the early ninth century makes more explicit the connection between divine order and medical theory with its biblical introduction. "In the beginning, God created heaven and earth. Then man was made, for whom all things were made. Therefore, it is said that the world consists of four elements, that is, fire, water, earth, and wind or air."[40] The treatise then proceeds to outline the four qualities (hot, cold, wet, dry), the four seasons, and the four humors "by which the healthy are ruled and by which the sick are struck down."[41] A subtler attempt to infuse the fourfold scheme with Christian tones is found in a compilation called *The Wisdom of the Art of Medicine*: "Four are the winds, four are the corners of heaven, four are the seasons (spring, summer, autumn and winter), four are the humors in the human body (yellow bile, black bile, blood, and phlegm)."[42] In its explication of the four fluids of the human body, the text draws directly on the *Letter to Pentadius*,[43] but its reference to the four corners (*anguli*) of heaven may be an allusion to the Book of Revelation's testimony regarding "four angels standing at the four corners of the earth, holding back the four winds of the earth [Rv 7:1]." In their attraction to a late antique fourfold interpretation of the body, the Carolingians evinced a desire to set classical medical knowledge within a framework of spiritual common sense. As artists crafted imposing illuminations of the fundamental harmony interlacing the four evangelists, four major prophets of the Old Testament, and four corners of heaven—depicted in the First Bible of Charles the Bald (see Figure 14)—so did scribes find theoretical significance in medical writings that alluded to the quadripartite unity between human microcosm and divine macrocosm.[44]

Such an attention to fourfold symbolism was not limited to monastic and ecclesiastical authors and artists, if Dhuoda's *Handbook* is an indication of lay beliefs more broadly. The work begins with a discussion of God, where Dhuoda expounds on the mystery of the letters in *Deus*, explaining that *D* (*delta*, the fourth letter of the Greek alphabet and the equivalent Greek numeral) "signifies four, the number of perfection." Moreover, it "refers to various groups of four—on the one hand the four characteristics of bodies, that is, hot, cold, wet, and dry; or the four virtues, that is, justice, strength, wisdom, and moderation; or the words of the four evangelists. Or this four means or refers to the four directions in the universe, that is, east, west, north, and south."[45] Vividly, we can see Dhuoda's intention to draw together knowledge related to the body (in the elements), the material world (in the four quadrants), the soul (in the virtues), and divine truth (in the evangelists) by means of numerical symbolism.

We can discern the same educational goal in the texts that were copied alongside one of three extant witnesses of Dhuoda's *Handbook*.[46] Cullen Chandler has suggested that this manuscript derives directly from a compilation of texts that the mother selected and sent to her son to further the moral program outlined in her manual.[47] Among the seven works found in the codex are Alcuin's *On the Virtues and Vices*, Isidore's *On the Differences of Things* (which includes a lengthy chapter on the elements of the body, the five senses, and the anatomy of the different organs), and a computus text on the

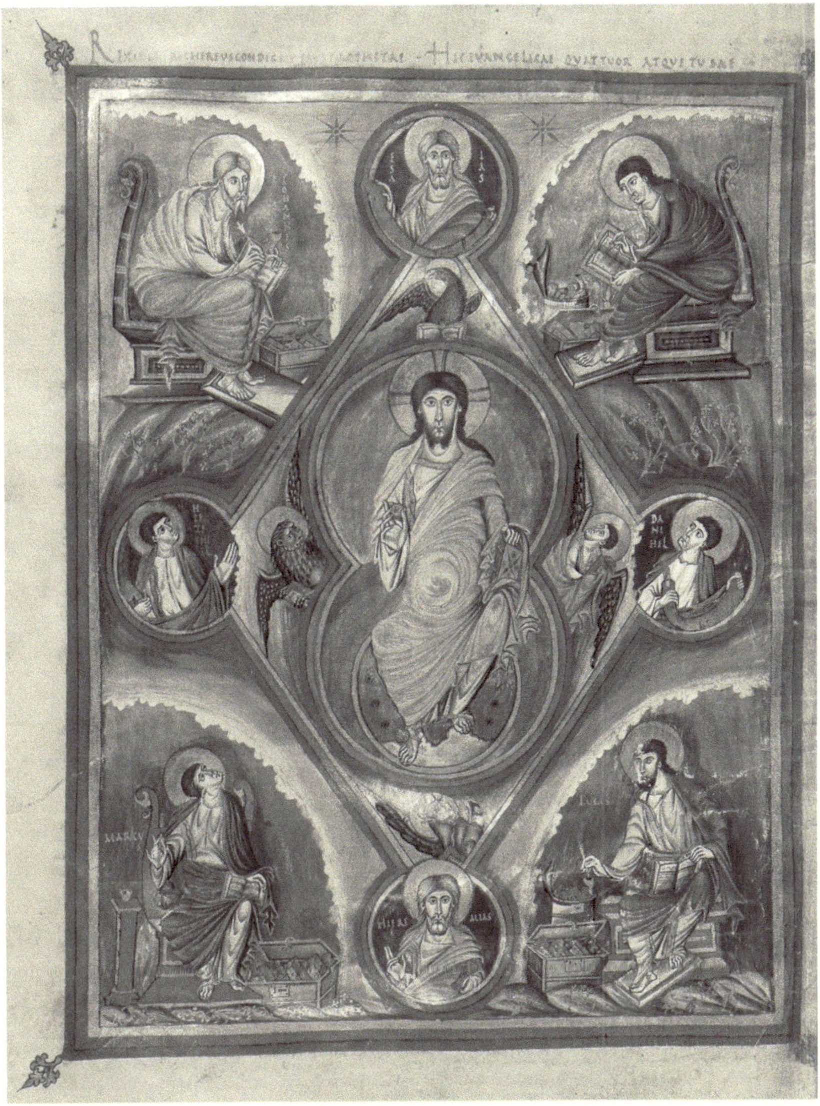

Figure 14. The frontispiece to the Gospels, with Christ in Majesty, the four evangelists, four prophets, four tetramorphs, and four corners of heaven, from the First Bible of Charles the Bald (the Vivian Bible). Paris, BnF lat. 1, f. 329v. By kind permission of the Bibliothèque nationale.

mathematical art, the units of time, and the reckoning of lunar and solar cycles.[48] One component of the latter is precisely the investigation of the "four parts of the year," a subject that plainly relates to Dhuoda's own fascination with numerical interpretations but also directs our attention to the connections between computus (the science of measuring time to determine the liturgical calendar) and the style of medicine practiced by the Carolingians.[49]

Even as computus was trained on a concrete end (resolving the date of Easter), it was intimately bound up with a Christian conviction that measuring and ordering the fluxes of the world brought human society closer to God's unfolding design.[50] The marking of time was a skill grounded in reckoning and observation and dependent upon calendars and temporal units that were classical in origin, but time itself was not deemed a secular phenomenon. Rather, the development of medieval computus was tightly fused with the belief that God existed outside of time and had established a natural order according to his will.[51] Consequently, the study of time was the study of divine reason permeating the years stretching between the first day of creation and the Last Judgment. Thus did Bede end *On the Reckoning of Time* with the eighth age, comparing "the fleeting and wave-tossed course of time" with the "eternal stability and stable eternity" of the future to come.[52] That future stability was already partially present in the highest reaches of the cosmos, where the stars stood fixed in the firmament and the planets, though moving, traced and retraced their heavenly paths. This pure heaven (as opposed to the earth's upper atmosphere) would not be consumed in the fire of the Last Days but would persist into timelessness.[53] As Eric Ramírez-Weaver says of a handbook created for the Carolingian royal family, astronomical diagrams were "signs of stability in a world of transience."[54]

It was against this backdrop that, just before 800, scholars in Charlemagne's inner circle took up the science of reckoning as a means to tackle practical matters related to the aims of *correctio*. This included establishing an accurate calendrical system to ensure liturgical uniformity across local churches and compiling a series of handbooks and encyclopedias intended to assist the clergy in performing computus calculations (as mandated in various capitularies).[55] Far from being novel, these efforts depended heavily on Irish and English scholarship, especially Bede's writings on the nature of time.[56]

By contrast, the marked fascination with astronomy that emerged in the 790s was more directly tied to Carolingian initiatives.[57] It reflected local interests (like that at the monastery of Corbie) as well as courtly curiosity associated with Charlemagne himself.[58] In his *Life of Charlemagne*, Einhard mentions computus and astronomy in succession, noting that the emperor "learned the art of calculation [arithmetic] and with deep purpose and great curiosity investigated the movement of the stars."[59] The epistolary correspondence between Alcuin and Charlemagne in the years before 800 abounds with discussions of both calendrical issues and lunar and planetary movements.[60] Naturally, an awareness that lunar and solar movements underpinned units of time (like years and months) had long been part of Christian computus, and texts like Gregory of Tours's *On the Course of the Stars* taught the constellations as a means to correctly mark monastic offices. Still, we find few attestations of Roman astronomical knowledge in the Merovingian period; yet by the middle of the ninth century, the Carolingians had acquired a set of authoritative ancient texts, elaborated upon them with commentaries, and created new diagrams of the heavens, which set the earth within the wider cosmos by picturing the intersecting paths of the various planetary bodies.[61] As Bruce Eastwood and Eric Ramírez-Weaver have demonstrated, this pursuit of knowledge extended beyond the needs of computus and signaled that astronomy was valuable in its own right as one of the liberal arts and as a path toward spiritual wisdom.[62]

Such developments intersected with medicine's incorporation into the liberal arts, but the two disciplines did not simply run parallel. Rather, as Faith Wallis has illuminated, the promotion of computus and astronomy amplified certain themes within ninth-century medicine, especially the relationship between bodies and the rhythms of time. This is evident in a capitulary of 805, where computus and medicine are mentioned in sequence (or even together), as well as in numerous extant manuscripts, which intermingled computistical and healing-oriented texts.[63]

Attention to the invisible patterns governing the cosmos quickly returns us to the example of the number four and its capacity to unite distinct fields of thought (medical, environmental, chronometric, and anagogical).[64] The legacy of Galen's endorsement of *On the Nature of Man* inclined medieval medical thinking toward the four humors, but this scheme also proved popular because it resonated with the Carolingian consensus that creation was imbued with a discernible, divine mathematical order.[65] That is a guiding principle throughout the twenty-eight figural poems of Hrabanus's *In Honor of the Holy Cross*, as Lynda Coon has demonstrated.[66] The majority of the poems are divided into quadrants, with the four sections partitioned by the arms of the cross, the members of Christ's body, or (in one case) the four elements, as symbolized by four circles.[67] Reflecting on the manner in which the cross partitions space, Hrabanus declares that "almost everyone is aware that a quaternion is a number sanctified by perfection."[68]

## Rationality and Prognostication

In a letter to Charlemagne from 797 regarding the cycles of the moon, Alcuin referred to his king as "a most wise researcher of the nature of things and a most devoted investigator into the rational account of every cause."[69] Formed in the image of God, the soul was reason (*ratio*) itself, according to the theological treatises examined in Chapter 1. It was also firmly fixed within its own proper body until (by divine will) it vacated its home, and the flesh returned to the elements. As spirit uniquely tied to matter, the soul constituted a crucial link between the utterly incorporeal God and the material world. Just as God was the lord of creation, so was the soul the governor of that beneath it (the body) in the cosmic hierarchy. The soul or mind, as Alcuin wrote to Charlemagne, was capable of discerning the *ratio* of nature, including the numerical and temporal rhythms of the *mundus* and the heavens, and it fell upon the soul to bring the body into harmony with those rhythms.[70]

Through the astronomical study of heavenly bodies, Carolingian scholars glimpsed that future age in which their own resurrected bodies would not be subject to disintegration or putrefaction but would remain secure in their eternal wholeness. As Lupus of Ferrières wrote to Gottschalk of Orbais, *then* the body will be "set free, not only from the vexation of entire corruption, but even the suggestion of it," and it will have "such harmony with the spirit, with which it is now in conflict, that it will henceforth neither wish nor be able to sin with it."[71] Though the present earthly union between soul and body was imperfect, as Lupus acknowledged, this did not invalidate efforts to perceive and respect the divine constancy imbuing the temporal world. Care of the body was not simply an expression of charity toward others but a form of pious self-governance.

The affinity between material person and material cosmos was strikingly visualized in a simple schematic found in copies of Isidore's *On the Nature of Things*. At the center of these diagrams, one finds not only *homo* (human) and *mundus* (world) but also *annus* (year)—three terms that clearly display the collision of body, time, and astronomy. Radiating from the center in a cross form are the humors, seasons, and elements, in that ascending order; and in the remaining arcs are the four qualities, two shared by each arm of the cross (see Figure 15).[72] The sphere both represents the cosmos and symbolizes the fundamental harmony pervading opposing pairs. As a mixture of the four elements, the body was constantly responding to the power of the planets, unseen yet observable in effects like the tides, the weather, and the lengthening and shortening of daylight. The diagrams made clear *why* health and sickness cycled back and forth within individual bodies; what they did not tackle was *when* this might occur or *what* could be done to treat and prevent such changes.

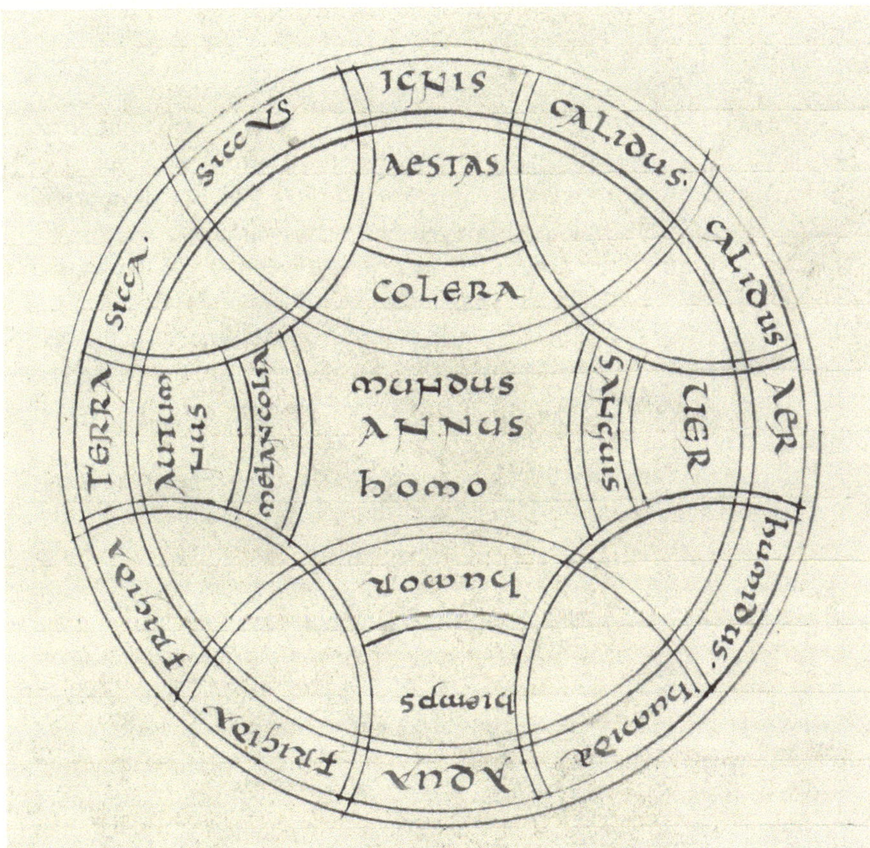


Figure 15. Isidorian *annus-mundus-homo* diagram, with the four seasons, elements, humors, and qualities, produced ca. 800 at Chelles Abbey. St. Gallen, Stiftsbibliothek, Cod. Sang. 240, p. 137. By kind permission of the Stiftsbibliothek.

On the one hand were patterns, on the other, predictions. If diagrams visualized the first, prognostics represented the second. Though "prognostics" were not a coherent genre in the early Middle Ages, this label is used to categorize texts concerned with future states of being and temporal calculations; they typically appear as lists, charts, or figures in manuscripts.[73] While often cast as evidence of medieval superstition, prognostics resembled many ancient approaches; the Hippocratic *Epidemics*, for example, stressed the importance of the weather, season, and stars in provoking sickness and urged the calculation of crises, paroxysms, and other temporal patterns in the treatment of disease.[74] Still, the ninth century was particularly important in galvanizing the circulation of prognostics—they are found in medical codices, computus collections, pastoral handbooks, and miscellanies from this time. Many health-related prognostics are first attested in Carolingian manuscripts.[75]

We can loosely divide prognostics that relate to bodily health into three categories.[76] First, there are those that answer simple, direct questions, such as whether a sick person will live or die. Second, those that provide information about outcomes according to specified times; the most popular here were *lunaria*, which indicated such things as the progression of an illness based on when in the lunar cycle the sickness began.[77] Third, those that offer instruction on what should be done (or avoided) in specific months of the year or on certain dates of the calendar; within this category are monthly dietetic guides and Egyptian Days (lists of unlucky days on which, for instance, phlebotomy was forbidden).[78]

Toward the end of the ninth century, a monk at the monastery of Saint-Gall might have come across the following diagram as he was leafing through the remedies found in *Pliny's Medicine* looking for a cure for another brother's sore spleen (see Figure 16).[79] Recognizing the name of the purported author of this diagram—the very same Apuleius Platonicus who composed a herbal of great fame—the monk would have learned that the sphere before him offered information "about life, about death, and all other troubles, and whatever else you wish to seek out."[80] He need only tally up the letters of the sick person's name (using the chart on the right), add to that the lunar day on which the person fell ill, and deduct 30 from that total until a final number between 1 and 30 was reached. This calculation would yield the crucial figure, which could then be sought in the diagram. If it was located in the top half of the sphere, the sick person would recover. But if the figure were found in the lower half, our monk carried grave news back to the sufferer, for that indicated this splenic pain would certainly lead to death.

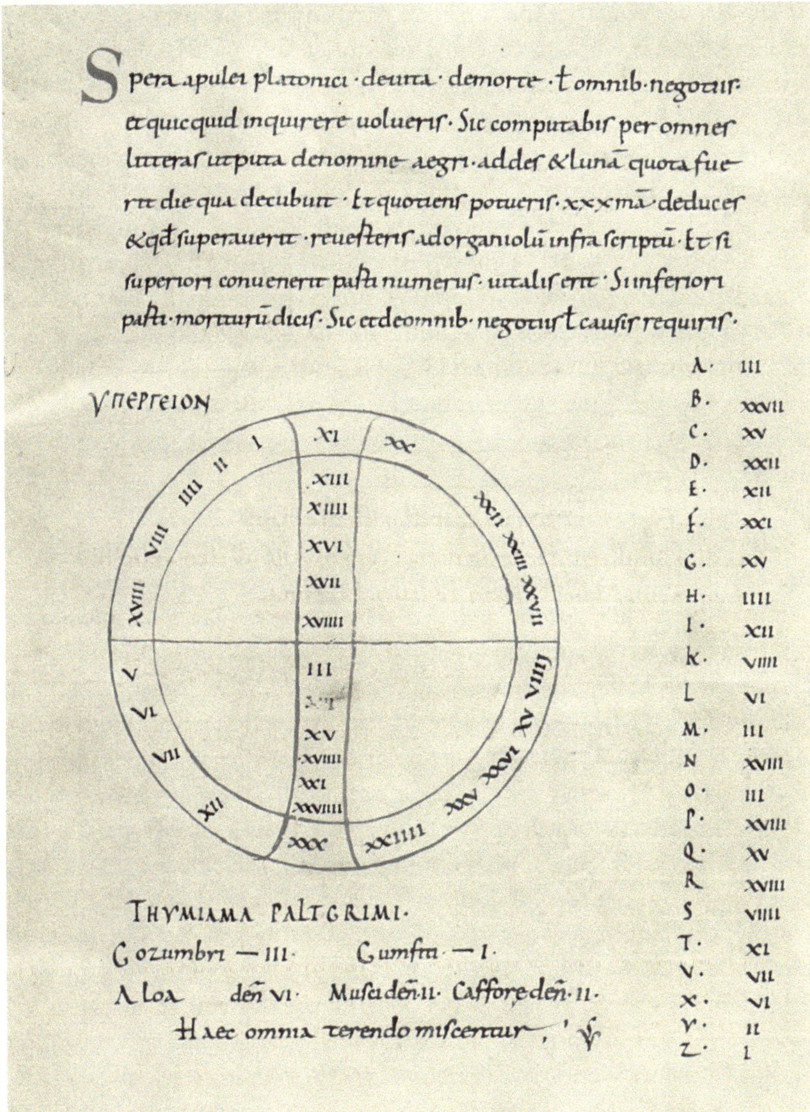


Figure 16. A medical prognostic: the Sphere of Apuleius. St. Gallen, Stiftsbibliothek, Cod. Sang. 752, p. 82. By kind permission of the Stiftsbibliothek.

Having learned from the Sphere of Apuleius that his patient would die, our monk might have then proceeded to consult a text labeled *A Letter of Prognostication* in another manuscript held in Saint-Gall's library.[81] This listed various signs of death under a preface that vividly described the text's ancient origins with the Greek philosopher Democritus.[82] Unlike the rough translation of the Hippocratic *Prognostics*, which focused on visible facial features and simply indicated which traits were "deadly" or "dangerous" in acute diseases, the "secret" signs of Democritus were far more specific.[83] If, for example, a sick individual is examined and "a pustule shaped like the louse of a pig appears under her tongue, and she desires to soak in a bath, she will die at the beginning of that illness."[84] This investigation involved not only peering under the patient's tongue but also judging whether any raised bump sufficiently resembled a tiny insect (the louse being approximately one sixteenth of an inch).[85] But the results yielded were relatively precise, as the text promised information on the time of death for each group of signs.

As our monk was preparing to return to his patient in order to inspect his body for these signs, imagine that he cast his eyes ten folios beyond the Democritus text and spotted a *lunare* for illness. Alongside each day of a thirty-day lunar cycle, *lunaria* listed the varying outcomes for the matter in question; those that addressed sickness often used terse expressions, such as "will rise quickly," "will not evade [death]," or "will be healed by physicians."[86] In this case, the monk consulted the lunar day on which his patient fell sick and then discovered that "he will convalesce slowly."[87] Relieved that his fellow brother would, after all, survive this particular ailment, our monk might have decided that treatment was necessary, namely a bloodletting of the little finger for inflammation of the spleen.[88] Hence, he turned to a list of Egyptian Days in that same codex to confirm that it was not one of the twenty-four dates in a year when phlebotomy or the taking of medication was forbidden because the patient would certainly die.[89] Likewise, he consulted another text that listed which lunar days (and which hours, in particular, on those days) were optimal for bloodletting.[90] With his research complete and a course of action coalescing in his mind, our monk returned to the infirmary.

I include this imaginary sequence because I believe it highlights many of the difficulties that are encountered in attempting to understand the role of prognostic material in the early medieval world.[91] *Lunaria* and Apuleian Spheres are possibly the strangest type of text one finds in extant Carolingian medical manuscripts. Given the evidence of prognostics being copied into ecclesiastical manuals, earlier notions that they were a type of folklore that slipped surreptitiously into written culture simply cannot be supported, as Carine van Rhijn has shown.[92] However, despite recent attention to these texts, scholars have reached little consensus on how they were understood, particularly given that their popularity appears to contradict injunctions not to observe omens or divine the future by consulting those who work with numbers (*cauculatores*) or charms (*incantatores*), as set forth in royal commands and penitentials.[93] Episcopal mandates, too, criticizing "those who observe months and times," echoed the denunciations of Church Fathers like Augustine, who had inveighed specifically against people who believed in Egyptian Days or lucky and unlucky positions of the stars.[94]

Of course, the Carolingian elite may have read such injunctions selectively. The difference between judging the likely course of a disease based on experience and blindly heeding a written prognostication was not necessarily clear.[95] Indeed, Augustine's own writings against astrology were far from precise—in the same letter, he both condemned the observation of the sun and moon to forecast success and praised farmers' useful scrutiny of the heavens in order to predict the weather.[96] Unsurprisingly then, Carolingian authors evinced some hesitancy about drawing direct predictions from astronomical events.[97] Both Charlemagne and Louis the Pious sought to divine the meaning of comets, eclipses, and planetary movements, but Dutton argues that in such cases "learned Carolingians were not so much actively prognosticating as reading what they thought had been forced on them."[98] The same may have been true of medicine. The moon's regular waxing and waning, after all, affected fluid levels in the body (just as with the tides), and some versions of the Egyptian Days went beyond the comment that they were ambiguously "unlucky" to explain that they were days when the body was especially laden with blood. In light of such correspondences between the heavens and earth, it might have been possible to treat *lunaria* as interpretations of God's will rather than divination.[99]

That said, unlike royal interest in astronomy, Carolingian medical prognostics (with the exception of signs of death) did not involve acts of interpretation. Rather, like Paschal tables, the calculations had already been worked out, and the results were presented in linear form or diagrams like the Sphere of Apuleius. The very graphic of the prognostic on the page might itself have symbolized to a viewer that stable rhythms governed the body's fluxes.[100]

The work of numerical calculation and the skill entailed in monitoring the moon, sun, and stars aligned the medical use of prognostics with liturgical activity and monastic timekeeping.[101] Accordingly, van Rhijn suggests that the acceptability of prognostication depended on *who* performed it, with the educated clergy possessing an expertise and legitimacy that distinguished their actions from those of future-tellers.[102] Several extant manuscripts, which were probably handbooks for bishops or local priests, contain texts on bloodletting, Egyptian Days, dietary calendars, *lunaria*, and prognostic spheres sandwiched among baptismal *ordines*, expositions on the Mass, computistic texts, penitentials, and canon law.[103] The ecclesiastical rites found in these manuscripts were meant to guarantee the health of the soul through the correct performance of sacraments from baptism to extreme unction; likewise, the therapeutic texts were intended to aid in the care of the body from birth to death by utilizing knowledge about the inherent order of the world. Roy Liuzza asserts that prognostics "offer a glimpse of cosmic order beneath the chaos of passing time," and it is in this vein, I believe, that Carolingian scribes eagerly copied such texts in close proximity to more overtly "religious" material.[104]

One mid-ninth-century medical compilation prefaced a series of *lunaria* and a prognostic entitled "Computus for the Sick" with an excerpt from the apocryphal *Life of Adam and Eve* that described God's creation of Adam's body from eight parts, six from nature (the mud of the earth, the ocean, the sun, the clouds of the sky, the winds, and the stones of the earth) and two divine (the Holy Spirit and Christ, the light of the world).[105] By drawing connections between God's construction of the flesh and prescriptions on how to treat the sick, this particular set of texts emphasized the divine mandate to heal and mend broken bodies. It also underscored the body's existence as an elemental composite, a fact that made its association with the planetary bodies "natural" rather than superstitious. We see such an acknowledgement in a West Frankish canon from around 900, which forbade Christians from observing "the day or the moon" for marriages or other endeavors yet allowed lunar calculations for the purposes of bloodletting and felling or planting trees because "the humors and juices of trees, and even the airs, accord with the movements of the moon and follow its nature."[106]

Health prognostics typically forecast outcomes important to a single individual. Even so, their circulation across society called attention to the individual as a member of a group, whether that was a group of people who fell sick on the same day or a group in need of phlebotomy during a proscribed time. This dynamic, as we have already observed, was also central to the theoretical treatises, which did not emphasize personal humoral complexion or gendered humoral "type" but rather the cycles by which *all* bodies were transformed throughout the day, year, and lifetime. A medical attention to the collective rather than the individual resonates strongly with the focus of the Carolingian monastic reforms. The uniform adoption of the Benedictine Rule (as expounded by Benedict of Aniane) was intended to ensure that the monks within a community operated according to a single schedule for eating, sleeping, working, reading, praying, and, probably, urinating and defecating.[107] Similarly, the texts that were included in ninth-century medical manuscripts implied that all people (whether lay or monastic) could physically move in harmony with the same universal temporal patterns. While a monastic context may have especially favored this approach to healthcare, we should recall the extent to which the lay manuals examined in chapter 2 assumed that monastic rules could apply to the laity as well. From this perspective, we can imagine how medical and computus texts were frequently brought together not only because they both dealt with numerical calculations but also because both shared a similar agenda—to enable all subjects to advance in time according to the same liturgical calendar and to govern themselves rationally in sync with this vision of Christian history.[108]

A close relationship between the popularity of prognostic texts and the Benedictine reforms of the ninth century is also proposed by Frederick Paxton, who argues that an intensified interest in forecasting death reflected the development of new monastic rituals for the dying.[109] He draws attention to manuscripts like the Burgundian codex prefaced by the *Passion of Cosmas and Damian*, where a medical *lunare* and signs of death may have been used in the same ritual context in which the *Passion* was read out over a suffering Christian.[110] Monastics needed to predict the time of death with accuracy, in anticipation of the final rites, and, Paxton suggests, prognostics offered them the means to do so.

Such a scenario assumes, I think, that medieval communities concluded that these inherited lists of signs functioned effectively. Assessing the efficacy of premodern healing techniques is notoriously problematic. However, one aspect here that we cannot ignore is the variety among the prognostics themselves. As in the imagined example, any one *lunare* might have contradicted the outcome forecast by a Sphere of Apuleius or that offered by another lunar chart.[111] Consequently, what can we say about whether the Carolingians themselves felt bound by these predictions? At first glance, prognostics appear to diminish human agency in healing, placing emphasis instead on predetermined patterns. However, many of the *lunaria* extant from the ninth century in fact predict death on a relatively small percentage of lunar days (on average four out of every thirty). And the other predictions—whether they state "suffers for long time [but evades death]," "will be healed by physicians," or "evades [death] if rises on the third day"—have the result of galvanizing action. This is especially evident in those lunar forecasts that describe a course of medical treatment by which the patient will be cured.[112] Similarly, in forbidding phlebotomy on approximately 6.5 percent of calendar dates, Egyptian Days imply that such medical therapy is condoned during the rest of the year.[113]

From this perspective, early medieval prognostics might have served both to call attention to the individual's place in broader communal, material, and divine patterns *and* to underscore human agency in treating disease. This is precisely the orientation of the numerous dietary calendars that survive in Carolingian medical, computus, and pastoral manuscripts.[114] These exceedingly popular texts urged readers to imprint upon their consumption habits the schedule of the year, not simply in terms of perceivable changes in weather and temperature but in regard to the precise and established demarcation of months.[115] The calendars run from January through December, or March through February, and employ similar language in their titles.[116] One, for instance, reads, "On food and drink that ought to be habitual for each month," while another states simply, "An account (*ratio*) of what we ought to do during each month," and still another, "Here is the character (*virtus*) of the twelve months, which ought to be observed for the health of the body, and this is the type of observation people ought to maintain."[117]

Certain of the calendars list only one or two items that ought to be ingested or avoided during each month, but others give longer entries that include not only food and drink but whether phlebotomy should be performed, purgatives and medicines should be taken, sex and bathing should be eschewed, and unguents should be used.[118] A version found in the *Lorscher Arzneibuch*, for example, recommends the following: "In the month of July, the flower of celery and wild grapes, that is the flowers of rustic vines. . . . In November, cinnamon."[119] A more extended entry, on the other hand, might read: "In the month of October, drink goat's or sheep's milk as you fast in order to sweeten the blood, break up stones [bladder or kidney], and heal the lungs. Take as many leeks as you are able to eat. Daily, take grapes and drink unfermented wine because it heals the body and purges it [as in a laxative]. Take a drink of clove and pepper."[120] The instructions are blunt and so concise as to be vague; even if they were not always easy to execute, that was not necessarily a problem, since the text suggests that general adherence (not perfect obedience) was the goal. Similarly, the focus of the text is on action, not comprehensive understanding. The *Letter to Antiochus* and *Letter to Pentadius* would have provided a basic explanation for why the rotation of the months dictated changes in routine; references to hot and cold substances in the calendars were, we can assume, supposed to make sense against this theoretical backdrop.[121] Not infrequently one finds a brief comment on counteracting phlegm, bile, black bile, or simply "humors."[122] But, in general, the calendars functioned as quick reference guides and offered few explanations.

While one might expect to find more emphasis on individual constitution and the role this ought to play in directing diet, this is not a prominent theme in the Carolingian dietary corpus.[123] Instead, what these medical texts foreground is all bodies being shaped in similar ways by the passage of time. Thus, dietary habits become both a communal activity and an individual mandate.[124] Despite the lack of a theoretical apparatus in the calendars themselves, their directives are justified by broader intellectual assumptions that the body must be brought into cosmic alignment by the soul's rational attention to the calendar. By framing the instructions according to month, not season, these texts emphasize a process of reading, recalling, enacting, rather than intuiting or feeling. We have here a clear case of mind over matter.

## Necessity as Interruption and Exception

Thus far, this chapter has concentrated on revealing the intersecting temporal, numerical, and astronomical patterns by which the body was bound to the material world. Yet, as much as medical manuscripts from the ninth century (as well as medical material in computus and pastoral manuals) sought to advance this theoretical framework, they also acknowledged that nature was only as consistent as God allowed it to be. God's inscrutable will and his hidden judgment could interrupt the cycles of the heavenly bodies and their timely advancement at any moment.[125] As a result of human sin, the *mundus* in which the human being now found itself was, as Peter Dendle has characterized it, "a caricature of what was at one time indeed a seamless, interrelated whole."[126] Thus, even religious experts could never be entirely confident that they would be able to predict changes in the atmosphere or explain the significance of unexpected natural phenomena. As

Dutton elucidates, Carolingian writers often recorded these phenomena but rarely explained how they intersected directly with human affairs. Rather, this act of witnessing was a statement of faith: "To isolate irregular and unpredictable happenings in the heavens was . . . to affirm God's power to do in the sky whatever he wished."[127]

Acute sickness was, in many respects, similar to the sudden burst of a comet across the night sky. The body's rhythms could be mapped and managed according to the calendar, but it was impossible to completely counter the instability of a material world beset by sin.[128] As the Lorsch apology declared, the cause and meaning of any particular illness might remain a mystery. Nevertheless, whether sickness resulted from nature or divine justice, humans were called upon to respond to the disorder of disease. On the one hand, prophylactic medical techniques were to be employed as spiritual exercises by the soul; these included, above all, the regulation of diet according to anticipated temporal fluctuations. On the other hand were the treatments that responded to unpredicted pain and injury; here, the use of medical remedies in a therapeutic sense was repeatedly justified with reference to the body entering a state of necessity. In ninth-century medical writings, *necessitas*—a term also found in contemporary penitential and legal works—emerges as a way to designate exceptional circumstances and, consequently, to distinguish between care of the body from need rather than from *luxuria* (extravagance).[129] The close correspondences between medical and moral uses of *necessitas* point to the development of a theory of bodily intervention, one that responded to the currents of penitential thought in the eighth and ninth centuries.

A text on bloodletting, attributed to Bede and extant in several ninth-century manuscripts, begins by asserting, "At all times of day and night, if necessity (*necessitas*) threatens in acute suffering, phlebotomy should be applied."[130] The treatise then outlines the annual regimens to be used to protect the body, including the calendar and lunar days on which phlebotomy was strongly discouraged. What becomes clear is that, except for three Egyptian Days on which it was absolutely forbidden to perform bloodletting or give medication, a condition of *necessitas* impelled the letting of blood during all other times of the year. That is, the term *necessitas* recurs at three points in this text to justify a course of action on the body that would not be condoned if the circumstances were different. We might think nothing of this coincidence in language, especially since *necessitas* may be translated simply as "need" or "exigency," a translation that makes sense in this case.

However, the appearance of this particular term in a number of other passages that justify medical cures should alert us to the possibility that a more complex principle is at play here.

Indeed, the Lorsch apology likewise includes three uses of the term *necessitas*. The first appears in its crucial reinterpretation of a biblical dictum: "Although Paul said, *make no provision for the body*, he immediately added *in its desires*. For what he prohibited in desire, he conceded, without doubt, in necessity."[131] The second invokes not Paul's but Christ's demonstration that "medicine and human comforts should not be refused in necessity."[132] And the third follows a string of authoritative quotations meant to underscore that "whoever does not seek medicine in necessity deserves to be called foolish and ignorant."[133] The repetition of this term suggests a concept that is not fully articulated. But the clear implication is that *necessitas* indicates a state of acute bodily suffering, a state that underpins a division between the legitimate and illegitimate use of medicine.

This exact application of *necessitas* appears in Hildemar of Civate's discussion of illness in his commentary on the Benedictine Rule (although the term never surfaces in Benedict of Nursia's original chapter). Here, in a section that outlines the baths and meat afforded to sick brothers, Hildemar alludes explicitly to the potential for medical cures to be associated with luxury. Yet, his aim is to remind his readers that medicine *is* sanctioned by God and the Rule and, thus, these allowances are legitimate exceptions to daily monastic practice. "Because divine scripture proscribes those things that relate to pleasures, not those things that relate to the support of human weakness and sickness, just as you have, *make no provision for the body in its desires*. See now, when he [Paul] says, *in its desires*, it is clear that he conceded that care ought to be shown to the body in its necessities (*necessitatibus*)."[134] The parallels between the Lorsch text and Hildemar's are striking.

Though the apology, unlike the commentary, does not treat the use of medicine in the context of prescribed rules of conduct, both texts assume that there is heightened spiritual danger surrounding medical intervention (as opposed to prophylactic regulation); they imply that treatments *could* be considered sinful except that a concession is triggered by a body in *necessitas*. This assumption closely follows an event described in the Gospel of Mark and further elaborated upon by Bede in his Marcan commentary. The episode centers on the Pharisees' rebuke of Christ's disciples for gathering corn on the Sabbath. To which Jesus responds by invoking the example of David, who, in contravention of Jewish law, ate the bread in the Temple (the bread of the presence) when he was hungry and in necessity.[135] Bede's exegesis focused in particular on Jesus's use of the term *necessitas*, drawing an explicit comparison between the imperatives of divine law and a state of necessity: "What was not permitted in law was made licit by the necessity of hunger."[136]

However, it was not Bede's *Commentary on Mark* but rather his *Commentary on Revelation* that likely inspired the Lorsch apologist. There (in an interpretation of the names of the twelve tribes of Israel), Bede states that "we shall confine our care of the body strictly to what is necessary for the human condition *and make no provision for the flesh in its desires*."[137] It is here, then, that we find the link between *necessitas* and Paul's letter to the Romans—and yet, we note that the emphasis differs between Bede and the Lorsch apologist. The former underscores the need to *limit* the care of the body, while the latter employs the same quotation to *expand* the possibilities for intervention in the body's well-being.

In their manipulation of language surrounding necessity, Bede, the Lorsch apologist, and Hildemar participated in a legalistic tradition that stretched back to the Gospel of Mark. The principle that *necessitas* created exceptions to divine law also entered penitential discourse, where it surfaced as a factor that mitigated or eliminated the penance required to atone for an illicit act. The *necessitas* of hunger or nakedness excused theft, violation of the Lenten fast, and the eating of unclean meat in various penitentials popular in the eighth and ninth centuries.[138] Following such penitential authority, in his harsh capitulary directed at the recently defeated Saxons, Charlemagne declared that any Saxon who ate meat during Lent would not face execution *if* it was ascertained that this was done "by reason of *necessitas*."[139] Similarly, in a diocesan capitulary, Heito Bishop of Basel (807–23) proclaimed that there were "legitimate times" to perform baptisms during the year but that nevertheless, "if necessity occurred," one ought to render assistance in performing an immediate baptism, no matter the time of year or day of the week.[140] The reasoning he provided was that "necessity scarcely has a law."[141] In his discussion of Roman legal cases, Seneca the Elder (d. 39 C.E.) had pronounced *necessitas* "the law of the moment," and, to a certain extent, medieval ecclesiastical authorities built on this notion of a temporary law external to the legal code.[142] However, as Heito's statement indicates, early medieval thought emphasized, above all, the belief that necessity created a situation of exemption—whether from adherence to royal law, strict standards in moral conduct, imperatives surrounding purity, or restrictions on things pleasurable to the body.[143]

Among ninth-century medical writings, the term *necessitas* appears with particular frequency in texts related to bloodletting. Two different phlebotomy treatises that circulated in the Carolingian period included lines from the Latin translation of Oribasius's *Synopsis* with an interpolation regarding necessity.[144] Thus, whereas Oribasius (following Galen) states that one can perform phlebotomy at any time of day and into the night, these two texts add that there must also exist a condition of *necessitas*, which compels bloodletting.[145] Similarly, the early medieval compilation *The Wisdom of the Art of Medicine* details the treatments appropriate for different stages of life, with reference to *necessitas*. Between the ages of fifteen (when yellow bile increases) and fifty-six (when heat starts to diminish), the text states that phlebotomy can be applied, but outside that age range purgatives should be utilized instead. Lest, however, the reader think that treatment always ought to hinge on a person's age, the text warns: "If *necessitas* occurs, do not ask about the [patient's] stage of life but act judiciously in accordance with what has been written."[146] Here, the term denotes urgency, the implication being that the physician cannot follow standard procedure but must act swiftly to counter the disease. So, too, a pseudonymous letter from Diocles to one Pamperius praises the utility of phlebotomy, asserting that "the soul is redeemed through the letting of blood, as the disease rushes to resist. *Necessitas* does not wait for a [certain] time."[147] The suggestion is that *necessitas* and *tempus* (time) are somehow opposed to each other: time proceeds linearly, in an expected and regular manner; *necessitas* interposes in time, being by nature unexpected and irregular.[148]

The Carolingian elite were clearly attuned to this understanding of *necessitas* because it appears in ninth-century conciliar statutes, which, as Mary Yearl has demonstrated, are the first references to monastic bloodletting in the West.[149] The Synod of Aachen from 816 declared that the monks "should not observe a specified time of bloodletting, but it should be granted to each according to what *necessitas* demands."[150] That is, rather than bloodletting being a periodic activity—as it would become in twelfth-century monastic houses, with timetables for bloodletting related to the liturgical calendar—Carolingian councils dictated that the irregularity and urgency of *necessitas* ought to check the practice.[151] There may have been a concern that phlebotomy itself was a bodily pleasure or that the food given after bloodletting was a luxury desired by monks. Whatever the impetus for this decree (and subsequent reiterations), Carolingian monasteries were evidently being encouraged to develop protocols for bloodletting, and these protocols aligned closely with the theory advanced in contemporaneous medical treatises.

This theory presented the body as precariously balanced between the predictable and the unpredictable. If Egyptian Days and monthly dietetic calendars situated the flesh in a steady, rational cycle of fluctuations, the term *necessitas* seems to have emerged as a counterpoint to these cycles. It signified the opacity of God's judgments, the mystery of events witnessed in nature, and the ubiquity of exception in a world that was never entirely stable. Human life on earth was always subject to necessity for the very reason that Adam and Eve brought pain, hunger, thirst, aging, and disease into existence with their first sin; in the ejection from Eden, the body became subject to time, an advance toward death, and erratic desires and catastrophes that periodically interposed along the way. Only with the resurrected body, as Augustine emphasized, would humans again exist "without necessity."[152] This sense of a body constantly beset resonates in the uses of *necessitas* in ninth-century medical texts.[153] Yet, in suggesting a state of exception or concession, *necessitas* captured something beyond the daily or unchanging needs of the body. This is apparent in the commentary on the Benedictine Rule by Smaragdus of Saint-Mihiel, who explains that baths are only to be granted readily to sick brothers for reasons of illness; once a brother has been restored to health he must return to his usual practice. For, he states, "Desire should not hold those who are now recovered there, where *necessitas* had bound them while they were infirm."[154]

Similarly, the *Letter of Arsenius*, a medical treatise that, as we saw in Chapter 5, sets forth a glowing description of the *medicus*'s character, ends by calling him "a sensor of internal things, a teacher or deliverer of health, and an expert craftsman, who is a warrior against necessity."[155] In fact, the last phrase differs slightly in various witnesses, with one asserting that the *medicus* "frees [people] from necessity."[156] The *medicus* cannot free people from the possibility of illness, since it is part of the fallen condition of humanity, but he can combat the effects of existing in this fallen state, and he acts with divine approval when he does so. Indeed, the language in the *Letter of Arsenius* recalls Old Testament prayers to God, which state that he alone possesses the power to "free his people from their necessities."[157] Consequently, although *necessitas* served as a tool to restrict the human physician's powers (he was sanctioned to intervene only when the patient was in necessity), it also endowed the *medicus* with a type of divine power—the ability to liberate, temporarily, the body from the worst features of a world of constant turbulence and decay.

If *necessitas* remained a somewhat ambiguous concept, this was not from lack of interest in theoretical frameworks. It was clearly central to the theology of medicine advanced by the Lorsch author, as well as to monastic discussions of sickness, bodily pleasure, and therapeutic protocols. That the concept is never defined in extant sources could suggest an intention for *necessitas* to remain a flexible and expansive guideline, capable of accommodating individual differences and unique circumstances as much as possible. The aim, after all, was to *enable*, not condemn, the use of medical treatments such as phlebotomy, baths, and special diets. The language of *necessitas* allowed for the body's starkest needs to supersede other spiritual concerns, and thus, the reiteration of necessity as a state of exception across many different genres in the Carolingian period points to an abiding interest in taking the health of the *corpus* seriously.

## Ending with an Example: Walafrid Strabo

Let us return here to a figure we met in Chapter 4: Walafrid Strabo (808–849), a monk of Reichenau, who later studied under Hrabanus at Fulda, became tutor to a young Charles the Bald, and then returned to Reichenau as its abbot.[158] Within the surviving corpus of Walafrid's prodigious scholarship is a manuscript that, according to Bernhard Bischoff, was the monk's personal handbook (*vademecum*), compiled piece by piece over the course of his life, with many pages written in Walafrid's own hand.[159] Designed for continual perusal, the handbook consists of excerpts of varying lengths on an array of subjects, including grammar, computus, natural science, Christian history, medicine, and poetry.[160] Many of the specific texts correspond precisely with treatises covered in this chapter; we find all of Bede's *On the Nature of Things* and selections from *On the Reckoning of Time*, the pseudo-Hippocratic *Letter to Antiochus*, a list of Egyptian Days, a few pages of medical recipes, a text on the best times for phlebotomy and purgatives, a dietary calendar, and various other snippets on food and drink (including a popular dietary treatise addressed in the next chapter).[161]

The editorial choices manifest in the *vademecum* are thus a powerful statement regarding the associations among bodily health, temporal calculations, and cosmic structures in the minds of the Carolingian elite. Computus bleeds into chronicle, chronicle into calendar, calendar into regimen and prognostic. There is a clear nod to the liberal arts as a framework for the handbook, and medicine is firmly established as equally important to grammar and astronomy within Walafrid's understanding of the *artes*.[162] Indeed, he even inserted a short proclamation on why "the discipline (*scientia*) of doctors is most useful for mortals." It is, he asserts, a "knowledge of healing, which thoroughly investigates the power of drugs and herbs and the juice of trees and the natures of nearly everything for the sake of the moderation and health of the body."[163]

Part of this definition is identical to that contained in the *Lorscher Arzneibuch*, but Walafrid added his own touch in emphasizing medicine's encompassing study of the natural world, of which the human body was only one component.[164] Medicine is presented not simply as the art of moderating the body but of moderating the relationship between cosmos and individual. This might help to explain why the majority of the treatises in the handbook center on the daily, prophylactic care of the body, rather than treatments for specific ailments.[165] In focusing on cosmic patterns, the texts illuminate the *ideal* to which the human body should strive but from which it was always falling short.

CHAPTER 7

# Habits for Health

> The senses of the body are horses; the soul is a charioteer.
> The body is a child; the soul is its teacher.
> We employ the soul to rule, the body rather to serve.
> Wine is a luxurious thing and drunkenness riotous;
> whoever is under their influence is not wise.
> We cannot give attention to wisdom if we are thinking
> about the abundance of the table.

These aphorisms are from Walafrid Strabo's *vademecum*, listed together on a page titled *On Struggle* (*De conflictu*). If the previous chapter noted the overlap between computus and medicine in the handbook, here I suggest that the presentation of these maxims offers a further layer to the way in which this source endowed medicine with spiritual meaning.

The ten aphorisms that Walafrid includes on this page all relate to the moral life, but several concentrate particularly on the soul-body relationship and strikingly resemble metaphors found in the Carolingian lay manuals. Many of them have a long history among classical authors, though Walafrid likely encountered them within the Christian ascetic tradition.[1] They emphasize the need for the soul to enforce a strict hierarchy by governing and restraining the body, some employing more aggressive imagery (the charioteer), and others more nurturing (the teacher-student relationship). Above all, these maxims highlight the supremacy of reason and reason's capacity to ensure moderation. They make clear that a chief method by which the rational soul enacts its governance is by regulating food and drink.

It is, then, surely no coincidence that only twenty pages after the aphorisms, one finds a series of dietary texts within the *vademecum*. Indeed, the manner in which the page of aphorisms is sandwiched roughly between statements concerning the utility of medical learning, a letter on fasting, and a popular treatise on healthy food draws attention to the moral implications of those texts drawn directly from the medical corpus of the ninth century. Medicine was rarely simply about healing physical ailments; it was consistently implicated in strategies for managing the relationship between body and soul.[2] This chapter assembles a cluster of comparisons between Carolingian medical and moral literature, giving special weight to each genre's treatment of the proper habits regarding food and drink. It thus pursues the question of individual responsibility for spiritual health across both the lay manuals and Benedictine commentaries examined in Chapter 2 and the prophylactic and therapeutic medical regimens analyzed in Chapter 6. These comparisons take us through the similarities in format evident in both genres, shared fears about the dangers of excess, and sustained preoccupations with the power of digestive processes to introduce corruption to the internal cavity. Throughout, we return to ideas sketched in Chapter 1 about the soul being diffused throughout the body yet especially present in certain members and fluids.

Ninth-century intellectuals conceptualized "ancient" medicine as one useful technique among many for controlling invisible, polluting forces within the social body. In encouraging fixed routines and daily habits, it purged bodies and souls and thereby uprooted the seeds of potential disorder. By evaluating traces of the lay ownership of medical writings, this chapter proposes that such routines and habits were understood to be proper for all Christians to cultivate, not only those pursuing the religious life. It thus challenges the dominance of *Mönchsmedizin* as a model for understanding early medieval healthcare, suggesting instead that, even if monasteries were the primary producers of medical knowledge, the laity also embraced the possibilities it advanced for self-care.[3] The interest in bodily regimens spanned the lay-monastic divide more seamlessly than has often been assumed, even if certain details differed within the cloister. And though the role of *medicus* may have been one associated with monks and clergy, medical erudition itself was valuable to ecclesiastics and laity, men and women, alike.

## The Lordship of the Stomach

In his verses on cultivating garden plants, addressed to Abbot Grimald of Saint-Gall, Walafrid Strabo referred to the stomach as "the king of the body" (*corporis rex*).[4] He did not, however, invent this epithet for the organ but appropriated it from that medical work so cherished by Charlemagne, the late antique poem by Quintus Serenus.[5] Other medical writings in circulation in the ninth century likewise accorded the stomach a regal status within the body. An anatomical treatise attributed to Vindicianus declared that "our stomach, which is the lord of the whole body, both holds and dispenses nourishment,"[6] while a treatise on digestion defined the stomach as "the steward of the whole body" on account of its role in receiving and distributing food and drink.[7]

Why this focus on the stomach, especially given the possible connections between the head and the soul or the heart and life? With the exception of the eyes, the stomach is the most frequently discussed organ when it comes to matters of health; it appears more prominently than the liver, heart, or brain in medical manuscripts from the ninth century. One explanation for its prominence comes from Alcuin's didactic dialogue for Charlemagne's son, where the question, "What is the stomach?" is answered with the definition, "The cooker of food."[8] Although it was understood that other organs participated in the digestive process, the stomach (as represented by various Latin terms) came to represent the overriding importance of food regulation to the body's well-being.[9]

The intense interest in managing digestion is witnessed by the popularity of a text that is extant in at least seven manuscripts from the ninth and tenth centuries.[10] Often entitled *A Letter on the Nature of the Belly or Inner Organs*, this treatise begins with a brief anatomical description of the chest area; we follow the esophagus, called "the mouth of the belly" (*os ventris*), to the crucial configuration of organs—the stomach (*ventriculus*), liver (*epar*), gallbladder (*vesica fellis rufi*), and spleen (*splen*).[11] Rather than dwelling on the unique attributes of each part, the anonymous author underscores the transformations that food undergoes at this nexus of organs and the relationship between consumption and disease.

First, the stomach loosens all food and drink into a milky juice with the assistance of heat produced by the liver and the gallbladder. From this mixture, the stomach takes some for its own sustenance, gives some to the liver, and transforms the thicker part of the juice into phlegm, which it transmits to the head "by some mystery of the art of nature."[12] The portion of the juice passed to the liver is cooked a second time and is turned into blood, which is fed into the heart and veins. A residual amount of blood, however, remains from this transformation and is cooked a third time by the heat of the gallbladder and turned into yellow bile.[13] This then crosses from the liver to the gallbladder and passes through a fourth cooking process by which it becomes black bile. The black bile, in turn, seems to be mixed with the dregs of blood from the liver, with the result that part becomes a "melancholic humor" and part is released to the spleen.[14] Thus, "the four-part elements of the body," as the text terms them, are each assigned a proper seat—phlegm in the head, blood in the liver, yellow bile in the gallbladder, and black bile in the spleen.[15] The stomach is not a seat but is the first processor and the regulator of the entire system.

*On the Nature of the Belly* promises to explain not only how the four humors are converted from food and where they primarily reside in the body but also how they acquire their powers (*vires*) and what happens when one humor dominates the others. It is this latter concern that links the processes of digestion with the mechanisms of illness and, consequently, with moral questions about overconsumption. The author suggests that a surplus of any three of the four humors obviously stands in direct relationship to the occurrence of quotidian, tertian, and quartan fevers.[16] That is, as phlegm is produced in the stomach every day, so an overabundance of phlegm is clearly the cause of a daily fever. As yellow bile results from the third cooking of ingested food, so is it the root of a tertian fever, which recurs every three days. Likewise, black bile, from the fourth cooking of food in the spleen, is responsible for a quartan fever, which arises every four days.[17] The account implicitly relies on Galen's attributions of quotidian, tertian, and quartan fevers to phlegm, yellow bile, and black bile, respectively, and then works backward from these associations to a system that, the author emphasizes, is inherently rational.[18] In doing so, the treatise manages to highlight the importance of the number four, asserting the existence of four concoction phases grounded in four close-knit organs.

The causal connection between digestion and fever emerges from the "cooking physiology." Under normal circumstances, each humor is constrained to its proper seat or location in the body, "except when the amount of one rises up beyond its norm, and this matter is so abundant that, as a result of the excess, a piercing heat is produced."[19] The text implies that an overabundance of one humor triggers a failure of the digestive process; the corresponding organ cannot contain the excess humor, and "when it pours out from its proper place through the rest of the body, the body shakes and grows cold from its biting force."[20] Because of the overabundance, the digestive organ cannot produce sufficient heat to properly cook the humor; as the liquid flows through the body it provokes chills and tremors, and the body responds by increasing its heat to consume the unpurified element. Thus, a fever follows the chills.

Rather than a survey of normal digestion, *On the Nature of the Belly* is primarily concerned with the ramifications of digestive failure. Although it offers no details on how to prevent gastronomical abundance, its typical arrangement within a codex containing appropriate dietary regimens leaves little doubt that the production of excess humor was recognized, here, as an ethical problem. While acknowledging that the internal production of the humors was somewhat mysterious, these compilations argued for an undeniable connection between an individual's dietary habits and the proper functioning of the digestive organs that ruled the body.

Certainly, this was the lesson imparted by the *Letter from Anthimus, vir illustris, count, and legate, to the most glorious Theuderic, king of the Franks.*[21] This treatise, which outlined in detail the benefits and dangers of various foods and provided instructions on their ideal preparation, circulated relatively widely in the ninth century. It is found in the *Lorscher Arzneibuch* and a contemporaneous medical codex from the vicinity of Paris or Auxerre. It is listed in a Lorsch library catalogue and a catalogue from Murbach, and it appears in the *vademecum* of Walafrid Strabo.[22] A twelfth-century copy of the letter also includes what may have been a ninth-century interpolation, an invocation to a "glorious and unconquered August King Charles."[23] It is tempting to suggest that this preserves a version intended for Charlemagne or Charles the Bald, one that mimicked the address of Anthimus's original letter to another king of the Franks.

Though the work is typically associated with the court of the Merovingian King Theuderic I (r. 511–533), its origins cannot be determined with any certainty. Anthimus *may* (as most scholars assert) have been a Greek physician exiled from the Byzantine Empire by Zeno, who then joined the court of Theodoric of Italy (r. 493–526) and served as his ambassador to the Merovingian king.[24] Yet, this assumption is speculative; all we know from the treatise itself is that the author comes from a distant (and warmer) region, considered himself a Greek-speaker, and does not seem to have identified as a Frank or Ostrogoth.[25] It is quite possible, as Yitzhak Hen proposes, that the author was an envoy sent from Constantinople, who framed the *Letter* within the culture of *romanitas* shared by Byzantines and Franks as a means of ingratiating himself with the Merovingian king.[26] Yet, his decision not to name Galen or any other Greek medical authority (although he claims to have on hand several medical texts) leaves open the possibility that Anthimus was not from eastern lands; furthermore, the increasing ubiquity of the title *legatarius* within seventh-century Frankish writings may point toward a later date for the treatise than previously assumed.[27]

With that said, the most reliable context in which we can situate the *Letter of Anthimus* is among the medical treatises with which it was (almost) exclusively transmitted in the Carolingian period.[28] Like the pseudo-Hippocratic *Letter to Antiochus*, it is framed as correspondence to an illustrious king. Indeed, titled as an *epistula*, it corresponds closely to the obvious preference for medicine-as-epistle witnessed in the compilations assembled by Carolingian scribes. Bonnie Effros keenly notes that there is no surviving reference to Anthimus's letter from the Merovingian world and speculates that his work did not appeal to sixth- and seventh-century lay elites, who deemed it inappropriate, or at least unnecessary, to discipline their bodies like monks. With the first witnesses to the text being manuscripts likely produced at Carolingian monasteries, Effros argues that its historical use was shaped by the monastic treatment of the sick.[29] And yet, Anthimus emphatically declared his text to be about *preventing* illness rather than prescribing techniques to treat it.

The learned author announces in his preface that he has provided "a rule of observation" (*ratio observationis*) for Theuderic, culled from the teachings of medical authors.[30] He seeks to cultivate a sense of urgency in the reader, warning him to pay personal heed to the selection and preparation of foods, since good digestion is the root of "distinguished health" (*prima sanitas*).[31] A prophylactic attention to bodily functions here becomes a display of reason, morality, and Christian teaching:

> We who drive ourselves with diverse foods, diverse delicacies, and diverse drinks must govern ourselves such that we are not weighed down by excess but obtain health by behaving more moderately. . . . It is right to attentively observe the [instructions] which we have pre-

> sented with the help of divine majesty and our lord Jesus Christ, by whose grace may we hold a longer life and extraordinary health.[32]

As civilized people, Anthimus implies, the Franks have access to a range of food and drink. Comparing other nations (*aliae gentes*) to wolves because they eat only one type of food, he suggests to Theuderic that the status of the Franks as a people is manifested by their self-control over their dietary choices in the face of such diversity.[33] God intends that individuals should enjoy excellent health, and they can, Anthimus asserts, by executing the instructions that follow. Genuine good health depends upon eating well-prepared foods in moderation, proportion, and proper sequence. To revive health through remedies is, according to Anthimus, a sign of bad choices; they are merely "quick fixes," and those who use them only *appear* healthy.[34] They lack true physical integrity because their bodies are not mirrors for the rational regulation of their habits. Similarly, those whose health rests on the scarceness of their diet are driven by circumstance and need, not cultivated practice; hence, Anthimus refuses to define their lifestyles as virtuous.[35] This is a treatise for the Frankish elite, a short handbook intended to be consulted frequently in order to maintain the body's health and stability in a turbulent world.[36]

The text addresses each category of food in turn (grain, meat, fowl, eggs, fish, vegetables, pulses, dairy, and fruit), detailing what is best from each category and how to prepare it.[37] Though these instructions are relatively detailed, the *Letter* includes almost no explanation of the digestive process. The basic premise is that the stomach is (as Alcuin said) a "cooker." Consequently, those foods that are already well-cooked before entering the body are more easily broken down by the stomach and turned into "good humors" (*humores boni*).[38] Raw food is to be avoided, as are overly cold foods that might dampen the heat of the stomach, or dense, dry, or heavy foods that might not cook properly.[39] For these reasons, Anthimus warns against eating unripe fruit; baked or boiled cheese (which turns hard as it cooks); too many oysters (which are chilling); boiled eggs (which do not cook evenly); salted meats and fish (which are dry); and meat roasted close to the fire (which burns on the outside but remains raw inside).[40] Conversely, he recommends garlic (which warms the stomach); hot, well-leavened bread; meat and fish that have been recently killed (which are lighter); steamed or boiled lamb and venison (which are softer); and warmed milk (which does not curdle in the stomach). It is among just such directives that we can set Einhard's statement about Charlemagne's physicians urging him to cease his consumption of roasted meat and eat boiled meat instead.[41]

While there is a logical framework to Anthimus's recipes and rules, it is not the fourfold humoral theory witnessed elsewhere.[42] He references sporadically a bad or "melancholic humor" (*melancholicus humor*) and people who are phlegmatic (*flegmaticus*), but he never alludes to four distinct substances and places more emphasis on the production of simply good or bad humors.[43] Similarly, he does not suggest that season, month, gender, or age ought to be considered in choosing food and drink.[44] Instead, Anthimus emphasizes a set of binaries implied by his key terms: heavy vs. light, indigestible vs. digestible, rotten/raw vs. cooked, and decay (*corruptilla*) vs. health. Less concerned with balancing two opposites than entirely avoiding anything corrupt, he declares that "if, at a meal, one item within a diverse mixture of good foods is raw and not appropriate, it destroys all the other good substances and does not permit the stomach to have good digestion."[45]

Despite its differing approach, Anthimus's *Letter* accords closely with other medical treatises in its central premise—"everything in excess is harmful."[46] Food or drink that overburdens the powers of the stomach results in corruption trapped deep in the internal cavity. Anthimus illuminates the signs that communicate whether digestion has occurred properly. He constantly invokes the feeling of "heaviness" (*gravitas*) that signals a problem in the stomach; accompanying it are gases that travel through the body, as well as vomiting and loose bowels.[47] Uncooked foods "generate raw humors (*crudos humores*), burning gases (*acidivas carbunculos*), and violent belching (*ructus gravissimos*). As a result, fumes rise into the head and typically cause sudden dizziness and heavy fog."[48] The noxious vapors given off by the stomach thus connect the belly with the highest reaches of the body—the head, a space associated with the senses as well as with reason and soul. An inability to govern the physical body is both a reflection of a lifestyle without *ratio* and a precursor to the loss of rational thought.

## Eating and Drinking as Moral Exercises

The *Letter of Anthimus* includes an invocation to Christ but does not otherwise reference the spiritual dimension of dietary regulation. As an edifying treatise addressed to members of the lay elite, it can, however, be set alongside other spiritually edifying handbooks popular with the Frankish nobility. With Anthimus, we can clearly see a trajectory in which Carolingian discourse amplified certain attitudes expressed by Merovingian authors. A desire to promote and sanctify the classical virtue of temperance was not new to the late eighth century, but the teachings proffered in countless Carolingian didactic works focused even more attention on this particular virtue as an essential element of Christian identity.[49] Speaking of earthly goods in general, Alcuin's textbook on grammar warned that anything exceeding moderate use weighs down (*gravare*) individuals. In two different formulations, he repeated the classical saying "not anything in excess," in one case mirroring the exact wording found in Anthimus's letter (*omnia nimia nocere*).[50]

If we return, here, to the lay manuals discussed in Chapter 2 (by Paulinus, Alcuin, Jonas, and Dhuoda), it becomes evident just how central the act of eating and drinking was for maintaining a healthy soul. We have already seen how Jonas of Orléans focused on consumption as a chief mechanism by which laypeople committed sins and defiled themselves, often unsuspectingly; they assumed that they could eat for pleasure rather than the necessity of the body. Jonas attempted to draw them back to the path of moderation by explaining that there were Christian rules governing dietary habits. His was not the only Carolingian handbook to do so. By narrowing our investigation to diet, we can envision how "medical" and "moral" letters reinforced similar mandates, even as they laid bare different internal processes.

It was through Adam's and Eve's desire to eat, as Paulinus explains to Duke Eric, that sin first corrupted humanity.[51] The devil was jealous of Adam, who was made in the image of God and ordered by temperance. The repercussion of the first couple's sin, then, was to render humanity intemperate and subject it to illness and death.[52] The language of temperance and disease that Paulinus employs to discuss the Fall is likewise the language that he uses to justify the regulation of food and drink in the life of a layman. Somewhat surprisingly, perhaps, it is through eating that Paulinus envisions the soul subjugating the body and *not*, as one might expect, through its governance of sexual acts between Eric and his wife. In explaining the move toward a stricter sexual code and monogamous marriage over the ninth century, modern scholars have often framed the lay manuals as responses to an anxiety surrounding the nobility's conjugal life; there is a tendency to read all the manuals through the lens of Jonas's work, which *does* focus on marriage and sex as central issues in lay morality. Paulinus and Alcuin, however, accord much more attention to habits of consumption than of sex (see Figure 17).[53]

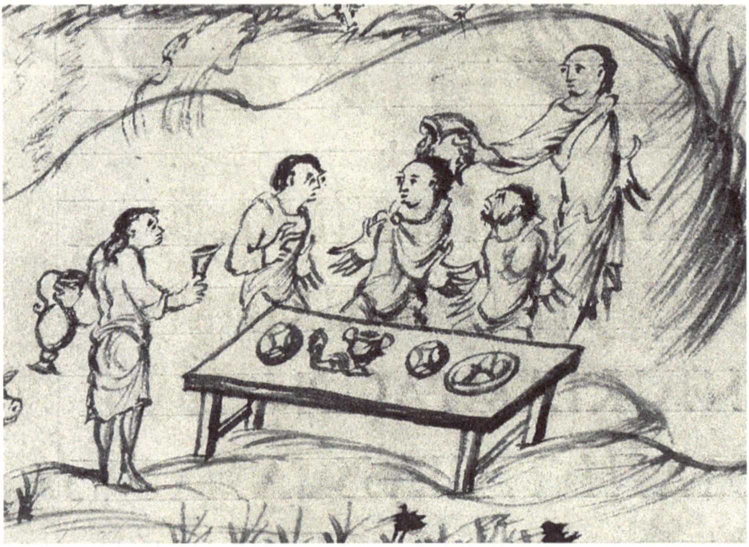

Figure 17. Men feasting with bread and wine around a table in the Utrecht Psalter (Ps 103:14–15). Utrecht, University Library, MS 32, f. 59v. By kind permission of the Universiteitsbibliotheek.

Paulinus says nothing at all about marriage.[54] But he does offer a short explanation of the physiological effects of food on the health of both the spiritual and physical components of the self.

> Too much food profoundly harms not only our souls but also our bodies and leads to infirmity. For the strength of the stomach (*stomachi fortitudo*) is typically shattered (*frangi*) through too much greed for food and intemperance in drink, and a large amount of food provokes an abundance of blood and bile and many sicknesses. Just as those things are contrary to the soul and body, thus the cure for both is moderation through fasting.[55]

Paulinus does not go into detail about the specific foods that Eric should avoid. Unlike Cassian (d. 435), for instance, he does not list substances that dry and cool the body for the purpose of dampening lust and preserving chastity.[56] This silence distinguishes Paulinus's approach from that of many late antique writers, who emphasized fasting and the control of food as key measures in the suppression of semen and nocturnal emissions.[57] Such writers, however, were composing works intended for a monastic or episcopal audience, as was the case with Cassian's *Institutes*. In fact, Paulinus derived this passage from a sixth-century work directed to the monks of Lérins.[58] There, the abbot warns the monks against excessive consumption amid instructions on conducting vigils; an abundance of food dulls a monk's senses and impedes his soul's ability to remain alert and awake. The body may be nourished by such food, the abbot states, but the soul is nourished by prayer and psalms, and thus, to fast while keeping vigil weakens the body and strengthens the soul.[59] By extracting the comments about excessive eating from a guide aimed at ascetics and dealing specifically with the need for vigilance during prayer, Paulinus adapted a focused set of rules into a precept for daily life and made it relevant to the lay and religious elite alike.

The passage draws attention to the ill effects of overconsumption on the body as well as the soul. The emphasis in Paulinus's *Book of Admonition* is not on the heaviness and sleepiness that come over the body after large meals (as in the source-text on vigils) but rather on the important role the stomach plays in maintaining health and on the relationship between indulgence and humoral superfluity. As in *On the Nature of the Belly*, an abundance of bile or blood is treated as a cause of sickness, and, as in the *Letter of Anthimus*, immoderate desire for food is linked with failure of the digestive system. Paulinus, however, makes explicit what Anthimus does not. He teaches his lay readers that one of their daily activities—which might appear to affect only the state of the body—in fact has bearing on the health of the soul.

In their manuals for Wido and Matfrid, Alcuin and Jonas took a similar approach, excerpting works for monastics and extending their stipulations about eating to the laity. Jonas used selections from Julian Pomerius's work for the clergy to argue that all people should habitually take food in moderation, not out of desire but for the body's needs. A layperson should maintain an acute awareness of the quality and quantity being ingested, he indicates, receiving enough to "rebuild the stomach" and avoiding delicate foods or overconsumption, which weaken and weigh down the body.[60]

Alcuin, likewise, suggests that gluttony derives not only from improper desire for luxurious or superfluous food but also from any choice that harms the healthy functioning of the body. The vice is present "when one desires to anticipate the canonical and established hour for the sake of gluttony, or orders that more exquisite food be prepared for him than the necessity of the body or the quality of his person demands, or takes in more food or drink on account of his intemperate desire than is beneficial for his health."[61] The implication for lay readers is that they can adopt the rules established within a monastery in order to set predetermined routines that regularize the repletion of the body. Instituting fixed times for meals, embracing a simpler diet, and judging amounts by reason rather than fullness are tools by which the lay noble can ensure the body's health and eschew customs that incite sin. With this assumption, Alcuin refers Wido to "a common rule for all healthy and infirm religious, that from whatever sort of food they never completely fill up their bellies."[62] Jonas, comparably, urges his readers to avoid pleasure by not eating "before time or . . . beyond moderate measure."[63] Directives such as these appear in the lay manuals in order to support the soul's rational governance of the body.

While Paulinus, Jonas, and Alcuin spoke in general terms about immoderate and irrational consumption being detrimental to an individual's spiritual and physical health, Smaragdus and Hildemar framed their guidelines on monastic dietary practices with more detailed physiological information. Benedict's original Rule stipulated that "above all, overconsumption (*crapula*) is to be avoided so that indigestion never steals up on a monk," but it offered no guidance on how to recognize overconsumption.[64] Smaragdus, however, clarifies that the word "*crapula* comes from the phrase raw food (*cruda epula*)," a connection that makes intuitive sense because the result of eating raw food is that "the heart is weighed down and the stomach suffers indigestion."[65] Indigestion, he then elaborates, refers to the lack of draining (*indeductio*) from the stomach.[66] Associating food that is not properly cooked with the burdening of the stomach, and indigestion with the failure of food to pass through to the other digestive organs, Smaragdus's explanation closely resembles Anthimus's linkage of rawness, heaviness, acidic surfeit, and noxious gases.[67] Smaragdus echoes the stress that Anthimus places on *gravitas* by frequently returning to the relationship among luxury, physical heaviness, and spiritual vacuity. The body's distention with food, he proclaims, "greatly dulls the sharpness of the mind" and "produces torpor in the body and soul, equally."[68] Whether or not he was familiar with Anthimus's *Letter*, the monk clearly believed that his peers would better avoid sinful indulgence by understanding something of the physiological processes at play.

Hildemar introduced his comments on Benedict's chapter "On the Measure of Food" by drawing a provocative comparison between the advice of a *medicus* and the mandates of God. "Just as a most skilled *medicus* says to his patient when he sees him sick: 'Abstain from this food and that food because unless you abstain from these foods you will fall into greater illness,' thus also the Lord said . . . 'Pay attention *lest your hearts be weighed down with overconsumption and drunkenness or temporal concerns* [Lk 21:34].'"[69] Given that Christians heed the earthly physician (*medicus terrenus*), how much more, Hildemar exclaims, should they heed the heavenly one (*medicus coelestis*)!

Hildemar appears, at first, to set up a distinction between bodily affairs and spiritual matters, the former concerned with a proper diet and the latter with a proper attention to eternal truths. However, he immediately follows this with a lengthy and technical description of the perils of overconsumption (*crapula*), focusing on the mechanics of the digestive process. In doing so, he moves away from his initial dualistic approach to body and soul toward an understanding of diet as sustaining physical *and* spiritual health.

> For the stomach (*stomachus*) of a person is a small sac (*ventriculus*), which is like a pot near the liver, and there food is stored, and it is cooked by the heat of the liver. But when food fills that sac beyond measure, it is not able to be [properly] cooked by the heat of the liver, and as a result, the smoke of the food ascends through the members to the head. Consequently, the person is weighed down and belches just as from an illness and grows so weak that she is not able to do any good work.[70]

Hildemar is not using dietary medicine as a metaphor for the Christian lifestyle here. Rather, like Paulinus and Smaragdus, he is explaining internal physiological processes as part of his warning against gluttony. Ultimately, he affirms the usefulness of the *medicus terrenus* and his dietary advice to the project of salvation.

This is no abstract narrative of temptation and the soul's need to master bodily impulse. It is a multilayered reflection on the relationship between bodily purity and spiritual health.[71] As Hildemar proceeds to elaborate, "owing to *crapula* one comes into gluttony, from gluttony into impurity, and then into the other vices."[72] One concern, then, is that gluttony acts as a gateway to other temptations. Yet, the physiological discussion has made clear that *crapula* produces real, material impurity in the body. It suggests that the polluted smoke and raw eruptions that rise from stomach to head affect the soul's functioning, which results in irrational and sinful decisions. Finally, as the text indicates, the physical illness resulting from indigestion impairs the individual's capacity to employ the body in performing good works (like divine offices and charitable labor). To be sure, Hildemar does not illustrate his points with lengthy citations from medical works. However, the shared language of excess, overflow, and corruption highlights how dietary guides, descriptions of digestive anatomy, and pastoral mirrors for the soul all fed into a common discourse on self-governance.

The physiological and dietary texts examined here emphasized that the roots of sickness lay in the overabundance of bodily fluids, fluids that gushed forth from their proper places and channels or were not appropriately transformed into useful matter when in excess. They implicitly urged the reader to be mindful of the inner self's potential to fluctuate between extremes. Even more important than balancing one humor against another was ensuring that no individual substance radically altered its quality, quantity, or location:

> As Hippocrates says, there are four humors in the human body. . . . If they do not exceed their measure, a person will enjoy perpetual health. If, however, they diminish or abound more than is fitting, or they are thickened or thinned or change their nature or become more bitter or leave their seats and occupy unnatural ones, they cause various sicknesses in people.[73]

Such brief, theoretical explanations of the causes of disease assumed their full meaning when read in the context of the many other texts that accompanied them in ninth-century codices—texts with instructions on bloodletting, on purgatives, on diets throughout the year, on diets for different infirmities, and on the properties of different natural substances. These materials affirmed that a rational soul could be trained to recognize the signs of excess and take steps to prevent or overcome it. From mirrors for princes to hagiographies, to grammars, to poetry, Carolingian intellectuals highlighted the virtue of temperance and knit together the physiological effects of immoderation with the spiritual dangers of luxury.[74]

## Early Medieval Food Safety

Medical writings, lay handbooks, and monastic rules were not, of course, the only genres that dealt with food and drink. There were also letters and sermons on fasting and sobriety, penitentials that repeated the requirement to "do penance on bread and water," and hagiographies that modeled the sacred life on severe abstention. But what medical treatises uniquely offered was a way to conceptualize the physiological meaning of spiritual practices like fasting. Indeed, fasting was not solely a penitential or ascetic exercise but also surfaced as an instruction in Hippocratic medicine: remedies often specified that a particular cure was to be taken "while fasting," or made fasting itself into a mode of treatment. Fasting, phlebotomy, and the taking of purgatives (such as emetics, laxatives, and diuretics) were all popular methods of purification that affected, above all, the constitution of fluids within the body, especially the blood. Notionally, they were a means of purification, not because they harmed or diminished the body, but because they purged excess and wiped the slate clean; one could then begin anew building up the inner life.[75] Food and drink were necessary but dangerous. The act of consumption could spur on immoderation and the victuals themselves could harbor a type of impurity that then tainted the inner cavity.

With fasting, vomiting, and diarrhea, the aim was to produce purity through tempered cycles of avoidance, purging, and replenishing. After bloodletting, one monastic guide specified that those treated were to be restored with Lenten fare, while those who were also given draughts for particular illnesses were to be allowed the meat of birds.[76] Even during Lent, fasting alternated with days of indulgence, when one enjoyed the fruits of God's creation.[77] A visionary text from the 820s about a monk named Wetti conveys this expectation that "potions" be followed by replenishment. Along with his brothers, as was the custom on Sundays, Wetti had taken a "drink for his health," but while this produced salubrious effects in the others, Wetti became so ill that he could not consume "the food that he ought to have taken to rebuild his body."[78] The issue was not that Wetti vomited "undigested food," because this, presumably, was one of the intended consequences of the drink; the issue was that proper nourishment did not ensue after vomiting, and it was this that caused his extreme illness.[79] The Plan of Saint-Gall indicates that phlebotomy and purgatives were to be administered in a room with a number of tables, where richer foods (prepared in a nearby kitchen) were served to those monks who had been voided of impurities. In these examples, we can see that careful attention was directed to how the body was replenished, based on the assumption that the right food could be used to nurture inner integrity. Similarly, the *Letter to Antiochus* urged fasting while gargling an acidic potion for head pain, abstinence while inducing vomiting for stomach pain, and moderate food and drink alternating with fasting and vomiting for chest pain.[80]

Although many of these examples surface in writings from the cloister and point to rules imposed on the monks by the dictates of obedience, a concern with managing bodily purity is also evident in the life of the laity. This is attested by the lay ownership of certain medical writings (considered below) as well as by a penitential tradition that emphasized both regular fasting and the elimination of polluted substances. Beliefs regarding physical pollution drew heavily on the laws of Leviticus—but we should keep in mind that it was possible to interpret these biblical passages along a continuum from the concrete to the allegorical. When it came to the minutiae of sexual relations in his manual for lay men and women, for example, Jonas acknowledged an exegetical tradition in which the Jewish law was understood spiritually by Christians, yet he insisted on a literal reading.[81] "There are certain things which Christian custom preserves even now according to the letter of the law, with a salvific mystical understanding, for the integrity and cleanliness of the body," he proclaimed.[82] According to Abigail Firey's analysis of Carolingian exegesis of Leviticus, "The objective . . . was always to move the audience to the spiritual frame, and to affirm that the condition of the soul has priority over the condition of the body."[83] However, while an exegete like Hrabanus recast the Levitican proscriptions against certain animal flesh as spiritual proscriptions against the interior vices, this was not Jonas's approach.[84] In his manual for the laity (contemporaneous to Hrabanus's commentary), it was the danger of tangible bodily pollution that worried the bishop of Orléans.

Even if Jonas took a more extreme position than other Carolingian theologians, a new emphasis on concrete bodily pollution certainly penetrated Carolingian culture, as Firey observes, with the diffusion of penitentials that echoed Old Testament attitudes toward impure food.[85] Just as in Jewish dietary laws, some penitential stipulations declared certain animal flesh to be categorically impure.[86] However, this was a minor detail in most early medieval collections, which instead located pollution in animals that had tasted human flesh, participated in coitus with humans, been lacerated or eaten by predators, or already died and begun to decay.[87] Similarly, the texts declared liquids (whether well water, soups, or porridges) to be impure if an animal had tasted them, excreted in them, or died in them. Rob Meens rightly states that it is difficult to detect a consistent rationale in these stipulations, but he speculates that fears of pollution centered upon substances that blurred boundaries—such as flesh eaten by both animals and humans or food contaminated by fluids that had escaped the body.[88]

The importance of cosmological boundaries surely does underpin penitential food restrictions, but we can also note the theoretical overlap between impure food in the penitentials and unhealthy food in the medical writings surveyed above. By far, the majority of penitential dietary prohibitions concern the danger of carrion and meat already torn by animals, which Firey and Meens have associated with taboos against blood pollution.[89] So, too, injunctions against consuming food that is "half-cooked" (*semicoctum*), found in a series of penitentials from the early eighth through the tenth centuries, can be read as stemming originally from anxieties about bloody meat.[90] However, as it appears in the texts, the prohibition encompasses not only fears about blood but about rawness more generally and, as with the approach to carrion, fits within a broader framework of taboos regarding spoiling and putrefaction. Anthimus's text, as we have seen, is pervaded by a concern about decay (*corruptilla*). While this is often attributed to raw or overly dense food that cannot be broken down, there is also danger in meat, poultry, or fish left lying around and not being eaten soon after it is killed.[91] Likewise, Anthimus warns that fruit picked while raw and left to soften for a few days does not tend toward ripeness but toward "putridity" and will produce noxious humors if consumed.[92]

Both medical and penitential traditions seem to assume an inevitability about bodily "exposure" and a corresponding tolerance toward those whose health was somewhat compromised. The scribes who put together medical collections presupposed that rules would be broken and thus interspersed preventative and therapeutic regimens. Penitentials, similarly, acknowledged a gray zone in which one might sit between pure and impure states. Those who ate carrion but did so unknowingly, for example, typically received a significantly lighter penance.[93] And, as we have already seen, the penitentials did not forbid polluted food at all costs—those in necessity were permitted to eat otherwise proscribed meat. Such gradations of penance seem to shift the emphasis from the material, bodily level to the moral, intangible one. From this perspective, Firey has proposed that the penitentials indicate an attention to *remedying*, rather than prohibiting, the pollutions that inexorably arose within human society. One could not, as she points out, prevent a curious mouse from leaping into a soup pot.[94] And yet, I would add, one could, for instance, keep soups covered to deter mice from falling in. In this sense, Firey's theory that the texts were intended primarily to *remedy* pollution rather than prevent it does not completely capture the extent to which the penitentials *did* urge greater attention and care toward the preparation of food. Just as medical treatises advocated, penitentials impelled Christian kitchens to test that food was fully cooked before serving it and to more vigorously guarantee that meat came to the table shortly after it was killed. This precise convergence of a medicalized and spiritualized discourse is expressed in Charlemagne citing "cleanliness" as the reason for the stewards on royal estates to keep a closer eye on those handling food products and to ensure that wine was crushed in a press and not by foot.[95]

In addition to those foods that provoked alarm because of their associations with blood, bodily fluids, animal defilement, decay, and generalized uncleanliness, the penitentials fostered an attitude of caution toward a substance that was, strictly according to its nature, neither polluting nor susceptible to putrefaction—wine.[96] Despite the ubiquity of wine as a drink at the royal table and within monastic houses, it was not treated as an innocuous substance. It occupied an unusual conceptional space because it was sacralized through association with Christ's blood but, at the same time, condemned for stimulating drunkenness and luxury.[97] Very few actions symbolized a rejection of moderation and an embrace of excess as much as inebriation. The Council of Mainz in 813 declared that drunkenness was the font of all vices and warranted excommunication until it had been absolved through penance.[98] Einhard observed that Charlemagne himself abhorred inebriation and consumed wine only in small amounts.[99] While on the one hand, the emperor urged the systematic production of wine on royal estates, on the other hand, he admonished the *seniores* of the realm to set a worthy example of sobriety for the rest of society.[100] Discretion in drink was thus in no way limited to those who had taken religious vows.

The sense of danger arose primarily because of the observable effect that wine had on the rational nature of the soul. In his dialogue on rhetoric, for instance, Alcuin remarked that memory is undermined by drunkenness, "which does the greatest possibly injury to all scholarly pursuits, undermining the health of the body, and also weakening the integrity of the soul."[101] On the other hand, Alcuin was certainly no teetotaler and apparently received wine supplies from none other than the royal *medicus* Wintar.[102] This was probably not a coincidence, as wine was commonly the substrate for brewed potions and was also treated as a medicine unto itself. An entire text on the *virtus* of wine, transmitted in a later ninth-century manuscript, describes how varietals with different properties have specific effects on the body, some salubrious and others adverse depending on whether one is sick or healthy.[103] Wine's intense nature meant that it needed to be employed carefully, for it was equally capable of strengthening the blood or of harming a patient too weak to handle strong food.[104] The same language of moderation found in moral literature was applied to wine, with the best for both hale and infirm being "in the middle" (neither old or young, nor dark or white, but a ripe, red variety).

Wine was known to keep the stomach in optimal condition, thereby enabling it to perform its role as guardian of the body. Two of the lay handbooks, the commentary by Smaragdus, and the Lorsch apology all articulated a similar position on the importance of wine, drawing authority from Paul's advice to Timothy (1 Tm 5:23) not to drink water but to take a little wine "on account of your stomach and your frequent infirmities." Jonas explained the difference between wine's innate properties and its misuse by human society: "It is an excessive consumption of wine, not its natural quality, that causes and nourishes luxury . . . since the moderate use of wine comforts an infirm stomach, but drunkenness debilitates the soul and body."[105] Implying that some of his contemporaries might disagree, Paulinus baldly declared to his lay readers that wine "was given to us as a cure for the body, thus let us not judge it something pernicious."[106]

Given the power of wine to corrupt the image of God in the soul—that is, the ruling, reasoning function—it could well have been categorized as a polluting, prohibited food. Instead, Carolingian reformers turned to the language of moderation in order to delineate its legitimate use. It is striking that these attempts to exonerate wine did not rely upon its liturgical function, highlighting its presence in the Mass. Rather, even in nonmedical genres, writers commonly invoked its curative properties and underscored the drink's fundamental place within a medical regimen for a healthy body.

## The Laity and Medicine

When we read about the effects of digestion in Hildemar's commentary on the Rule, we can assume that he himself likely had access to medical codices at the library of Corbie and that some of his monastic readers might have been motivated to pursue further study on the topic.[107] But can we say the same about the lay nobles who encountered Paulinus's comments about the stomach? Given that three of the four manuals for the laity emphasized the importance of regulating food and drink, one would expect dietary medicine to figure notably in discussions of Carolingian moral reforms. However, the periodization of early medieval medicine as *Mönchsmedizin* has cast a long shadow, and the role that both prophylactic and acute medicine played in the life of the Carolingian laity has rarely been considered (even on the battlefield). For the most part, due to the assigned production of extant medical manuscripts to monastic scriptoria, learned (or written) medicine has been associated solely with monasteries and a few episcopal centers.[108] Scholars have acknowledged the presence of court physicians but have not speculated on healthcare for the rest of the laity. Indeed, the typical assumption has been that monastic infirmaries cared solely for those within the cloister, as stipulated in the Benedictine Rule.

While acknowledging the lack of firm evidence, I want to suggest that part of the ninth-century reimagining of medical practice as a Christian art involved individual laypeople assuming a new level of medical responsibility. Monastics were already subject to a regimented and communal mode of life, within which the adoption of seasonal routines or dietetic calendars fit easily. The fact that ecclesiastical authors were recommending to their lay peers a heightened attentiveness to eating (both in content and manner) may well point to the increasing value of medical treatises outside the cloister. Certainly, the laity would have grown accustomed to the notion of external regulation of diet through imperial fasts, which, beginning in the late 770s, ordered all healthy subjects to abstain from meat, wine, and beer for two or three days.[109] What, though, can be said about the laity's daily, habitual practices? Here, I explore three different avenues for clues regarding the lay participation in so-called *Mönchsmedizin*: first, the emphasis on "self-help" within the medical corpus; second, the evidence for lay ownership of medical material; and third, the penetration of monastic space for the sake of healing.

In the *Handbook* sent to her son, Dhuoda evocatively impressed upon William the personalized nature of the advice therein. She hoped that by infusing her own maternal voice in the text and crafting a work suited to William's particular circumstances, the handbook could act as substitute for her physical presence.[110]

> I rejoice that, even if I am apart from you in body, the little book before you may remind you, when you read it, of what you should do on my behalf. . . . Even if you eventually have many more books, read this little work of mine often. May you, with God's help, be able to understand it to your own profit. You will find in it all you may wish to know in compact form.[111]

Although Dhuoda intended her handbook to circulate beyond her family to other members of the Carolingian elite (as we saw in Chapter 2), she did not believe that these expressions of personal devotion would detract from the appeal of her work.

This should not surprise us. The prefaces of ninth-century spiritual handbooks and treatises within ninth-century medical compendia both noticeably incline toward the personal. They seek to establish an intimate relationship between writer and reader. Calling attention to the unassuming style of the work, the authors underscore how daily consultation of the text serves to bring two people together in thought and purpose, despite distances in time and space. Take, for example, the opening to a popular medical treatise entitled the *Letter of Hippocrates to Maecenas*, where the tone is that of someone writing to a cherished friend.[112]

> Showing every care, I have sent this arrangement, a most reliable guardian of your health, which you ought to consider as diligently as it was written. And for the healing of your body everything has been explored, which I verified through my experience and quickly summed up. . . . Therefore, you will have me with you [in essence], if you handle and read often my little book, which will be able to impart council to you in all matters even while I am absent.[113]

Both Dhuoda and "Hippocrates" draw attention to the status of the text as an in-situ counselor or guardian. They emphasize that their works are handbooks: relatively short in length, condensed in content, and designed to be read frequently.

The other lay manuals may not have been as personalized as Dhuoda's, but these, too, presented themselves as fashioned for one individual. Still, we know that they were acquired and used by many more. Similarly, numerous early medieval medical texts appeared as "letters," even if this was apparent only in a title that indicated the sender and recipient. Apart from the herbal or head-to-toe remedy collection, the epistle was the most common format in ninth-century medical codices.[114] To some extent, this reveals earlier developments: Marcellus of Bordeaux prefaced his *Book of Medications* (ca. 400) with seven different letters from Greco-Roman authorities in addition to his own short dedication to his sons;[115] and scholars have argued for the existence of two other letter-collections (*Briefcorpus* I and II) that traveled as units in the early Middle Ages.[116] But ninth-century scribal work also furnishes examples of epistolary-enthusiasm: the prefaces to late antique medical writings being detached and presented as stand-alone letters, of nonletters being turned into letters as they were copied, and of shorter treatises being titled as *epistolae* and grouped together under the label *Book of Letters*.[117] Since most of these do not adhere strictly to an epistolary form, it appears that merely the superficial presentation of texts as letters served an important purpose.[118] The epistolary mode was a marker of authority and efficacy; though the medical advice espoused therein was broadly applicable, the familiar and confidential tone cast it as personally tailored. Health was an intimate matter. We have already discussed (in Chapter 3) how medical and moral literature shared a similar vocabulary. Here, we can observe how the very format through which ninth-century readers approached advice concerning the *salus* of body and soul likewise shared many parallels.

We should also note the emphasis on brevity in many of these treatises. Just as Jonas assured Matfrid that he had skimmed through volumes of scripture and patristic writings to glean what was most relevant, so did medical writers emphasize that they had distilled a vast amount of potentially relevant information into a (relatively) brief summary.[119] This reflects a late antique (specifically, post-Galen) trend toward encyclopedic organization.[120] But it also evinces, as Wallis has eloquently demonstrated, an early medieval "indifference to textual authenticity" when it came to medicine.[121] Scribes freely mixed-and-matched authors, titles, and snippets of text to create new synopses (often arranged into reader-friendly books and chapters).

It is equally interesting that many medical treatises popular with the Carolingians were originally composed for a lay practitioner or nonexpert. The only authentic Galenic text to circulate widely in Latin, for example, was *On the Method of Healing to Glaucon*, originally composed for Galen's friend, a philosopher taking a long journey who desired a medical handbook to carry with him.[122] Likewise, the *Letter to Pentadius* claimed to be a familial passing-down of knowledge from Vindicianus to his nephew.[123] And of the two works by Oribasius translated into Latin, one was a collection of relatively simple medicines for his friend, the philosopher Eunapius, and the other (addressed to his son Eustathius) declared itself useful both to those unlearned in medicine and to physicians.[124] *Pliny's Medicine*, meanwhile, began with the author's recollection of being swindled by doctors and promised to provide a handbook of common remedies for the self-sufficient traveler.[125]

Such works manifestly draw attention to their conciseness and appropriateness for a broad, unspecialized audience.[126] The prefaces reiterate that the knowledge and remedies that follow will enable the reader to heal himself (or herself, as the advice is rarely gender-specific) without the assistance of professional physicians and often using local, easily obtainable substances. In just this vein, the author of *On the Nature of the Belly* states explicitly that s/he has brought together this information for the nonspecialist as well as expert, and thus the physiological explanation is not abstruse but "is easily understood by a wise man."[127] Marcellus, likewise, tells his sons that his collection "will furnish you with the necessary aid and remedies without the intervention of a *medicus*."[128] And, finally, the exceedingly popular *Letter to Antiochus* ends with the promise that if "you use all these things at their proper times, you will accomplish complete health without the help of any *medici*."[129] These texts repeatedly affirm the possibility of self-care, implying that every intelligent individual is capable of understanding and regulating the inner movements of the body and its frequent infirmities.

If numerous medical texts circulating in the Carolingian period were designated as suitable for a learned but untrained audience who practiced healing in domestic or rural settings, what can be said about the evidence for the use of medical manuscripts outside the monastery? None survive that can be fixed to the Carolingian court (though recall that Charlemagne ordered his court notary to copy the remedies of Quintus Serenus). However, there is the folded medical codex that ended up at Saint-Gall and may have been used by an itinerant *medicus*, and Clare Pilsworth suggests that two pocket-sized codices (one containing remedies and the Hippocratic *Aphorisms*, and the other, part of a psalter, two recipes, and a pseudo-Galenic pharmaceutical text) might have been equally appropriate for an educated layperson as for a cleric or monk.[130] Consider also a manuscript produced in Tours, which contains a monthly dietetic guide, a *lunare*, and remedies for purging the stomach, alongside selections from the *Etymologies*, the *Lex Salica*, excerpts from Visigothic law, a list of Frankish kings, and a letter to those going to war. There is every likelihood that this is the type of collection that was deemed useful for a Carolingian lay noble in the fulfillment of his secular and spiritual duties.[131]

Two extant wills of Carolingian noble families survive from the ninth century, and these offer comparatively strong evidence for lay interest in medical works.[132] The first was drawn up around 863 by Eberhard, count of Friuli, and his wife Gisela, the daughter of Louis the Pious; the second was written in 876 for the nobleman Eccard, count of Mâcon.[133] Among other goods, both designate the bequeathal of books, of which Eberhard owned around fifty and Eccard somewhat fewer. Eccard bequeathed to Theutberga, the widow of Lothar II and lay abbess of Aveney, a manuscript that he termed simply "one book of medicine" (*medicinalis liber I*).[134] He also owned two books of prognostics (*pronosticorum libri II*), which he gave to Bishop Raganfridus of Meaux.[135] Eberhard and Gisela owned a book of beasts (*liber bestiarum*), which they gave to their eldest son, Unroch, and a manuscript they termed the *Physionomia Lopi medici*, which they bequeathed to their son Rodolphus (their daughter Judith, meanwhile, received a copy of Alcuin's *On the Virtues and Vices*).[136]

Although we cannot identify with certainty the contents of these codices, both wills undoubtably testify to a lay familiarity with medicine.[137] Pierre Riché suggests that the bestiary was the *Physiologus* (a set of moralized beast tales that survives in eight manuscripts from the eighth and ninth centuries), yet a pharmaceutical work with that precise title (*Liber bestiarum*) appears in a medical codex from the early ninth century.[138] The two books of prognostics may have been Julian of Toledo's *Prognosticum* (as Riché proposes), but they were more likely a collection of various medical and weather prognostics, especially as they are listed with "another [book] on agriculture."[139] The ambiguously titled *Liber medicinalis* was most likely a standard compilation of medical treatises, herbals, and remedies, as listed in monastic library catalogues and attested by the majority of extant manuscripts. Finally, Sébastien Bricout makes a persuasive case for identifying the *Physionomia Lopi medici* as the late antique *Book of Physiognomy*.[140] While physiognomy is not a subject raised in any extant medical compendium of the ninth century, its concern with studying signs exhibited by the body implicitly associated it with the art of medicine and the fundamentals of prognostication.[141] That Eberhard and Gisela themselves considered it a medical work is evident in the title they gave to the codex, listing a *medicus* as the author. Medical works may have constituted a small percentage of each noble family's collection—as they did within monastic libraries—but they nevertheless stood beside the psalms, many works of the Church Fathers, and narratives of Christian history as a genre that was valued by the Carolingian laity.

Unfortunately, no extant manuscript can be securely linked with the medical books mentioned by Eccard or Eberhard. However, two medical manuscripts preserved at the monasteries of Reichenau and Saint-Gall might conceivably have been intended for, or owned by, a noble family.[142] The first is a collection of medical material most likely produced in northern Italy in the second half of the ninth century and brought north of the Alps shortly afterward. The codex contains bloodletting treatises, recipes, prognostics, an herbal, a list of head-to-toe conditions, the poem of Quintus Serenus, Oribasius's work for Eustathius, the *Letter to Antiochus*, the *Letter to Pentadius*, and numerous texts on diet (including a heavily redacted version of the *Letter of Anthimus*).[143] Indeed, the compiler of this manuscript seemingly decided to make diet and the health of the stomach the dominant theme across this (relatively lengthy) medical volume.[144] Scribbled in the upper border of a page in the middle of the compilation a note reads: "In the name of Christ, Alberic, count by the grace of God and of the lord emperor. . . ."[145] Though there was an Albrich who was a count in the upper Rhine region in the mid-ninth century, there is no evidence that links the note to him. Still, even without more clarity about the meaning of the marginalia, the mention of a *comes* (count) inclines one to consider lay engagement with the codex.[146] Undoubtedly, it is exactly the type of manuscript that could have constituted the *Liber medicinalis* in Eccard's will.

Certainly, several decades earlier, Alcuin assumed that a lay nobleman would be familiar with practical dietary medicine, the kind used while traveling in order to prevent illness. Writing to Count Chrodgar about his impending expedition to Benevento as part of a military campaign under Charlemagne's son Pippin, Alcuin inserted a warning about bodily health in the midst of his spiritual counsel. "You know very well what type of danger threatens you there [in Benevento] on account of the pestilential air of that region."[147] The count needed to remain vigilant in Italy, Alcuin stressed, repeating advice that he had also imparted to a pupil traveling there: "Italy is an unhealthy land and produces harmful foods; therefore, take the greatest care in deciding what, when, how and what types of food to enjoy. And, most importantly, avoid repeated intoxication because intense fever often overcomes the incautious as a result of wine's heat."[148]

The second manuscript for which I propose a lay audience is a compilation of computus texts, works on logic and grammar, a moral manual, and medical writings, possibly put together at Reichenau in the first half of the ninth century.[149] As it stands now, the manuscript is neatly bookended by texts devoted to the interpretation of time, with selections from Bede's *On the Reckoning of Time* at the start and various medical writings focused on temporal change at the end. These writings include the *Letter to Antiochus*, a treatise on the four humors, a prognostic on signs of death, an illness *lunare*, a list of Egyptian Days, two pages of various recipes, and a text titled *On Moderation during the Times of the Year*, which discusses bloodletting or purging in relation to different seasons and regions.[150] Unique to this manuscript is the combination of medical treatises with a lay spiritual manual, the *Book for Gregoria*.[151] This is a conduct manual, written for a fifth-century Roman noblewoman, which describes the Christian life as a battle between virtues and vices, just like Alcuin's work for Wido.[152] Gregoria is forcefully reminded that her soul has no gender, and thus, even as a member of the weaker sex, she must become a soldier of Christ. Above all, she is urged to cultivate patience and stability of mind in carrying out her marital duties.

The inclusion of this manual for a Christian laywoman suggests the codex may have been compiled for a noble family.[153] The explicit to the "little book" announces that it covers "wifely duties, or what a wife ought to do with regard to the omnipotent God and what with regard to her husband."[154] It would hardly be surprising to find this work among the libraries of the Carolingian laity, just as Eberhard and Gisela bequeathed their copy of Alcuin's *On the Virtues and Vices* to their daughter. As the household manager, a wife may well have overseen the domestic care of the sick and found the medical texts in the codex to be of use in that duty.[155] The variety of subjects covered in the manuscript may also have offered an education in the liberal arts (similar to that obtained by Dhuoda), with the *Book for Gregoria* imparting guidance on the health of the soul just as the medical texts addressed the health of the body.

That said, we should not assume that any manuscript geared toward a laywoman would have been out of place in a monastic setting. Historians have puzzled over the presence of gynecological treatises in codices that were owned by male monasteries; most often, they gloss over the issue, perhaps unsure whether to interpret said texts as evidence of male monks finding titillation in descriptions of the "unknown" female body. Zubin Mistry, however, has offered the bold suggestion that these texts were valued because they did exactly what they claimed to do—assist with problems of fertility, female reproductive health, and the dangers of childbearing. Monasteries lay at the intersection of many different networks (familial, spiritual, economic, and charitable), any of which may have precipitated a healing encounter.[156] We can imagine monks offering masses for barrenness, dispensing medical counsel to female noblewomen (who may have been their sisters, cousins, or mothers), and treating the reproductive issues of their servile tenants.[157] The stability of the monastery, after all, depended on its lay labor force and its lay patrons.

Mistry's arguments are novel in large part because of an entrenched resistance to considering *Mönchsmedizin* as a phenomenon that crossed the boundaries of the cloister wall. It is certainly true that Benedict's Rule only specified care for other sick brothers, and no ninth-century source explicitly reveals the treatment of laypeople within the monastery. Furthermore, the Carolingian councils of the early ninth century endowed the purity of the cloister with new significance, seeking to draw firmer boundaries between the polluted affairs of the world and the sacred contemplative life within, even as monasteries became ever larger economic engines.[158] Total separation was impossible, however, and thus a monastery needed to accommodate both constant transgression of its borders and an inner sanctum open only to the monks.[159]

Although never conceived as an architectural blueprint, the Plan of Saint-Gall, created by monks at Reichenau around 830, expresses imagined possibilities for how this accommodation might be achieved.[160] In surveying the entire plan, one sees that a significant percentage of the building space (especially if the gardens, livestock, and workshops are excluded) is devoted to medical care (see Figure 18).[161] In the northeastern quadrant of the monastic complex, there is a secluded cloister and chapel for infirm brothers, with a storeroom, refectory, warming room, dormitory, room for the very sick, and dwelling for the master of the sick. Nearby stands a building called "the house of the *medici*," with another bedroom for the very sick, a pharmacy, and "quarters for the *medicus* himself" (generally thought to be the head physician). Separated by a fence (with a passage) is a building for bloodletting, the taking of medications, and replenishment.[162] Beside it is a small bathhouse and a kitchen dedicated to preparing meals for the infirm and the phlebotomized.[163] Clearly, this highly specialized series of rooms, with their accompanying treatments, goes far beyond Benedict of Nursia's stipulation that a separate room, attendant, baths, and meat be provided for sick brothers.

The authors of the plan say nothing about the people designated as *medici*. They may have envisioned them as monks, but the fact that their house is distinct from the cloister of the sick and in a corner distant from the abbey church suggests they may be outsiders, possibly clergy or even laymen.[164] The existence of two rooms for the "very sick" could allude to different degrees or types of illness, but it could also imply that nonmonks might be housed in the physicians' quarters.[165] The fence between the physicians' house and the treatment area could be to segregate the physicians or to mark off polluted spaces, including a kitchen where meat was cooked and a building designated for patients producing effluvia. What is apparent from the diagram is that the technical medical spaces are aligned directly above other

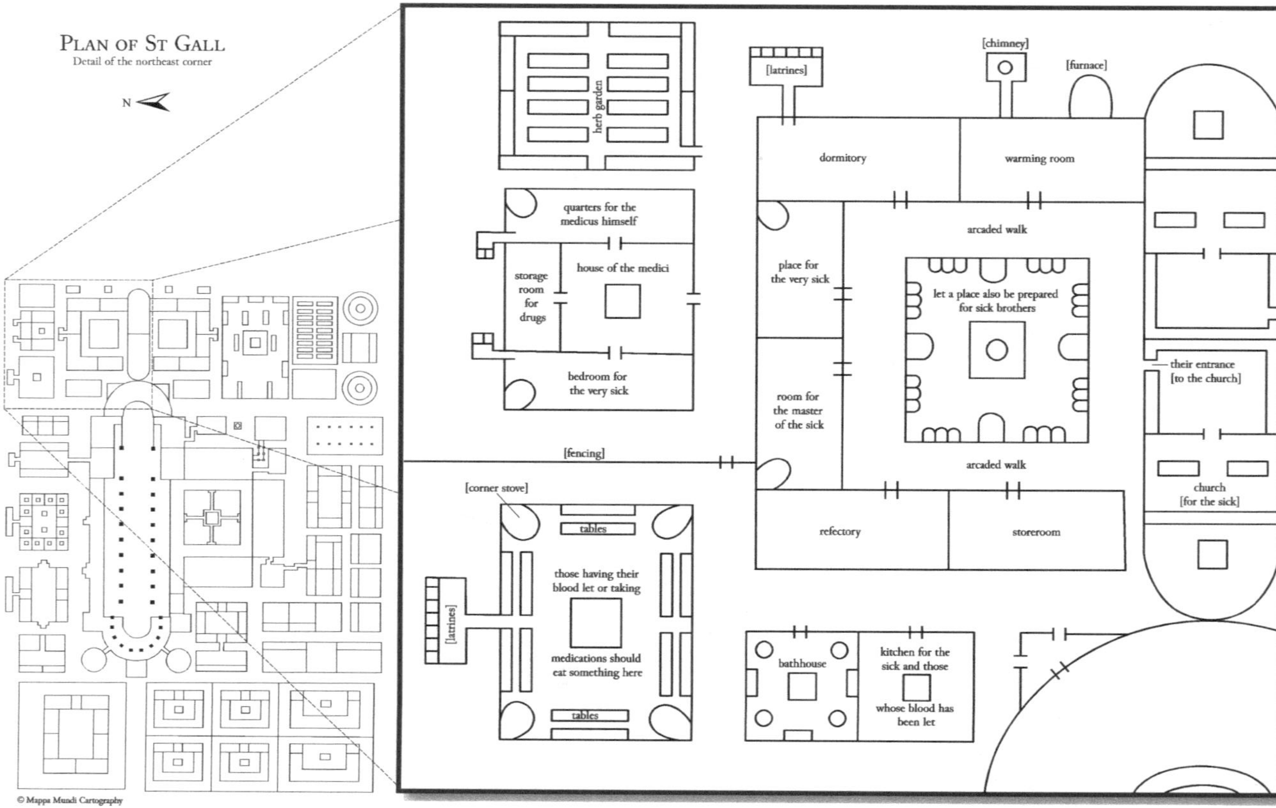


Figure 18. Healthcare corner of the Plan of Saint-Gall (St. Gallen, Stiftsbibliothek, Cod. Sang. 1092), with translations of the Latin inscriptions. Drawing by Erik Goosmann, Mappa Mundi Cartography.

sites in the monastery in which laypeople might be found, such as the school, the guest house, and quarters for the servants of the abbot. Furthermore, we know from charter evidence that the housing and care of elderly laypeople could take place within the monastic walls (usually in exchange for donations of property). Thus, although the plan offers insight only into architectural concepts and not necessarily realities, it seems far from speculative to suggest that sick laypersons among an institution's patrons, dependents, and neighbors assumed the possibility of being admitted within the monastery for treatment, the prescription of drugs, and the receipt of expert medical advice.[166]

## Blood, Balance, and Soul

The *Book of Physiognomy* owned by Eberhard and Gisela was likely a head-to-toe description of how to read different parts of the body in order to ascertain a person's character.[167] Traversing such parts as the head, eyes, nose, neck, belly, back, and legs, it details how particular colors, shapes, and sizes of different features indicate a person who is angry, foolish, shameless, stupid, violent, of good habits, temperate, or spiteful (and so forth). For our purposes, the most striking aspect of the text is the underlying logic used to account for the connection between physical appearance and character. This, in the words of Loxus/Lopus the *medicus*, lies in the fact that the blood is "the seat of the soul," and thus the purpose of physiognomy is:[168]

> To observe and investigate from the quality of the body the quality of the soul. For Loxus established that blood is the dwelling place (*habitaculum*) of the soul and that the whole body as well as its individual parts (those capable of signifying) give forth diverse signs concerning the strength or weakness of the blood and whether it is thick or thin and whether it follows easy and direct channels or is restricted and awry in its course.[169]

There is no extended explanation of how the soul is lodged within the blood and, apart from general comments that abundant blood furnishes a strong body but a weak mind (and vice versa for scant blood), there is no attempt to link individual traits with a certain quality of the blood.[170] Nevertheless, this text presents a clear link between the literature on the soul examined in

Chapter 1 and the lay manuals (one of which was owned by Eberhard's family) analyzed in Chapter 2.[171] The *Book of Physiognomy* suggests that the vices and virtues that warred within a person's inner self were made manifest on the external body and could there be scrutinized by a discerning observer.[172] This was because the spiritual health of the individual was directly linked to the state of the blood, with the suggestion that the nature of the soul could be influenced by the condition of the humor that flowed throughout the *corpus*.

If the principles central to physiognomy allude to the importance of "managing" the blood, such an approach is explicitly endorsed in Carolingian legislation, which stands as the first documented instance of regularized bloodletting within the monastic life. The earliest, albeit oblique, reference is found in a capitulary from 789, which indicates some concern with the pallor of nuns who had received bloodletting.[173] The second stems from various documents produced in connection with the reforming synods held at Aachen in 816, 817, and 818/19, which mandated emendations to the rules governing Benedictine monasteries. These announced that phlebotomy should be allowed to anyone in need and special food and drink granted afterward.[174] Statutes from Corbie monastery (ca. 826) dictated that reading be performed during the letting of blood, implying that the therapy might have had a contemplative angle as well as a tactile one.[175]

In charting the development of periodic bloodletting within Western monasticism, Mary Yearl suggests that phlebotomy was a medical practice that took on spiritual meaning because blood was known to constitute flesh and semen and was thus intimately associated with the causes of sin; as "the flesh lusts against the spirit [Gal 5:17]," so was bloodletting a means of diminishing the danger of corporeal vigor.[176] Textual traditions in the ninth century, however, present a different reading of the consequence of bloodletting.[177] If the soul was housed in the blood, phlebotomy offered an avenue by which the manipulation of the body could directly affect spiritual well-being. The medical *Letter to Maecenas* includes a lengthy description of the relationship between the health of the blood and that of the soul. "When the blood is sound (*integer*), without doubt it strengthens the soul," the author asserts. But too much food and drink corrupts the blood with rawness, and "when [the blood] strays beyond the path of nature, it introduces all sorts of vices into the body. . . . And so blood also damages the soul." As we saw above, overabundance or rawness (*cruditas*) is said to contaminate the blood and create a physical environment inconducive to the well-being of the soul.[178]

Certainly, Carolingian theologians never *equated* the soul with the blood; yet they emphasized the soul's diffusion throughout all the parts of the body, a fact that correlated with the natural disposition of the blood. Isidore himself had declared that "blood is the possession of a soul."[179] And medical writings like the *Letter to Maecenas*, the *Book of Physiognomy* and the *Dispute of Plato and Aristotle* (examined in Chapter 1) spoke to the belief that the soul was ambiguously embedded within the blood.[180] Indeed, all but one of the extant copies of the *Dispute* survive immediately alongside instructions on how to perform phlebotomy.[181] A conscious thread was thus created between theory and action, with the one text addressing where the soul was located and the other providing the technical and anatomical information needed to manage the soul's well-being within the body.

According to broad models of medical development, the premodern period adhered to a Hippocratic notion of "health" as a balance among the various humors that constituted the core bodily elements.[182] Yet, texts from the ninth century—the first moment at which a medieval medical tradition comes into view—speak less about balance and much more about moderation (and its binary, extravagance). One could see balance and moderation as two sides of the same coin, but I believe the terminology matters here, primarily because the latter highlights the fear of excess that historians such as Shigehisa Kuriyama have argued was a persistent strain of premodern humoral mentalities.[183]

A passage in the *Book of Physiognomy* betrays this assumption. The author begins, "We have said many times that excesses (*nimietates*) are full of vice and the middle (*medietatem*) is optimal." But s/he then reflects on the impossibility of ever knowing the true middle point and questions whether this should be the universal paradigm. "Sometimes a mixture (*temperamentum*) is to be judged optimal, not when it is set in the middle between two extremes, but when it verges more to one side."[184] What we find here is not the belief that flawless health rests in the perfect equalization of opposing qualities; rather, this text gives voice to an overriding preoccupation with the dangers of excess.

Ninth-century moralists insisted that an individual could maintain a moderate lifestyle, such that a body of tempered features would give witness to a perfect soul within.[185] In light of these beliefs, it should not strike us as incongruous that the treatise on the soul which Alcuin composed for Charlemagne's cousin may have been bound together with one of the extant Carolingian copies of the *Letter of Anthimus* as well as a late antique work on agriculture and a theological tract on the Holy Trinity.[186] This codex suggests an understanding of ninth-century "practical" knowledge that was not at all restricted to the visible world but encompassed everything from agricultural techniques to trinitarian doctrine, with medicine for the body and meditation on the nature of the soul occupying a central position.

# CONCLUSION

This book began with a recipe for removing hair and drying out the humors supposedly endorsed by one Pardulus of Laon, bishop from 848 to 856. The very same Pardulus left a record of his own medical expertise in a letter to Archbishop Hincmar of Reims (author of one of the soul treatises discussed in Chapter 1), in the wake of the latter's recovery from a particularly bad illness. Pardulus urged his superior to show greater care for his body than he had done in the past, underscoring the way in which the ecclesiastical order's well-being was intertwined with Hincmar's.[1] "If you despise yourself in your accustomed manner and, for that reason, care very little for the health of your body [you fail your faithful flock]. Instead, you ought to be mindful of them and studiously guard the health restored to you through divine grace and abstain thoroughly from everything that is contrary to [combatting] your infirmity."[2] As a role model with weighty responsibilities, Hincmar should have known that he was to regulate his body carefully, maintaining its vigor and not pursuing illness in the name of asceticism.

Although Pardulus points to divine grace as the facilitator of Hincmar's recovery, he by no means ignores human agency; rather, he writes specifically to instruct the archbishop about the therapeutic steps he ought to take to maintain his body and avoid future sickness. What is particularly interesting about this letter is that Pardulus follows his reference to abstention with a detailed dietary regimen. He instructs Hincmar not to fast excessively, not to eat tiny fishes, and not to consume any raw foods. He explains that fish and meat should be eaten a little while after they are slaughtered because that allows time for them to be properly gutted and the flesh to be dried out with salt. He advises the archbishop to select wine of a medium strength, to take cooked beans to clear out any phlegm lurking in the body, and to use both bacon and red meat to revive his stomach.

Some details may vary, but we observe here a number of parallels between Pardulus's recommendations and those found in dietary texts like

Anthimus's, which proved to be some of the most popular medical writings among the Carolingian elite. Unlike Latin regimen literature from the twelfth century onward, which was grounded in the regulation of the six non-naturals (air, food, exercise, sleep, excretions, and emotions), similar texts from the early Middle Ages focused predominantly on food and drink.[3] It was through daily attention to the time of eating and the preparation, quantity, and type of sustenance that the soul's dominion over the body became manifest and was constantly reinforced. Pardulus was clear that physical *sanitas* undergirded the individual's ability to perform good works, but he also implied that bodily integrity had a spiritual role beyond the functional: health manifested the individual's attention to the forces of the inner cavity and a desire to burnish the image of God through the exercise of rational governance.

Despite being Hincmar's subordinate, Pardulus seems to have been comfortable rebuking the archbishop in a manner similar to that which an abbot might use toward a monk fasting to excess. He did so by drawing on language that emphasized the pursuit of the common good and suppression of personal desire. In his reflection on the monastic life, Smaragdus of Saint-Mihiel succinctly summed up a Christian mandate to find a "middle way," one that could preserve the health of the individual and of the broader community:

> But the physical needs of the flesh are to be discreetly regulated, so that it be neither completely destroyed nor immoderately relaxed. For the weakness of the body breaks the powers of the soul and causes the natural capacity of the mind to grow feeble. Whatever is done with moderation fosters the health of body and soul.[4]

Alongside the idealized ascetic, whose flesh had been subdued and mortified in order to elevate the spiritual, we must also recognize the exemplar of a healthy religious, who regulated and stabilized the *corpus* using techniques of moderation. Both were "types" that competed for relevance in the Carolingian world, and works of admonition were as likely to feature prompts to fortify the body as to chastise it.

Nor was disciplined self-monitoring thought to be applicable only to those in a monastery. Moderation was essential for bishops and kings, monks and laypeople, men and women alike. Carolingian nobles were avid collectors of a diversity of Latin writings, and the assemblage of texts found in certain ninth-century codices, as we saw in Chapter 7, offers the strong impression of a lay audience. The governance of the body was not a private matter but a duty, as Pardulus seems to have assumed, that fell under the public eye and ought to invite commentary from those tasked with admonishing both the powerful and the lowly. Such an attitude emerges in Einhard's *Life of Charlemagne*, when the author subtly criticizes the emperor for failing to stick to a diet of boiled meats after his physicians repeatedly condemned the unwholesomeness of his predilection for roasts. For the sake of good order within the realm, it was especially important that the emperor give due attention to his bodily state, monitoring his health and making appropriate preparations for his death. But Charlemagne did neither, Einhard reports. He stubbornly refused to give credence to omens predicting his death and, when it came to sustenance, neglected his constitution in pursuit of pleasure.[5] Even when it came to a great and virtuous leader, the *Life* suggests, moderation was not necessarily an easy path but was a daily battle against small temptations. That made it all the more important for a responsible Christian to use acquired knowledge to develop habits and techniques by which the body's necessities could be met without straying into luxury or excess.

Historians of humoral medicine have often explained its enduring attraction over the centuries by underscoring its focus on the individual. Every person was distinguished by a unique constitution, and a productive healing encounter was thought to be grounded in an intimate relationship between patient and doctor. Details of a patient's lifestyle, demeanor, physical features, emotions, and environment all contributed to a flexible notion of one's complexion or temperament and played a significant role in diagnosis and treatment. Unlike modern clinical medicine, then, the focus was not on subsuming the individual within a larger statistical grouping but on discovering and maintaining a distinct set of bodily fluids and rhythms through adherence to a personalized regimen.

A particularly significant inflection point in the development of this "complexional" model was the growing popularity of *regimen sanitatis* literature (in both poetry and prose) across Europe in the thirteenth and fourteenth centuries, much of it accessible in a new form as it was translated into the vernaculars. Yet, as the foregoing chapters have argued, there was an intensifying interest in regimens well before the thirteenth century, as witnessed in many ninth-century medical manuscripts, alongside extant wills and library catalogues. It is beyond the scope of this book to say whether this trend outlasted the Carolingian era, yet its coherence in the period studied here testifies to a turn toward self-care and highlights an engagement with the interior life that, until recently, has long been deemed lacking in the early Middle Ages. A fascination with evaluating and preserving idiosyncratic humoral complexions has typically been associated with the supposed turn toward introspection that accompanied the "discovery of the individual" in the twelfth century.

This book joins many other studies in challenging such binaries, arguing that the Carolingian reforms spurred on a lively engagement with different forms of introspection.[6] In exploring how the boundaries of the "self" might be conceived, it has focused on assumptions about the building blocks of individual identity—the materiality of the soul and its interface with the flesh, the forces or virtues that structured the hidden space of this interface, and the means by which purity or pollution could be maintained, eradicated, and monitored through attention to the continuous processes of recomposition within the body. The goal was not "health" as an abstract norm or teleological summit but rather as the manifestation of conscious, rational choices. Medicine was one strategy or tool to be employed in the continual, labored transformation of the self.

In this struggle for salvation, bodily regimens were useful because they were seen as an ideal means of linking text with practice and thought with expression, binaries that surface again and again in the literature of the Carolingian *correctio*. Fundamental to the lay mirrors' designation as mirrors was the conviction that reflection on the soul would stimulate new modes of outward behavior, which could then be imitated by others. Yet the authors also assumed that the same evolution could run in the opposite direction: habitual action could cultivate inner awareness, the external could be internalized. Even if their approaches diverged, all four lay manuals offered to their audience a toolbox of spiritual technologies for cultivating mindfulness through external prompts. In this way, the act of eating, just like the act of praying, could stimulate a focus on the divine by directing attention to the functioning of the internal organs, an opaque realm in which food became flesh and fluid and shaped the physical boundaries of the ethereal soul as it coursed through the body.

What distinguishes the interest in regimens (and, indeed, medicine more broadly) in the ninth century from that manifested in the high Middle Ages is the fact that the desired outcome was not simply the care of the self or the familial unit but a deeper melding of personal health with broad understandings of the purity of the realm. Caring for the body was only partly about recognizing a state of personal difference regarding what lay under the skin—much more important was subverting that difference so as to bring the body within the parameters of a universal program. As Renie Choy has argued in regard to prayer, a defining feature of the Carolingian reforms was a focus on the "un-uniqueness" of the monk, whose intercession was not an expression of personal power but was grounded in a common liturgical schedule and participation in a shared social project.[7] This same monastic interest in the humility of "un-uniqueness" seems to have inflected the medical impulses of the ninth century, with its attention to collective temporal patterns and unexceptional bodily problems.

Overwhelmingly, the medical texts copied by Carolingian scribes favored a language of uniformity and standardization—all bodies were formed of the same materials, they became healthy or sick according to the same processes, and they ought to follow a schema in which all moved according to the same temporal rhythms. This basic outlook contrasts sharply with, for example, Hildegard of Bingen's approach to health, as found in her twelfth-century medical work *Causes and Cures*. There, the theoretical framework posits the existence of various humoral types, which are differentiated according to the two sexes and correspond with specific personality traits and moral inclinations.[8] Hildegard emphasizes that not all bodies are affected in the same way by habits surrounding chastity, arousal, menstruation, and emotional upheaval and is particularly attuned to the way in which maleness and femaleness are imprinted on the physical form (from the nature of the skull to the susceptibility to hernias).[9]

Of course, sex and age were also factors that shaped the trajectory of the body's movements in the medical texts advanced by the Carolingians, and, to a certain extent, medical treatises *did* recognize a difference between male and female bodies, most particularly in terms of the gynecological conditions and pains that women suffered.[10] However, neither the regimen nor the prognostic literature so favored by the elite indicated that women's bodies were subject to different temporal movements, that digestion produced unique humors in women, or that remedies might be conditioned by the sex of the patient.[11] It was entirely possible, in the ninth century, to produce a medical compilation that did not allude to gender distinctions when it came to physiology or treatment. Nevertheless, it cannot simply be assumed that the type of self-care advanced by Carolingian writings included all selves within this initiative. The oaths that imperial subjects had to swear applied only to men, and almost all of the treatises, letters, and handbooks we have examined over the course of this book were addressed to men (whether real or imagined).

These factors must have influenced the way in which the care of the body was gendered, as must the fact that the role of the *medicus* was implicitly restricted to men.

Yet, the starting point in managing the body was understanding the nature of one's soul—and Carolingian theological discourse concurred, in critical fashion, that women's souls were no different than men's. Women, just like men, needed to cultivate the image of God in their souls: by training the soul to exert its rational control over the body, medicine was a means of confirming the proper hierarchical relationship between the spiritual and material components of identity. As husbands and wives, the Carolingian laity were encouraged to follow a model of governance that set the man as the ruler over his wife and household, just like the soul over its body. But, as individuals, every lay person was supposed to conceptualize his/her own discrete soul as the lord of the body and the ruler over its members.[12] Within this theological framework, medical knowledge could function as a technique of the body that disrupted or transcended sex rather than reinforced it.

In broad strokes, then, although Hildegard's *Causes and Cures* was part of the same monastic milieu as the ninth-century manuscripts examined throughout this book, to categorize all early medieval practice as a uniform manifestation of *Mönchsmedizin* overlooks the intriguing discontinuities that shaped the transmission of classical medical knowledge across this period.[13] Hildegard had at least limited access to the new translations from Arabic being produced in southern Italy, and it is perhaps for this reason that her work seems to anticipate some of the assumptions of a later, complexional focus within humoral thought.[14] The shift in emphasis from universal rhythms to personalized physiology between early medieval and scholastic medical discourse highlights the (still underappreciated) fact that humoralism itself underwent continual transformations, even as the Hippocratic and Galenic framework of thought remained authoritative.[15]

At the same time that it is possible to locate disparities between the style of humoralism characteristic of the Carolingian period and that popular several centuries later, it is undeniable that strong continuities shaped the history of premodern medicine. Many of the themes charted throughout this book were not new to the ninth century but reflected concerns of Late Antiquity (if not earlier)—the importance of moderation, the need to investigate the body's mysterious internal cavity, the mandate to govern and monitor the self as a precondition to social responsibility. How, then, to avoid collapsing the early Middle Ages into one long story centered on the transmission of ideas "original" to classical Greek authors? Rather than searching for a specific text or theory that is original to the ninth century, we must recognize how a unique set of assumptions galvanized the selective clustering of texts and ideas. In an early contribution to the history of the body, Judith Perkins studied such clusters in the second century and concluded that discourse across the Roman Empire at that time gravitated toward an understanding of the individual as "a suffering self."[16] By contrast, I would argue, it was the self as rationally regulated harmony, balanced at a point of mutual benefit to both body and soul, that fueled the ninth-century imagination. It was also the body as one member of the body of Christ—a mode of thought that united secular and religious spheres and highlighted the individual's contribution to the ideal of an ordered, smoothly functioning society in which the integrity of the whole depended upon the purity of its parts.

As elites pondered the relationship between the temporal empire and the eternal city of God, the body served as a productive focal point for exploring notions of political incorporation and social cohesion. This was manifest most explicitly in endeavors to transpose the Pauline notion of the Church (*ecclesia*) as the body of Christ to the Carolingian Empire and its diversity of peoples.[17] The *ecclesia* could refer in a more limited sense to ecclesiastical personnel or in the broadest sense to all faithful Christians elected by God. But around the turn of the ninth century it increasingly became a way to conceptualize the specific Carolingian polity and the belief that each officeholder within that society occupied an assigned role necessary to the health of the entire community.[18] In the 830s, Jonas of Orléans launched his treatise on kingship with the assumption that "the universal *ecclesia* is the body of Christ and its head is Christ himself, and in it [the *ecclesia*] there are chiefly two preeminent persons, namely the priestly and the royal."[19] At other points in the treatise, however, the difference between the universal Church and the Carolingian body politic appears to collapse. When, for instance, Jonas speaks of every faithful man rendering aid to the ruler for the honor of the kingdom, "just as a member gives appropriate help to the head [of the body]," the implication is that the emperor stands in the position of Christ, at the crown of the Christian faithful, rather than one member among them.[20] Likewise did Hrabanus address Louis the German as the "rector of the members of the true king, Christ."[21]

Louis the Pious himself, in a capitulary issued in the mid-820s, adapted Paul's image of the ecclesial body of Christ to present a model of Carolingian politics in which all *fideles* of the realm were reminded that they possessed their own particular responsibilities in maintaining an empire pleasing to God; the ruler was to direct, exhort, and assist the members, thereby ensuring the cooperative functioning of the greater whole.[22] In this way, the state might have a multitude of offices held by a large number of individuals, but there could be one primary agenda, with discrete actions flowing into a single operation. In all of these metaphorical schemes, the main emphasis was on the way in which unity was created from diversity: there were many members, all with distinctive characteristics, but there was only one body. The members were of differing degrees of dignity, but all were necessary, with the function of the body dependent on even the humblest part.[23]

Such body-talk in the ninth century was in some sense metaphorical, but there was a literal understanding that underpinned the reflections. When Alcuin praised Charlemagne for the fact that he "rules and governs the city of perpetual peace constructed by the blood of Christ," he both linked Augustine's City of God with the Carolingian realm and highlighted the essential role of the sacraments in forging a political unity.[24] The consumption of the Eucharist was, of course, the most palpable way in which all the faithful were joined to the body of Christ. Though there was disagreement about whether Christ's historical, incarnate body was physically present in the bread and wine, the very fact that the ninth century witnessed the first extended deliberation on this subject within Latin Christianity points to the particular salience of corporeal visions of community among Carolingian intellectuals.[25] Staking out one position, Paschasius Radbertus declared that "we receive from him [Christ] and by him his flesh, while he remains whole and entire in it. This indeed is his very flesh, and the fruit of that flesh remains always the same, feeding all those who are in his body."[26] In taking the bread and the wine, an individual became part of both the body that died in the Passion and the resurrected body, and thus, for Paschasius, there was a literal meaning to the idea that the Church was formed *from his flesh and bones* (Eph 5:30).[27] He and his contemporaries saw the union offered through the Eucharist as a direct continuance of that incorporation as a member of Christ which was first conferred in baptism.[28] This sacrament, which so consumed the attention of Charlemagne and his advisers, began with a series of preparatory rites that directed attention toward priming the flesh for its membership with Christ: blowing out the breath deeply, receiving salt in the mouth, anointing the nostrils, breast, and shoulders, and performing an exorcism.[29] The intention was to flush out the devil and cleanse an internal space for God—gestures, then, that transformed the body even as they symbolized the invisible work of saving the soul.

If political unity was effected through processes that called upon visions of an integrated body—one that was necessarily vigorous, functional, and healthy—this opened the way to a medicalized discourse about the state.[30] Just so, we find that assumptions about the dangers that threatened the physical constitution of the flesh were projected onto the body of the realm, writ large. The diseased body clearly resonated with Carolingian intellectuals attempting to comment upon current affairs, for a wayward member that disrupted the equilibrium of the empire was what was greatly feared. This aligned closely with ninth-century models of sickness by which the improper domination of one substance or a dysfunctional rhythm throughout the system of organs produced a corruption that generated sores, fevers, and other life-threatening pains.

The Astronomer demonstrates a particular proclivity for thinking about the well-being of the realm as a type of body, describing the discontent brewing against Emperor Louis as "creeping like a cancer," with lesions that finally burst forth in the rebellions of 830 and 833.[31] Charlemagne himself had reportedly used a similar metaphor at the Council of Frankfurt when it met in 794 to address Adoptionism. Decrying the threat of this heresy, the ruler exclaimed, "What do you see? For the past year, the madness of this pestilence, like a weeping sore of faithlessness, has begun to spill forth and spread."[32] The Astronomer was not the only writer to frame the disorder under Louis the Pious in terms of physical putrefaction. A leading participant in the rebellion of 833, Bishop Agobard of Lyon invoked several such analogies, justifying the actions of his faction as being a necessary response to the "wound of iniquity" besetting the kingdom. Those who were truly loyal and God-fearing subjects would, Agobard insisted, correct the Emperor Louis and thereby enable a scar to seal the wound without any further effusion of blood and before impurity could take root.[33] By the late ninth century, as he contemplated the fragmentation of the empire and the end of Carolingian rule, Regino of Prüm despaired that the body could ever be made whole again. The power (*virtus*) of the Franks had become infirm (*infirmata*), and the various lords had torn apart the unity of the bodily framework, each seeking to create a separate kingdom from the body's "own inner organs."[34]

These metaphors had power because their authors could assume that contemporaries would be able to understand their implicit message. The disarray they charted cried out for a wise *medicus*, someone who could diagnosis the hidden tumor growing within, who could repair the wound of the *ecclesia* without further pain or loss of life, who could bring harmony to the various bodily members and their relationship with the ruling soul. We might recall from Chapter 5 that the *Letter of Arsenius* described the *medicus* as being able to illuminate the darkness, revive the soul, and bring the present, future, and eternal into alignment. The way in which his work impinged on both inner and outer worlds made him an especially suggestive figure in a society looking to unite various peoples through a form of pastoral power.

The pervasiveness of bodily imagery thus posited the *medicus* as the conceptual colleague of numerous figures of authority within Carolingian politics. Their common expertise was an ability to discern and decode external symptoms in order to discover what sickness lurked within the self (and society) and how best to remedy it. New genres of moral literature, such as Jonas's *On Lay Instruction*, sought to establish the importance of this "medicalized" form of authority in the minds of the Carolingian elite, broadly conceived. Jonas stressed that effective eradication of sin hinged on consulting "a most learned physician of the soul," because only such a bishop or priest could penetrate the layers of the self, identify the malady, and apply the appropriate penance.[35] A diseased sinner needed help in order to avoid self-deception.[36] However, even as Jonas elevated ecclesiastical authority, he also promoted a mode of self-care among the laity. It was this same twinned approach that we have observed in ninth-century medical manuscripts. While there was a concerted move to fashion the *medicus* as a righteous and wise expert who could direct Christians in the care of their souls as well as their bodies, there was also a clear favoring of treatises addressed to the nonexpert (do-it-yourself guides that could be used in the daily management of health). Similarly, at the level of the state and its disorders, the solution was to be found through a hierarchy of expertise and responsibility but also an emphasis on mutual accountability among the greater and lesser members.

* * *

This book has proposed that around the turn of the ninth century intellectuals began to stress more forcefully that it was morally right to seek to alleviate suffering and to do so through the acquired techniques of human medicine. From the crafting of the *Lorscher Arzneibuch* in 800, to the compilation of medical letters put together at Saint-Denis, to the ascription of a codex on anatomy and the soul to the Evangelist and physician Luke, we see a growing momentum behind the incorporation of medical learning as part of the virtuous Christian life. This was marked by an ever closer association between matters medical and moral, in which impulses to pursue physical health operated in an imaginative nexus together with ideas about the body's necessary processes, its material containment of the soul, and the ongoing struggle between virtues and vices for control over the inner space of the individual.

The significance of this development becomes especially clear if we consider a number of potential alternatives to this historical trajectory. Ninth-century intellectuals could have sanctioned medicine only as charity, an act that conferred spiritual benefit to the one who offered solace. But, although writings certainly underscored the importance of the doctor treating the needy for free and caring for all as if they were Christ, justifications of medicine's value went far beyond the embodiment of charity. The goals of treatment were cures, not simply comfort. Or medical intervention could have been categorized, as the Greek Father Origen suggested, as a recourse appropriate for the average Christian but not for those seeking the purest and holiest form of life. This also did not happen: medicine was not designated a secular matter, a technique relegated to the battlefield or birthing room as a remedy for dangers inherent in the life of a lay noble. Rather, the study of medicine seems to have been an experiment within Carolingian monasteries that was then taken up by the laity. Finally, medical *scientia* could have emerged from the theological discussions propelled by the reforms as a discipline treated with hostility and skepticism or simply indifference. This would have involved a heightened stress on the attitude exhibited in hagiography and the anointing of the sick—the belief that the only complete cures came from God through his saints and ministers, just as in the time of Christ and his apostles. Such a belief is rarely evident in Carolingian sources.

When they seized power from the long-reigning Merovingians and cemented that power by inciting a critique of contemporary norms, the Carolingian family fostered a sense of disjuncture between present and past. With regard to the care of the body, this disjuncture was marked by the elevation of the medical art, not its disparagement. This does not mean that there was a revolution in the overall health of ninth-century imperial subjects. While trade may have brought new medicinal ingredients, the circulation of texts may have produced more effective remedies, and changes in climate and agricultural production may have yielded more food, it is doubtful that the

Carolingian populace was significantly healthier than their Merovingian ancestors. However, that fact does not undermine the impact of medicine's elevation. The interest in, and audience for, medical learning witnessed in the energetic translation movement of the eleventh century and the foundation of new university structures that followed owed much to ninth-century efforts to foster an environment in which the practice of medicine was a valuable endeavor with wide-reaching benefits.

# ABBREVIATIONS

| | |
|---|---|
| *AGM / SAGM* | *Archiv für Geschichte der Medizin / Sudhoffs Archiv für Geschichte der Medizin* |
| Alcuin, *DRA* | Alcuin, *De ratione animae* |
| Alcuin, *DVV* | Alcuin, *De virtutibus et vitiis* |
| Anthimus, *DOC* | Anthimus, *De observatione ciborum ad Theodoricum regem Francorum epistula* |
| *ARF* | *Annales regni Francorum* |
| BA | Biblioteca Ambrosiana |
| BAV | Biblioteca Apostolica Vaticana |
| Bede, *DTR* | Bede, *De temporum ratione* |
| BL | British Library |
| BLB | Badische Landesbibliothek |
| BM | Bibliothèque municipale |
| BnF | Bibliothèque nationale de France |
| BR | Bibliothèque royale de Belgique |
| *BTML* | Guy Sabbah, Pierre-Paul Corsetti, Klaus-Dietrich Fischer, *Bibliographie des textes médicaux latins: Antiquité et haut moyen âge* |
| CCCM | Corpus Christianorum, Continuatio Mediaevalis |
| CCM | Corpus Consuetudinum Monasticarum, ed. K. Hallinger |
| CCSL | Corpus Christianorum, Series Latina |
| *CLA* | *Codices Latini Antiquiores*, ed. E. A. Lowe |
| CML | Corpus Medicorum Latinorum |
| *Codici* | Augusto Beccaria, *I codici di medicina del periodo presalernitano (secoli IX, X e XI)*. Citations are given by entry number. |
| CSEL | Corpus Scriptorum Ecclesiasticorum Latinorum |
| Dhuoda, *LM* | Dhuoda, *Liber manualis* |

| | |
|---|---|
| *EME* | *Early Medieval Europe* |
| Häse, *MBKL* | Angelika Häse, *Mittelalterliche Bücherverzeichnisse aus Kloster Lorsch: Einleitung, Edition und Kommentar* |
| Hincmar, *DAR* | Hincmar of Reims, *De diversa et multiplici animae ratione ad Carolum calvum regem* |
| Hrabanus, *DRN* | Hrabanus Maurus, *De rerum naturis* [often known as the *De universo*] |
| Hrabanus, *TDA* | Hrabanus Maurus, *Tractatus de anima* |
| Isidore, *Etymologiae* | Isidore, *Etymologiarum sive originum libri XX*, ed. W. M. Lindsay |
| Jonas, *DIL* | Jonas of Orléans, *De institutione laicali* |
| *JHMAS* | *Journal of the History of Medicine and Allied Sciences* |
| *Katalog* | Bernhard Bischoff, *Katalog der festländischen Handschriften des neunten Jahrhunderts*, 3 vols. Citations are given with volume number. entry number. |
| *LAB* | *Das Lorscher Arzneibuch: Ein medizinisches Kompendium des 8. Jahrhunderts (Codex Bambergensis medicinalis 1)*, ed. Ulrich Stoll. Available online at https://nbn-resolving.org/urn:nbn:de:bvb:22-dtl-0000018117 (accessed July 2021). Citations are given with the folio number and page number in Stoll. |
| LB | Landesbibliothek |
| Lehmann, *MBDS* | Paul Lehmann, *Mittelalterliche Bibliothekskataloge Deutschlands und der Schweiz, vol. 1: Die Bistümer Konstanz und Chur* |
| MGH | *Monumenta Germaniae Historica* |
| Capit. | Capitularia regum Francorum |
| Capit. episc. | Capitula episcoporum |
| Conc. | Concilia |
| Epp. | Epistolae |
| Epp. sel. | Epistolae selectae |
| Form | Formulae Merowingici et Karolini aevi |
| LL. nat. Germ. | Leges nationum Germanicarum |
| Poetae | Poetae Latini medii aevi |

| | |
|---|---|
| SS | Scriptores, in folio |
| SS rer. Germ. | Scriptores rerum Germanicarum in usum scholarum separatim editi |
| SS rer. Merov. | Scriptores rerum Merovingicarum |
| SS rer. Germ. N.S. | Scriptores rerum Germanicarum, Nova series |
| *MS* | *Mittelalterliche Studien* (collected essays of Bernhard Bischoff), 3 vols. |
| Paulinus, *LE* | Paulinus of Aquilea, *Liber exhortationis* |
| PG | Patrologiae Cursus Completus, Series Graeca, ed. J.-P. Migne. 161 vols. Paris, 1857–1866. |
| PL | Patrologiae Cursus Completus, Series Latina, ed. J.-P. Migne. 221 vols. Paris, 1844–1864. |
| SC | Sources Chrétiennes |
| SB | Stiftsbibliothek |
| *SHM* | *Social History of Medicine* |
| UL | University Library |

# NOTES

## Introduction

1. See Einhard, *Vita Karoli* 1, ed. Holder-Egger, 3.

2. On the Merovingians' long hair, see Diesenberger, "Hair, Sacrality and Symbolic Capital," who questions any association between hair and supernatural power.

3. Dutton, *Charlemagne's Mustache*, 3–42.

4. *LAB*, ff. 37r, 43v, 49v, ed. Stoll, 216, 246, 276. On this manuscript, see Chapter 4.

5. This is the *vademecum* of Walafrid Strabo: St. Gall, SB 878, pp. 331–32. On this manuscript's attribution and contents, see Chapter 6.

6. See Contreni's discussion of the recipe (which survives in several twelfth- and thirteenth-century manuscripts): "Masters and Medicine," 335.

7. Individuals named in the recipe are Bishop Pardulus of Laon, Fergus the Grammarian, and John Scottus Eriugena, according to Contreni, "Masters and Medicine," 335.

8. The unguent, labeled *psilotrum*, is edited by Contreni in "Masters and Medicine," 347–48.

9. On Charles the Bald's hair, see Nelson, *Charles the Bald*, 13; Dutton, *Charlemagne's Mustache*, 36–38.

10. For an overview of the Carolingian renaissance, see Contreni, "Carolingian Renaissance"; Brown, "Introduction"; Nelson, "On the Limits"; Sullivan, "Context of Cultural Activity"; Depreux, "Ambitions et limites"; Noble, "Carolingian Religion." On improvement through education, see van Rhijn, "Local Church"; Scholz, "Bemerkungen zur Bildungsentwicklung."

11. On the terms *corrigere* and *emendare* (in place of renaissance or reform), see Smith, "Emending Evil Ways," 189–92, 214–15; Rose, "*Emendatio* and *effectus*"; Hillner, *Prison*, 38–44, 66–70, 96–109; Barrow, "Ideas and Applications," 353–58; cf. van Rhijn, "Introduction," who rightly critiques how *correctio* implies top-down initiatives.

12. Alcuin, *DRA* 1, ed. Curry, 39.

13. Under the umbrella "Carolingian medical manuscripts" I include codices with *solely* and those with *some* medical material but exclude those written in Insular or Beneventan script.

14. The crucial work of identifying extant manuscripts was carried out in the 1950–60s by Augusto Beccaria (*I codici* covers all manuscripts from the ninth through eleventh centuries) and Ernest Wickersheimer (*Manuscrits latins* covers manuscripts from the seventh through twelfth centuries now held in French libraries). However, a new project, "Beyond Beccaria," dedicated to producing an updateable "living" catalogue of early medieval medical manuscripts, is underway, and preliminary findings suggest that Beccaria and Wickersheimer missed a significant number (for example, while Beccaria lists 145 manuscripts, there are, at

the time of writing, 404 in this new catalogue). Consequently, I hesitate to give a new estimate, given how unrepresentative these older numbers may prove in the long term. Most of the pre-Carolingian manuscripts are listed in the *CLA* and will be included in the "Beyond Beccaria" catalogue when it appears.

15. On issues of manuscript survival (such as the transition from papyrus to parchment), see Costambeys et al., *Carolingian World*, 16–18.

16. On the significance of this event and its relationship to reforms from the 780s onward, see McKitterick, *Charlemagne*, 114–18, 292–315; Gantner, McKitterick, and Meeder, *Resources of the Past*.

17. This problematic characterization of Carolingian theology is rebutted by Chazelle, *Crucified God*, 2–3. For an approach to medical texts, see Wallis, "Experience of the Book."

18. On self-knowledge, see Morrison, "Know Thyself," 373–88, 420–24; Rosenwein, *Generations of Feeling*, 68–85.

19. For the history of Lorsch, see Innes, "Kings, Monks and Patrons."

20. On this ambivalence, see Nees, *Tainted Mantle*; Teeuwen, "Seduced by Pagan Poets."

21. On the language of "technique," see Mauss, "Techniques of the Body."

22. On the "spiritual weight" of the body, see Halkias, "From Reflections to Membranes," 8.

23. On this council and its language of governance, see Moore, *Sacred Kingdom*, 319, 341, 354–58; Anton, *Fürstenspiegel*, 231–34. On the Gelasian two-powers model (cited as two "persons" in the 829 Council of Paris), see Robinson, "Church and Papacy," 288–99; Toubert, "La doctrine gélasienne," 526–33. In his exegesis of the two swords in Lk 22:38 (later said to designate royal and papal power), Alcuin claimed they represented soul and body and the need for both to be in harmony: Alberi, "Sword Which You Hold," 125–31.

24. *Yütz bei Diedenhofen* 2, ed. Hartmann, Conc. 3, 31.

25. Brown, *Ransom of the Soul*; Moreira, *Heaven's Purge*; Carozzi, *Le voyage de l'âme*; Meens, *Penance*; McLaughlin, *Consorting with Saints*; Effros, *Caring for Body and Soul*; Kreiner, "Autopsies and Philosophies"; Fort, "Penitents and Their Proxies." On the Celtic Mediterranean, see Brown, *Rise of Western Christendom*, 16.

26. On powerhouses of prayer, see Brown, *Rise of Western Christendom*, 219–31; de Jong, "Carolingian Monasticism." On local priests, see van Rhijn, *Shepherds of the Lord*.

27. For a recent assessment of regional difference, see Davis, *Charlemagne's Practice*.

28. On these themes, see Nelson, "Voice of Charlemagne," 81–85; Choy, *Intercessory Prayer*; Romig, *Perfect Man*; Phelan, *Formation*; Koziol, "Leadership"; Pohl, "Introduction: Ego Trouble"; Innes, "Place of Discipline."

29. Booker, *Past Convictions*; Firey, *Contrite Heart*; de Jong, *Penitential State*. See also Moore, *Sacred Kingdom*; Patzold, *Episcopus*.

30. On monastic purity across the early Middle Ages, see Diem, *Das monastische Experiment*.

31. On saints' bodies, see Smith, "Portable Christianity."

32. For a comparable assessment of scholarship on Jesus's corporeality, see Coon, "Gendering Dark Age Jesus," 8–9.

33. Coon, *Dark Age Bodies*; Chazelle, *Crucified God*; Nelson, "England and the Continent"; Airlie, "Private Bodies." See also Appleby, "Beautiful on the Cross"; Oliver, *Body Legal*; Palazzo, "Art, Liturgy, and the Five Senses"; Diem, "On Opening and Closing the Body"; Skinner, *Living with Disfigurement*; Coon, "What Is the Word."

34. See Coon, "Somatic Styles," 464–65, who suggests that studying the ancient-Dark Ages transition may offer a historical methodology (for the history of the body) useful in demolishing the premodern-modern divide.

35. Particularly influential on my thought have been: Park, *Secrets of Women*; Pouchelle, *Body and Surgery*; Rankin, *Panaceia's Daughters*; Pomata, *Contracting a Cure*; McVaugh, *Medicine Before the Plague*; Demaitre, *Medieval Medicine*; Green, *Making Women's Medicine*; Cohen-Hanegbi, *Caring for the Living Soul*; Biller and Ziegler, *Religion and Medicine*.

36. Early medieval English medicine has fared better, in part because the survival of vernacular medical codices has encouraged more diverse questions. Synthetic studies include: Cameron, *Anglo-Saxon Medicine*; Kesling, *Medical Texts*; Jolly, *Popular Religion*; van Arsdall, *Medieval Herbal Remedies*; Meaney, "Practice of Medicine."

37. See Horden, "Medieval Medicine," 50: "Derogation of the early Middle Ages, by comparison with a classical past and a later medieval future (a university future), remains implicit in even the best scholarship."

38. Horden, "What's Wrong"; Glaze, "Perforated Wall"; Wallis, "Experience of the Book."

39. On the dominance of Galen's thought, see Kaye, *History of Balance*, 128–35.

40. Galen's *De methodo medendi ad Glauconem* circulated in an abridged Latin translation, with a pseudonymous third book (the *Liber tertius*); see Fischer, "Die spätlateinische Übersetzung." Milan, BA, G.108 inf. (s.IX$^{2}$, Milan) preserves commentaries on Galen's *De sectis*, *Ars medica*, *De pulsibus*, and *De methodo medendi*, and Karlsruhe, BLB 120 (s.IX$^{2/4}$, northern Italy) preserves the commentary to the *De sectis* in a fragmentary form; on these, see *Katalog* 1.1650 and 2.2620; *Codici* 56 and 92. On the many pseudo-Galenic texts in the early Middle Ages, see *BTML*, 82–89.

41. See the classic study by Temkin, *Galenism*; Nutton, "Fortunes of Galen."

42. For an overview of medicine under the Abbasids, see Pormann and Savage-Smith, *Medieval Islamic Medicine*.

43. But see Goldberg, *Manner of the Franks*, 155–57, who has recently suggested that a veterinary treatise for hawks (likely composed by Grimald of Saint-Gall (d. 872) may contain material translated from Arabic or Greek into Latin and given to the Carolingians as a diplomatic gift. On the intersections among spices, incense, and drugs in the ninth century, and the ways in which increased long-distance trade may have shaped Carolingian recipe collections and healing practices, see Burridge, "Incense." On the trade in expensive *pigmenta* from Arab regions, see also Cameron, "Bald's 'Leechbook'"; McCormick, *Origins*, 708–16.

44. For comparative studies of the two empires, see Tor, *'Abbasid and Carolingian Empires*; Drews, *Die Karolinger und die Abbasiden*.

45. On the Abbasid translation movement, see Gutas, *Greek Thought*; cf. Saliba, *Islamic Science*.

46. On Italian medical traditions, see below. Bischoff, "Paläographie und frühmittelalterliche Klassikerüberlieferung," in *MS*, 3:55–72, at 69, points to Charlemagne's conquest of Ravenna and Pavia and his patronage of Italian scholars as routes of transmission for classical texts. In another article, "Italienische Handschriften," 189, he suggests that there was an exodus of medical manuscripts out of Italy and names Fleury, Laon, and Reichenau as places to which these manuscripts traveled. English and Irish connections are suggested especially by some of the prognostic material copied by the Carolingians (see Chapter 6).

47. Mavroudi, "Translations from Greek," at 39–44, highlighting the speed with which certain Byzantine texts seem to have been used by authors writing in Arabic, Old Church Slavonic, Syriac, and Latin. Much of early Arabic medical scholarship was undertaken not by Muslims but by Nestorian Christians patronized by the Abbasids.

48. On similar processes of appropriation, see the essays in Gantner, McKitterick, and Meeder, *Resources of the Past.*

49. Airlie, "Palace of Memory."

50. Reimitz, "Transformations of Late Antiquity," 263.

51. Even while discussing innovation in the early Middle Ages, for example, Keil speaks of a "Christian-monastic filter" that weeded out much of classical medicine. "Möglichkeiten und Grenzen," at 226.

52. On the role that trade in exotic, Arabic substances played in stimulating Salernitan medical scholarship, see Glaze, "Salerno's Lombard Prince."

53. Recent studies are challenging this narrative: see Kwakkel and Newton, *Medicine at Monte Cassino*; Green, "Medical Books." On Constantine's life and work, see Burnett and Jacquart, *Constantine the African*; Burnett, "Legend of Constantine"; Newton, "Arabic Medicine."

54. Glaze, "Perforated Wall," 187–261; Green, "Rethinking the Manuscript Basis." Both consider not only Constantine's work but also various forms of southern Italian medical scholarship, proposing transmission routes that included monastic networks, the movement of teachers and students, and Anglo-Norman political connections. An ongoing project to catalogue all Latin medical manuscripts from the "long twelfth century" is summarized in Green, "Medical Books."

55. On schooling, see McKitterick, *Frankish Kingdoms*, 146–52; Hildebrandt, *External School.* On the adoption (and adaptation) of the Benedictine Rule, see Kramer, *Rethinking Authority*; de Jong, "Carolingian Monasticism"; Diem, "Carolingians and the *Regula Benedicti.*"

56. Contreni, "Masters and Medicine," 333. See also, with similar conclusions, Touati, "Raban Maur."

57. See Charlemagne's emphasis on correct action as a product of correct knowledge in his *Epistola de litteris colendis* (ca. 784–790), ed. Boretius, MGH, Capit. 1, 79.

58. This is a point reiterated several times: Rudolf, *Vita Leobae* 7, 8, 11, ed. Waitz, 124–26.

59. Dhuoda, *LM* Incipit, ed. Riché, 66; trans. Neel, 1.

60. They discuss specifically how mathematics and astronomy were reoriented toward the science of *computus*: Wallis, *Bede: Reckoning of Time*, xxvi–xxvii; Englisch, "Realitätsorientierte Wissenschaft."

61. On the broader late antique shift toward the production of encyclopedias and epitomes, which summarized and condensed scientific knowledge, favoring the practical over the theoretical, see Beagon, "Science and Medicine"; Slaveva-Griffin, "Byzantine Medical Encyclopedias"; Nutton, "From Galen to Alexander"; Baader, "Lehrbrief und Kurztraktat."

62. On Alcuin, see Alberi, "Mystery." On medicine's integration into the liberal arts, I have benefited greatly from an unpublished paper shared by Faith Wallis, "Is There a 'Carolingian Medicine'?"

63. The liberal arts are discussed in Chapters 4 and 5.

64. Indispensable guides are the *BTML* and its supplements (in print and online) by Fischer; Kibre, *Hippocrates Latinus*; Wickersheimer, *Manuscrits latins*; Beccaria, *I codici.* Hippocratic texts translated into Latin and circulated in the early Middle Ages include: the

*Aphorismi*; *Prognostica*; *De aëre, aquis et locis*; *De septimanis*; *De mulierum affectibus*; *De natura hominis* (only a fragment survives); and adapted versions of *De victus ratione*.

65. Wallis, "Experience of the Book," 107.

66. Here I should note the difficulty of producing critical editions when each witness is so different. For the work of these scholars (building on that of Rose, Sudhoff, and Sigerist), please see the bibliography.

67. The exact phrasing varies slightly but appears in catalogues from Lorsch, Reichenau, Murbach, Saint-Gall, and Montecassino. See Häse, *MBKL*, A116, Ca12–14; Lehmann, *MBDS*, 82, 87, 89, 248, 261; Milde, *Der Bibliothekskatalog*, 48 no. 334; *Chronica monasterii Casinensis*, ed. Hoffmann, 89–90. The best reference here is the table of library catalogue listings compiled by Glaze, "Perforated Wall," 268–96, with a discussion on using catalogues as a source for medical history at 71–79, 192–201, 222–40. For a general introduction to the Carolingian catalogues, see McKitterick, *Carolingians and the Written Word*, 169–210. The phrase "in libro medicinali" is also used by Hincmar, *De cavendis vitiis*, ed. Nachtmann, 108.

68. Surprisingly, Hippocrates's name does not appear in any ninth-century catalogue entry.

69. See, for example, the ninth-century codex of Einhard's letters, which includes a medical recipe on f. 2v (Paris, BnF lat. 11379).

70. Green, "Medical Books," 279, finds the same for medical codices from the long twelfth century. Sometimes codices consist of sections with different genres, but here the medical material is typically a distinct unit. A key exception, as discussed in Chapter 6, is *computus* collections, as demonstrated by Wallis, "Medicine in Medieval Calendar Manuscripts."

71. Häse, *MBKL*, A118, Ca368, D253. Also listed is Caelius Aurelianus's work on chronic diseases (A117, Ca369, D254), which does not survive in any early medieval witness, though three leaves of this text (Zwickau, Ratsschulbibliothek Fragm. CL a+b) have been dated to the ninth century and identified as a Lorsch hand; see Drabkin, *On Acute Diseases*, xii. Other authors noted in the catalogues include Galen, Apuleius, Alexander, Vindicianus, and Vegetius.

72. In the case of Quintus Serenus, the Murbach catalogue listed his work under "pagan poets" rather than "the art of medicine," and it survives in several manuscripts that are collections of verse. Milde, *Der Bibliothekskatalog*, 48 no. 328 and nos. 331–35. But this cannot be taken to mean that it was consistently seen as a literary (rather than medical) text; cf. Wallis, "Experience of the Book," 108.

73. The Reichenau catalogue (821/22) lists under "De opusculis Boetii" various works on the liberal arts, including one book on the art of medicine: Lehmann, *MBDS*, 250; Glaze, "Perforated Wall," 91–92.

74. Lehmann, *MBDS*, 248.

75. Glaze, "Perforated Wall," 78. Burridge's analysis of a group of recipes for incense likewise points to a lively exchange that has yet to be recognized: "Incense," at 248.

76. On the ways in which oral knowledge and apprenticeship must have established a framework for understanding many of these texts, see van Arsdall, *Medieval Herbal Remedies*, 80–100.

77. St. Gall, SB 217. See Bischoff, "Über gefaltete Handschriften, vornehmlich hagiographischen Inhalts," in *MS*, 1:95–100, at 99.

78. On what follows, see Sigerist, "Latin Medical Literature"; Baader, "Early Medieval Latin Adaptations"; Nutton, *Ancient Medicine*, 293–309; Touwaide, "Legacy of Classical Antiquity"; Fischer, "*Ex occidente lux*"; Cilliers, "Medical Writing."

79. I avoid using the term "theoretical" here because scholars have almost uniformly cast early medieval Latin medicine as untheoretical. Glaze is one of the few to truly challenge this notion, and her study of the *Epistola peri hereseon* has demonstrated the lines of continuity between a more Greek- and Galenic-focused medical tradition in sixth-century Ravenna and the presence of this material in Carolingian monasteries. The *Epistola* outlines a series of different definitions of the art of medicine, naming various ancient philosophers and physicians as well as the three Roman medical sects (rational, empirical, and methodist). Its mode of cataloguing the art's four actions (theoretical, practical, acquisitive, and telic) and of subdividing medicine into two parts (theory and practice, the former of which is then further subdivided until one arrives at the various bodily humors, senses, and faculties) resembles the approach found in Islamic Galenism. However, texts such as the *Epistola* are rare in ninth-century manuscripts. See Glaze, "Master-Student," who demonstrates that the sources of the *Epistola* included the introductory lectures on Galen's works attributed to one Agnellus the Iatrosophist (themselves likely derived from sixth-century Greek Alexandrian commentaries). On these lectures, see Agnellus of Ravenna, *Lectures on Galen's De sectis*, ed. Westerink. On Agnellus (likely an Alexandrian living in Ravenna), see Palmieri, "Nouvelles remarques," 237–43; Herrin, *Ravenna*, 239–44.

80. For example, Fischer, "Dr Monk's"; Fischer, "*Isagoge* of Pseudo-Soranus"; Wlaschky, "*Sapientia artis medicinae*"; Laux, "*Ars medicinae*."

81. This situation can be contrasted against the emergence in the twelfth century of the *Articella*, a canon of teaching texts, which would become the standard curriculum at European universities.

82. Cassiodorus, *Institutiones* 1.31, ed. Mynors, 78–79; Sigerist, "Latin Medical Literature," 131–34; cf. Courcelle, *Late Latin Writers*, 403–9.

83. Various Latin translations of Dioscorides's *De materia medica* circulated, but more popular was a heavily reworked version known as the *Ex herbis femininis*; see Riddle, "Pseudo-Dioscorides'." Cassiodorus also referred to a work by Caelius Aurelius, likely one of the translations of a Greek text by Soranus of Ephesus (the *De morbis acutis et chronicis* by Caelius Aurelianus, or the bundled *Liber Aurelii* and *Liber Esculapii*); see Fischer, "Dr Monk's," 247–48, 250–51.

84. Foucault, "What Is an Author?" 125–26.

85. Voigts, "Anglo-Saxon Plant Remedies"; Riddle, "Theory and Practice."

86. Nutton, *Ancient Medicine*, 174–77, 292–301; Collins, *Medieval Herbals*, 148–238; Sigerist, "Latin Medical Literature"; Fischer, "Pre-Salernitan Medical Manuals"; Kai Brodersen, "Introduction," in *Medicina Plinii*, trans. Hunt, 1–10.

87. On Oribasius's life, see Baldwin, "Career of Oribasius." On his *Euporista* and *Synopsis* (both translated into Latin), see Mørland, *Oribasius Latinus* and *Die lateinischen Oribasiusübersetzungen*. Uncial and half-uncial manuscripts with the Latin Oribasius include Paris, BnF lat. 10233 + Bern, Burgerbibliothek F. 219 III; Paris, BnF nouv. acq. lat. 1619; Vatican, BAV Urb. lat. 293; on these, see *CLA* 1:116, 5:592, 5:688.

88. One key difference being that Marcellus's *Liber de medicamentis* may have become available to his near-contemporary Theodorus Priscianus in North Africa. See Opsomer and Halleux, "Marcellus"; Stannard, "Marcellus of Bordeaux."

89. Those who wrote originally in Latin or produced Latin translations of Greek texts include: Celsus (fl. 25 C.E.), Pliny (d. 79), Gargilius Martialis (fl. 250), Vindicianus (d. ca. 400), Marcellus of Bordeaux (fl. 400), Theodorus Priscianus (fl. 400), Caelius Aurelianus (fl. 400),

Cassius Felix (fl. 450), Muscio (ca. 500?). Those whose Greek works were translated (at least in part) include: the Hippocratic Corpus, Dioscorides (fl. 70), Soranus (fl. 100), Galen (d. ca. 210), Oribasius (d. ca. 400), Alexander of Tralles (fl. 525), Paul of Aegina (fl. 650).

90. Crucial pieces of evidence are a Ravenna papyrus from 572 that refers to a *medicus* "ab schola Graeca" and Milan, BA, G.108 inf. with three Hippocratic texts (likely translated in Ravenna) and the Galenic commentaries attributed to Agnellus of Ravenna (n79 above). See Mørland, *Die lateinischen Oribasiusübersetzungen*, 43–51, 187–94, on sixth-century Ravenna as the site of two Latin translations of Oribasius's *Synopsis* and *Euporista*; cf. Adams, *Regional Diversification*, 472–511, on attributing translations to northern Italy, not specifically Ravenna; Vázquez Buján, "Problemas generales," 641–80, on the importance of southern over northern Italy. For further discussion, see Palmieri, "Nouvelles remarques," 209–46; Mazzini and Palmieri, "L'école médicale de Ravenne"; Beccaria, "Sulle tracce," I, II, and III.

91. Everett, *Alphabet of Galen*, 23n49. Jouanna, *Greek Medicine*, 356n54, rightly critiques the tendency to firmly date Latin medical texts of ambiguous origin.

92. MacKinney, *Early Medieval Medicine*, 80–81, 103–4; Horden, "What's Wrong," 17.

93. On Anthimus's dietary treatise, see Chapter 7. On the veterinary text, see Goldberg, "Hunt Belongs to Man," 43–45; *Le* Liber accipitrum *de Grimaldus*, ed. Smets. On Walafrid's verse, see Chapter 4.

94. For example, though knowledge of Greek was rare in early medieval Francia, at least minimal levels of translation must have been possible before 800 if the following are taken as clues: a Greek to Latin translation of the *Apocalypse of Pseudo-Methodius* (ca. 700, southern France); a bilingual glossary (ca. 750, at Tours); a bilingual copy of the Pauline epistles (ca. 750, at Corbie); a number of Greek texts sent to Pippin III by the pope (758–63); a Greek to Latin translation of a chronicle known as the *Excerpta barbari* (ca. 775, completed at Corbie); a Greek to Latin translation, and then further revision, of an astronomical poem, the *Aratus Latinus* (ca. 735 and 790, completed at Corbie). These suggest the importance of Corbie, a monastery Beccaria likewise hints *may* have witnessed an early translation of the Hippocratic *Aphorisms*. Knowledge of Greek picked up in the ninth century with the arrival of several scholars from Ireland trained in Greek; the works of Pseudo-Dionysius the Areopagite (gifted by the Byzantine emperor in 827) were translated twice from Greek into Latin, once by Hilduin of Saint-Denis and once by John Scottus Eriugena. On these developments, see Beccaria, "Sulle tracce II," 22–23; Kibre, *Hippocrates Latinus*, 29–35; Berschin, *Greek Letters*, 102–56; Kaczynski, *Greek in the Carolingian Age*; Le Bourdellès, *L'Aratus Latinus*; Burgess, "*Excerpta latina barbari*"; Gastgeber, "Aristotle of Pippin III"; Ramírez-Weaver, *Saving Science*, 50, 74–75, 169–75; Lapidge, *Hilduin of Saint-Denis*, 64–80; Herren, "Pelasgian Fountains."

95. See the defense of the "scribal author" by Fisher, *Scribal Authorship*; Conti, "Scribes as Authors." For the Carolingians, see Shimahara, *Haymon d'Auxerre*; Lifshitz, *Religious Women*.

96. A comparison is Firey's use of the term "jurists," which she states (*Contrite Heart*, 2) is "intended to embrace the unknown range of Carolingian personnel who may have been involved in shaping the legal discourse of the era."

97. On networks of scholars, teachers, and students during this period, see Steckel, *Kulturen des Lehrens*.

98. See, for example, Reimitz, *History*; McKitterick, *History and Memory*.

99. Kühnel, *End of Time*; Collins, *Medieval Herbals*, esp. 188; Fricke and Holler, "Rosenrot," esp. 115; see also Jones, "Image, Word, and Medicine," 5; Kitzinger, *Cross*, 51–55; Ramírez-Weaver, *Saving Science*.

100. On the training girls may have received, see Garver, *Women*, 122–45, who suggests that laywomen may have been gifted such moral literature as a tool for educating their sons. On the audiences for spiritual advice, see Kramer, *Rethinking Authority*, 130–61.

101. Key studies of how duty was gendered in the Carolingian period include: Garver, *Women*; Brubaker and Smith, *Gender*; Stone, *Morality*; Smith, "Gender and Ideology"; Nelson, *Courts, Elites*; Le Jan, *Femmes, pouvoir.*

102. Partial translations of the Hippocratic *Diseases of Women* and Soranus's *Gynecology* circulated in the early Middle Ages, but while the former did discuss women's moistness and porous flesh, the focus of early medieval gynecology was on practical responses to specific conditions, not theory. Thus, the classical scheme in which women are wet/cold and men are dry/hot is difficult to find, though one could argue that it remained an implicit reference point. See Totelin, "Old Recipes"; Green, "Transmission of Ancient Theories."

103. Naturally, a focus on childbirth, pregnancy, menstruation, and male/female fertility might yield a different perspective, and this is not a topic covered in the book; for an overview, see Garver, "Childbearing and Infancy."

104. By focusing on medical literature, this work presents a different, though not contradictory, perspective to Coon, *Dark Age Bodies*, whose research on the cloistered monk illuminates a stark binary between the loose, soft, and penetrable lay body (gendered as female) and the bounded, hard, and hot monastic body (gendered as male).

105. Bynum, "Why All the Fuss," 6–8. On the diversity of the early medieval body, see also Coon, "Somatic Styles."

106. MacKinney, *Early Medieval Medicine*. The best synoptic view since MacKinney is Glaze, "Perforated Wall." Little synthetic work has yet been done to use archeology and paleopathology to widen our understanding of healing and disease during this time, but see the overview by Lee, "Disease"; Banham, "Anglo-Saxon *materia medica*"; Skinner, *Health and Medicine*; Pilsworth, *Healthcare*, 48–62; and forthcoming research by Claire Burridge.

107. Caciola, *Afterlives*, 21. This offers a stimulating synthesis of medical and theological ideas of death but one that (in a time-honored model) leaps from the patristics to the twelfth century, declaring that (82), "investigations into the physiology of life and death first emerged in the twelfth-century monastic milieu."

## Chapter 1

1. *Visio Baronti* 4, ed. Levison, 380; trans. Hillgarth, *Christianity*, 196. On the text, see Hen, "Structure and Aims"; Contreni, "Building Mansions"; Ciccarese, "La *Visio Baronti*."

2. In connection with Pelagianism, Christians like Claudianus Mamertus and Faustus of Riez disputed the corporeality of the soul in fifth-century southern Gaul: Mathisen, *Ecclesiastical Factionalism*, 235–72; Brown, *Ransom of the Soul*, 132–37; di Marco, *La polemica sull'anima*.

3. On problems of accessibility, see Alcuin's complaint (*DRA* 8) that he lacks certain works by Augustine and wonders if they might be found in Charlemagne's library.

4. See Dal Santo, *Debating*, on Gregory the Great's *Dialogi* as a response to contemporaneous Byzantine debates about the soul's postmortem existence.

5. On Adoptionism (concerning the unity of Christ's natures), see Cavadini, *Last Christology*. On Iconoclasm (concerning the role of material objects in worship), see Noble, *Images*. On predestination, see below. On new conceptions of the afterlife, personal sin, and

individualized judgment, see Brown, "End of the Ancient Otherworld"; Moreira, *Heaven's Purge*.

6. Smaragdus, *Expositio* 1.2, ed. Spannagel, 75; trans. Barry, 144.

7. On Carolingian references to Plato, see Marenbon, "Platonism," 71–77.

8. Five ninth-century manuscripts contain the *Disputatio Platonis et Aristotelis*, one with two versions; it is also extant in London, BL Sloane 2839 (*s*.XI/XII), whose contents give every impression of being a copy of an early medieval medical codex (at least from ff. 7–112). On the witnesses, see Schmitt and Knox, *Pseudo-Aristoteles Latinus*, 28. The two editions by Normann, "*Disputatio*," 68–73, are based on three witnesses, but a clearer reading is sometimes offered by other manuscripts (as below).

9. *Disputatio*, ed. Normann, 68–69. Plato's support for a tripartite division recalls his teaching in the *Republic* of the threefold soul: rational, spirited, and appetitive.

10. *Disputatio*, in Paris, BnF lat. 11218 (*s*.$VIII^{ex}/IX^{in}$), ff. 33r–v: "Sanguis ipsi quod et factus est frigidus effectus humor a sanguinem segregatum. Cooperuit levitatem suam sicut oleo super aqua natans, ita humor super sanguinem."

11. *Disputatio*, in Paris, BnF lat. 11218, f. 33v: "Tunc dicit Platon hubi est doctrina tua Aristotilis? Non dicebas quod sanguis esset anima et ipse contexit omnem fabrice? Sic dixi humor est sanguinem peragrat de quo dicit poenemon, hoc est spiritus [punctuation added]." What is meant by *poenemon* (Normann, 69, supplies *pneuma* here, based on *penetumon* and *penionem* in his witnesses), and how Plato became associated with this teaching, are beyond the scope of this chapter. On *pneuma* and soul in late antique medicine, see von Staden, "Body, Soul, and Nerves," 92–116.

12. *Disputatio*, ed. Normann, 70. Aristotle never argued that the soul was blood, but the association may lie in his classification as a cardiocentrist. See van der Eijk, "The Heart."

13. Discussed in Chapter 5.

14. Paris, BnF lat. 4883, ff. 6v–7v (*s*.$IX^{ex}$) and Brussels, BR 3701-15, ff. 3v–4v (*s*.$IX^{2/3}$); these witnesses are not directly related. Normann edits the Brussels witness and calls it *die christliche Fassung*.

15. *De disputatione*, ed. Normann, 71 (emphasis mine, with certain readings influenced by Paris, BnF lat. 4883).

16. *De disputatione*, ed. Normann, 72 (punctuation mine).

17. On the development of cautery images, see Jones, *Medieval Medicine*, 77–78. On London, BL Sloane 2839 (*s*.XI/XII, England), see *Codici* 81; Glaze, "Master-Student," 476–78, 485–89.

18. *De disputatione*, ed. Normann, 72.

19. *De disputatione*, ed. Normann, 71.

20. On Galen's attempt to distance the soul from corporeality, see Holmes, "Disturbing Connections," 147–76.

21. *Epistula ad Maecenatem* (a pseudo-Hippocratic letter discussed in Chapter 6), in Marcellus, *De medicamentis*, ed. Niedermann, 1:26. Compare with Wlaschky's edition of an early medieval medical compilation, "*Sapientia artis medicinae*," 105: "Sanguis gubernat animam, anima autem vitam, spiritus autem aëris est."

22. Brussels, BR 3701-15, f. 1r: "Cor in pectore, anima in corde, mens in anima, fides in mente, Christus in fide." The text lacks its opening but appears as *epistula* 9 in a collection where the original *Disputatio* is *epistula* 13 and the revised 14.

23. Paris, BnF lat. 4883 (*s*.IX$^{\text{ex}}$): ff. 1r–3r contain the beginning of Orosius's *Historiae adversus paganos*; ff. 3r–7v shift abruptly to medical material; ff. 9r–32v (added later, *s*.XII) contain two texts by Augustine. Bischoff suggests an origin in northern Francia, but Andrés Sanz notes that the Orosian fragment closely imitates a Breton witness (Vatican, BAV Reg. lat. 296, *s*.IX$^{1}$) in its use of the phrase "Incipit liber Orosii de ormesta mundi"; this might point to an origin in Brittany or connections with Bobbio (the site of diffusion of manuscripts with *ormesta*). On Paris 4883, see *Codici* 21; *Katalog* 3.4343; Wickersheimer, *Manuscrits latins*, 63–64; Andrés Sanz, "Isidoro de Sevilla," 50–51, 60. On manuscripts of the *Adversus paganos*, see Arnaud-Lindet, *Orose*, xiii–xiv, lxxiv, lxxx–lxxxiv.

24. Paris, BnF lat. 4883, f. 6v: "Istam ergo ordinationem humani corporis Lucas demonstrat. Explicit."

25. First one finds an anonymous *Textus libri* attributed to Augustine (ff. 3r–3v); then material loosely based on Isidore's *Liber differentiarum* (ff. 3v–5v); next a copy of Vindicianus's *Gynaecia* (ff. 5v–6v); finally, the *Disputatio*, titled *Disser<ta>tio de anima hominis*. Here, the *Gynaecia* 1, ed. Rose, in *Theodori Prisciani*, 429.

26. *Textus libri*, Paris, BnF lat. 4883, ff. 3r–3v. This draws on numerical symbolism in Augustine's *De diversis quaestionibus octoginta tribus* but is addressed directly to a *medicus* ("Vide ergo tu medice mysterium operis dei"). On theories of embryology in circulation, see Elsakkers, "Vocabulary of Abortion," esp. 383–84.

27. Paris, BnF lat. 4883, f. 6v: "iii mense quia tunc prius formatus invenitur infans conceptus inspirante deo accipit animam."

28. As far as I have been able to determine from the ten witnesses of the *Gynaecia* dated *s*.VIII–X. See the seven witnesses in Vindicianus, *Gynaecia* 20, ed. Rose, in *Theodori Prisciani*, 452–55, 465; and the (partial) list of manuscripts in Cilliers, "Vindicianus's *Gynaecia*," 155–56, which does not include London, BL Add. 8928 (*s*.X), Glasgow, UL Hunter 404 (*s*.X), or Paris, BnF nouv. acq. lat. 203 (*s*.VIII$^{\text{ex}}$/IX$^{\text{in}}$), the last noted by James Palmer.

29. This begins with the line at Paris, BnF lat. 4883, f. 4v: "Est et alia sedis anime in inguine que si incisa fuerit vitam perdet."

30. Paris, BnF lat. 4883, ff. 4v–5r: "Est ergo anima invisibilis ad immaginem dei condita. Non habens colorem neque pondus sed ex nichilo condita est a deo et inmortalis . . . Quae non est flatus, non est fumus, non est ignis, non est sanguis, neque pars divine substantiae." Compare Isidore, *Liber differentiarum* 2.25–28, ed. Andrés Sanz, 57–65.

31. Alcuin draws on the *Liber differentiarum* 2.25, 2.27, 2.28 in *DRA* 6, ed. Curry, 54–56.

32. Paris, BnF lat. 4883, f. 3v: "Hic ex diversis constat substantiis, id est corpus mortale et anima inmortale." Augustine's *De quantitate animae* is in the form of a dialogue, so this may also have influenced its placement after the dialogue of Plato and Aristotle.

33. See Normann, "*Disputatio*," who titles the first version *die heidnische Fassung*.

34. On the first, Paris, BnF lat. 11218 (*Epistola conflictus duorum filosoforum* at ff. 33r–34v), see Chapter 5. On the second, see St. Gall, SB 762, p. 270.

35. Brussels, BR 3701-15, ff. 2v–4v.

36. Thanks to James Palmer for this point. For a comparable example of "false" and "true" texts side by side, see Booker, "New Prologue," 94–96.

37. On early medieval understandings of nature, see Kreiner, *Legions of Pigs*, 44–77; Squatriti, *Landscape*, 91–121; Anna Dorofeeva, *Reading Nature in the Early Middle Ages: Writing, Language and Creation in the Latin Physiologus, ca. 700–1000* (Arc Humanities Press, forthcoming).

38. Note that both topics might be approached through the form of the *disputatio*. On a false debate (ca. 450) between Jerome and Augustine about creationism vs. traducianism (a text found in Carolingian libraries), see Hennings, "*Disputatio de origine animae*."

39. For the Carolingians, see Lockett, *Psychologies*, 281–312; Mathon, "L'anthropologie," vol. 2; Marenbon, *Circle of Alcuin*, 31–70; Luscombe, *Medieval Thought*, 30–33; and the Italian translations of various treatises by Tolomio, *L'anima dell'uomo*.

40. Partly, this reflects more robust scholarship on the soul within Anglo-Saxon studies.

41. On the dating of Alcuin's *DRA* (Ep. 309) to 801–804 while Alcuin was abbot of Saint-Martin at Tours, see Bullough, *Alcuin*, 246. The letter is addressed to one Eulalia, a nickname Alcuin gave to Gundrada, just as he gave them to many students and friends: Garrison, "Social World." On Alcuin's correspondence with Gundrada, see Scheck, *Reform and Resistance*, 57–71.

42. Alcuin, *DRA* 1, ed. Curry, 39. The situation resembles that in 798, when Alcuin was asked to answer an exegetical problem posed by a layman at court: Ep. 136, ed. Dümmler, 205. Gundrada was a chaste, consecrated woman who resided at court and held significant influence with Charlemagne: Nelson, "Gendering Courts," 191.

43. Alcuin, *DRA* 1, ed. Curry, 41. The metaphor of head/brain as acropolis is discussed by Wright, "Brain as Treasury," 544–46.

44. Alcuin also wrote to Gundrada detailing his arguments against Adoptionism and encouraging her to use dialectic to challenge this heresy: Ep. 204, ed. Dümmler, 337–40. On Gundrada as the recipient, see Bullough, *Alcuin*, 76–77. On dialectic, see van Renswoude, "Art of Disputation," 48–49. Alcuin wrote three treatises refuting Adoptionism and participated in the Synods of Frankfurt (794) and Aachen (799) called by Charlemagne to condemn its teachings.

45. See Szarmach, "A Preface." On the *DRA* as part of a theological instructional manual for the laity, see Matter, "A Carolingian Schoolbook?"

46. On his vocabulary, see Curry, "*De ratione animae*," 23–29.

47. Alcuin, *DRA* 1, ed. and trans. Curry, 39 and 73.

48. See Alcuin, *DRA* 1, ed. Curry, 40–41.

49. Alcuin, *DRA* 2, ed. Curry, 43.

50. Alcuin, *DRA* 1 and 10, ed. Curry, 41 and 66.

51. Alcuin, *DRA* 3, ed. Curry, 45. On the self as rational mind throughout the *DRA*, and especially in the prayer that concludes the work, see Choy, "The Brother," 109–13.

52. See Godden, "Anglo-Saxons on the Mind," 271–74.

53. For the terms *spiritus, sensus, animus, ratio, voluntas, memoria*, see Alcuin, *DRA* 6, ed. Curry, 55–56.

54. Alcuin, *DRA* 6, ed. Curry, 56. See Isidore, *Liber differentiarum* 2.27, ed. Andrés Sanz, 61.

55. This is from Cassian's *Collationes* and Isidore's *Liber differentiarum* (Curry, "*De ratione animae*," 6–7). The various schemata were intended as examples of how previous writers had divided the unitary soul by its functions. Cf. Lockett, *Psychologies*, 284–86.

56. Alcuin, *DRA* 3, ed. Curry, 47. Serralda, *La philosophie*, 139–48, argues that in adapting the language from Augustine's *De Trinitate*, Alcuin replaced Augustine's view that intellect, memory, and will were the substance of the soul in favor of the belief that the soul possesses (*habet*) these three faculties.

57. Cf. Lockett, *Psychologies*, 284–85, who suggests that Alcuin sought to teach Gundrada about the Trinity through the *DRA*. The *DRA* was often transmitted together with Alcuin's treatise *De fidei Sanctae Trinitatis*: Szarmach, "A Preface," 398.

58. On Alcuin's sources, which also included several works by Isidore, see Curry, "*De ratione animae*," 5–9.

59. Lockett argues for two dominant perspectives on the soul in the early Middle Ages: an immaterial soul grounded in Platonism, and a material soul grounded in Stoicism. The latter had a more lasting influence (and a greater prevalence in English libraries) than has previously been recognized: Lockett, *Psychologies*, 9–15, 180–227.

60. For Alcuin, the soul does not simply animate a material framework but plays a role in shaping that very framework. Alcuin, *DRA* 2, ed. Curry, 41: "imperare quid, per quae, vel quando, vel ubi, vel quomodo faciat membra et considerare diligenter quid cui membro imperet faciendum." Serralda argues that Alcuin ignores Augustine's claim (grounded in Aristotle) that the soul creates an intermediary *species* for the body, preferring the immediacy of the soul creating the body: Serralda, *La philosophie*, 102–4. On Augustine's commitment to an Aristotelian view, see Byers, "Augustine and the Philosophers," 176–80.

61. On Augustine and late antique "corporealist" theories of God, see Griffin and Paulsen, "Augustine and the Corporeality of God." For an incisive example of Alcuin's "subtle but significant departures" from Augustine in the *DRA*, see Choy, "The Brother," 110–11.

62. Alcuin, *DRA* 6, ed. Curry, 54. Lockett, *Psychologies*, 288, lists as possible sources Augustine's *De Trinitate*, Isidore's *Liber differentiarum*, and Claudianus Mamertus's *De statu animae*, but Alcuin's text resembles these very little verbatim.

63. Cf. Lockett, *Psychologies*, 289: "Alcuin took the trouble to crystallize the esoteric notion of the incorporeal soul into a prominent point of orthodox doctrine." (But p. 293 notes that Alcuin uses *incorporalis* only once.)

64. See Cristiani, "L'espace de l'âme," 156–60.

65. At Alcuin *DRA* 7, ed. Curry, 57. Alcuin mentions that the soul guides the body by the refined materials of light and air, drawing on Augustine's *De Genesi ad litteram*, but he does not include Augustine's statements concerning the differences between corporeal and incorporeal natures.

66. On Candidus Wizo (d. 804?), see Jones, "Candidus Wizo"; Marenbon, *Circle of Alcuin*, 33–61. Candidus discussed the soul in a response to an anonymous monk's question about whether Christ could see God with his bodily eyes: Ep. 39, "Num Christus," ed. Dümmler, 557–61. Cf. Chazelle, *Crucified God*, 191n106, who suggests the author was Candidus Bruun (d. 845) and links the letter with midcentury discussions.

67. Candidus Wizo, "Num Christus," ed. Dümmler, 558 (emphases mine).

68. A passage on the soul known as the *Dicta Candidi de imagine Dei* (likely composed by Candidus Wizo) similarly emphasizes that the soul can be compared to its Creator but falls far short of God's perfection. On this text, see Marenbon, *Circle of Alcuin*, 37–61, 161–63; Ineichen-Eder, "Authenticity of the *Dicta Candidi*"; Lebech and McEvoy, "*De dignitate conditionis humanae*."

69. Candidus Wizo, "Num Christus," ed. Dümmler, 558.

70. On the similarity between Candidus's ideas and those of the fifth-century semi-Pelagians, see Lockett, *Psychologies*, 283, 301–10. On the influence of the semi-Pelagians, see Brown, *Ransom of the Soul*, 132–37, 176, 187.

71. Alcuin, *DRA* 8, ed. Curry, 58–59, states that God alone knows the origin of souls and that people are foolish to pursue this question. But earlier in his life he was more willing to speculate on it. For Alcuin's change of opinion, see Serralda, *La philosophie*, 105–7. For the

suggestion that Alcuin's *DRA* consciously glossed over controversies about the origins of the soul, see Lockett, *Psychologies*, 296.

72. The phrase came from a work of Fredegisus's that is now lost. On Fredegisus (d. 833), see Marenbon, *Circle of Alcuin*, 62–66; Haverkamp, "Making Something from Nothing," 1–5, 110–25. Marenbon, 63–64, dates the start of the dispute to the late 820s and believes this letter to be Agobard's second response to Fredegisus.

73. On Agobard's understanding of his duties as a bishop, see Airlie, "I, Agobard"; Booker, *Past Convictions*, 133–75. On his cascade of admonitory letters from 822–829, see van Renswoude, *Free Speech*, 215–24.

74. Agobard, Ep. 13 (ca. 830), ed. Dümmler, 217. Fredegisus's belief in the soul's preexistence may have stemmed from the Neoplatonic eternal cycle of *processio* and *reditus* from the world-soul: Nauta, "Preexistence of the Soul," 106–7.

75. Agobard, Ep. 13, ed. Dümmler, 217 (citing Isidore's *Sententiae* according to Mathon, "L'anthropologie," 2:339).

76. Citing Eccl 11:5, Agobard compares humans' ignorance about the soul's creation to their lack of knowledge about how bones are joined in the womb to make a child. Similarly, in his writings against Adoptionism, Alcuin stated that the joining of soul and body in the womb was as ineffable to humans as the joining of Christ's two natures in one person: see Cavadini, *Last Christology*, 97–99.

77. Fredegisus was no stranger to controversy as the author of *De substantia nihili et tenebrarum*, a treatise about the nature of nothing, which was not well received or understood at Charlemagne's court: Haverkamp, "Making Something from Nothing," 110–28.

78. In the 840s, Gottschalk began preaching a theory of double predestination (to hell as well as to heaven) based on Augustine's writings; he was condemned in 848 and confined to a monastery at the Council of Quierzy in 849, but the issue did not subside for the next decade. On Gottschalk's life and teaching, see Ganz, "Debate on Predestination"; Chazelle, *Crucified God*, 165–208; Pezé, *Virus de l'erreur*; Gillis, *Heresy and Dissent*.

79. As Gillis and Pezé have argued, during his imprisonment Gottschalk smuggled out writings to interested parties (likely young monks and clerics around Reims). What survives on the soul's origin are four separate pamphlets (*schedulae*): one introducing the problem, a second with patristic excerpts, a third with a brief solution, and a fourth with a more extended defense. These are all grouped under *Quaestiones de anima* [XXI], ed. Lambot, in *Oeuvres théologiques*, 283–94. See Pezé, "Débat doctrinal," 38, 67–68; Gillis, *Heresy and Dissent*, 147–58, 210–11.

80. Gottschalk, *Quaestiones de anima*, ed. Lambot, 288–89.

81. Augustine's Ep. 166 to Jerome (cited by Gottschalk) laid out four possibilities for the origin of the soul but stated that he could not be certain which was correct: Ep. 166, ed. Goldbacher, in *Epistulae III*, 545–85. On Gottschalk's beliefs about the soul within the context of the Carolingian reception of Augustine, see Mathon, "Les attitudes," 41–44.

82. Gottschalk, *Quaestiones de anima*, ed. Lambot, 289–91 (referencing the story about a worm in Augustine's *De quantitate animae* but drawing a lesson from it that Augustine does not countenance).

83. Gottschalk, *Quaestiones de anima*, ed. Lambot, 291.

84. Gottschalk, *Quaestiones de anima*, ed. Lambot, 291 (emphasis mine).

85. Gottschalk states that God mandated human ignorance on the soul's origins as punishment for original sin, but that he (Gottschalk) received a divine revelation (six years before

the date of writing) that allowed him to answer what other theologians had been unable to resolve. He asks his supporters to keep his writings secret until he is released: *Quaestiones de anima*, ed. Lambot, 290. Gillis, *Heresy and Dissent*, 191, argues that Gottschalk began using prophecy as a strategy against his opponents after 853, which may suggest a date for this *schedula*.

86. In the treatise discussed below, Hrabanus does not dismiss traducianism but suggests it might be one explanation for the soul's origins; this suggests Gottschalk's teaching may not have been as controversial as he himself implies.

87. Gillis, *Heresy and Dissent*, 185, notes that Gottschalk intended his pamphlets to circulate beyond the young monks and clerics for whom they were written.

88. See Dutton, "Carolingian Invisibles"; Marenbon, *Early Medieval Philosophy*, 55–58; Chazelle, *Crucified God*, 191–95, 211–38; Pezé, "Doctrinal Debate."

89. On theological works composed for Charles, see McKitterick, "Charles the Bald," 32–36; Pezé, "Autorité royale."

90. On correspondences, see Cristiani, "L'espace de l'âme."

91. The letter (so called at *DAR*, col. 947D) cannot be definitively ascribed to Hincmar: Jacques Sirmond (d. 1651) edited the text from a manuscript (now lost) at the monastery of Saint-Rémi in Reims, in which the text was attributed to a "quidam sapiens." Devisse, *Hincmar*, 1:20–21, argues against Hincmar's authorship based on the form of address to Charles and the biblical and patristic citations used. Mathon, "L'anthropologie," 2:247–51, observes that Étienne Baluze (d. 1718) saw the text among Hincmar's letters in a different manuscript and that Hincmar himself listed "quod anima non sit in corpore" among contemporary theological controversies in his *De praedestinatione* 31, col. 296D. This exact phrase is a heading in the Reims manuscript (col. 948A), and it is not found in other extant soul treatises. Thus, I follow Mathon that it seems most likely the work was composed at Reims, if not by Hincmar then under his supervision. The use of the Virgilian "te, o bone rex" (col. 931A) is a rare form of address and may be worthy of further investigation for clues as to authorship. Comparable examples appear in the Vivian Bible and Sedulius Scottus (both to Charles), Smaragdus (to Louis the Pious), and Jonas of Orléans (to Pippin).

92. The headings are numbers x–xiii and xv in Gottschalk's *Responsa de diversis* [VI], ed. Lambot, in *Oeuvres théologiques*, 131. Gillis, *Heresy and Dissent*, 150, 185, believes that this work was composed for Abbot Haudoin of Hautvillers after 853 based on a series of questions posed to Gottschalk by an anonymous monk. Pezé, "Débat doctrinal," 31–32, believes that the *Responsa* were composed in relation to a larger debate about the soul in 850.

93. Scholars have proposed a range of scenarios, from Charles soliciting opinions on the soul after the Council of Quierzy in 849, to Eriugena's *De praedestinatione* prompting a controversy on the nature of angels that raised uncertainties about the soul, to Hincmar intercepting correspondence on the soul from Gottschalk, which then set off a chain of events. On these scenarios (which remain speculative), see Wilmart, "L'opuscule," 208; Cappuyns, *Jean Scot Érigène*, 91–93; Mathon, "L'anthropologie," 2:282–92; Bouhot, *Ratramne*, 41–50.

94. Hincmar, *DAR*, col. 931D. Though the text lacks identifiers, Charles is definitively the recipient, with reference to his eponymous grandfather and his pious father (col. 931C–D). This emphasis on his name's inherent association with Charlemagne suggests a date after 845, when poets and artists increasingly invoked such comparisons: see Diebold, "Artistic Patronage," 291–315.

95. Ratramnus, *De anima*, ed. Wilmart, 210. The text survives in two twelfth-century manuscripts.

96. All three take up the term *localis* and the issue of incorporeality; Hincmar and Ratramnus both discuss the soul's movement through space and time, while Hincmar and Gottschalk (like Candidus) consider the resurrected body's perception of God.

97. On the insults exchanged, especially between Hincmar and Gottschalk, see Gillis, *Heresy and Dissent*, 182–98.

98. See, likewise, Ratramnus's use of Boethius to explain universals in a work refuting the existence of a world-soul: *Ad Odonem* 2 and 9, ed. Lambot, 27–33, 130–31; Marenbon, *Early Medieval Philosophy*, 53–56; Delhaye, *Une controverse sur l'âme*, 43–50.

99. Ratramnus, *De anima*, ed. Wilmart, 210: "As much as [these matters] ought to be scrutinized by the learned so ought they to be concealed from those less intelligent because bread gives life to the elderly but harms those who should be nourished with milk."

100. Ratramnus's *De praedestinatione* and *De corpore et sanguine Domini* both date to around 850 and were directed to Charles; their arguments pitted him against Hrabanus, Hincmar, and Paschasius Radbertus, the former abbot of Corbie. See Chazelle, *Crucified God*, 211–15; Chazelle, "Exegesis." On Ratramnus's life and works, see Bouhot, *Ratramne*.

101. Authorities cited in the treatise include Ambrose, Augustine, Claudianus Mamertus, Cassiodorus, and Isidore.

102. Ratramnus, *De anima*, ed. Wilmart, 211.

103. Alcuin, *DRA* 6, ed. Curry, 54: "circumscriptus in singulis suae carnis membris totus." Cf. Ratramnus, *De anima*, ed. Wilmart, 210–11, 215–16.

104. Ratramnus, *De anima*, ed. Wilmart, 211: "non est circumscripta, quoniam nullo corporis fine concluditur." Ratramnus does allow that every created thing can be called *circumscripta* because it is a distinct entity, but this does not mean that it is circumscribed by physical limits.

105. Mathon, "Les attitudes," 38–41.

106. Ratramnus, *De anima*, ed. Wilmart, 211: "Ideoque qualitatibus suis, non fine corporis circumscribitur." Cristiani, "L'espace de l'âme," 158–59, explains that, unlike earlier authors, Ratramnus escaped the equation of space with corporeality by saying that the soul was bound not by the body but by its own essential properties; thus, the nature of the soul was not circumscribed, although it was found in a physical space.

107. Ratramnus, *De anima*, ed. Wilmart, 213.

108. Both Alcuin and Ratramnus cited Augustine's *De Genesi ad litteram* for their descriptions of how the soul communicates with the body, but they focused on different ideas within it to suit their own purposes.

109. Ratramnus, *De anima*, ed. Wilmart, 219.

110. Given his rejection of circumscription, it was perhaps historical justice that Ratramnus was asked to refute a monk's teachings about a single world-soul in a controversy from the early 860s. On this, see Ratramnus, *Ad Odonem*, ed. Lambot; Delhaye, *Une controverse sur l'âme*; Bouhot, *Ratramne*, 57–59.

111. Hrabanus, *TDA*, cols. 1109B–1120C; preface as Ep. 57, ed. Dümmler, 514–15. The method of address indicates Lothar II as the recipient: Garipzanov, *Symbolic Language*, 117. On Hrabanus's use of Cassiodorus's *De anima*, see Mathon, "L'anthropologie," 2:236–39.

112. Hincmar, *DAR*, col. 931A. As with earlier authors, Hincmar uses both *animus* and *anima* for the soul.

113. Hincmar, *DAR*, col. 931C.

114. A misunderstanding in the Latin leads Hincmar to answer "whether the soul alone is moved by time," instead of what must have been intended (whether the soul is moved by time alone, or by time and space).

115. These shared citations support the belief that the two authors were writing as part of the same conversation. They cite the same passages in Augustine's *De Genesi ad litteram* and Ambrose's *Hexameron*. On the use of the same authorities to argue different theological positions, see Chazelle's discussion of the Eucharistic controversy: "Glorified Body," at 36.

116. Mathon, "Les attitudes," 38–41, points to a difference between Hincmar's and Ratramnus's approaches but judges them primarily according to their adherence to Augustine. In describing the writings of the 850s as the "second failure" of Augustinian thought (the first being in the fifth century), Mathon suggests that, like the predestination debate, controversy on the soul was grounded in interpretative problems posed by Augustine's texts rather than pastoral concerns: "L'anthropologie," 2:330–32.

117. Hincmar, *DAR* 1, col. 932A.

118. Hincmar, *DAR* 1, col. 933B.

119. Augustine, *De anima et eius origine* 4.18.26, ed. Urba and Zycha, 406.

120. Hincmar, *DAR* 1, col. 933C: "In his namque, etsi non corpus quod non est ipsa cernitur, tamen similitudinem corpoream habere creditur." The phrasing here resembles Candidus's letter, although it is not sufficiently close to suggest a direct influence.

121. Hincmar, *DAR* 4, col. 939B.

122. Hincmar, *DAR* 2, col. 935D. See Gregory, *Moralia in Iob* 5.34.61, ed. Adriaen, 262.

123. Like Ratramnus, in discussing how the soul moves the body through space, Hincmar (*DAR* 7, col. 942D) borrows language from Augustine to describe the soul directing the body by means of its immobile "nods" or commands.

124. Hincmar, *DAR* 3, col. 936D.

125. Hincmar, *DAR* 2, col. 933C. At the end of Hincmar's *DAR* in the lost manuscript witness was a collection of quotations from Augustine's works under the title *Quod anima sit in corpore*. This may suggest that the manuscript was a working copy of a treatise still under revision; in either case, the title indicates the *DAR*'s central argument.

126. Quoting Cassiodorus's *De anima*, Hincmar states that when the body is wounded, the soul cannot depart except when God allows it, which accounts for why one person dies and another lives even if both have the same injury: *DAR* 2, col. 936B. On whether the soul can exceed the corporeal boundaries of the body, Hincmar notes that this happens when the soul extends further than the bodily eyes, nose, and ears in seeing, smelling, and hearing: *DAR* 5, col. 939C–D.

127. Hincmar, *DAR* 2, col. 936B: "Ecce quot et qualibus non argumentis, sed documentis ostenditur nobis animas corporibus vel indutas, vel colligatas, vel vinctas. Quorum auctoritati periculosum videtur nobis refragari" (punctuation mine in the translation).

128. The last chapter of Hincmar's *DAR* deals with the beatific vision (a subject on which Hrabanus, Gottschalk, and Eriugena also wrote), but this is not its main focus. On the vision of God, see Dutton, "Carolingian Invisibles"; Chazelle, *Crucified Body*, 191–93, 208.

129. There is no suggestion that Lothar solicited this work.

130. See de Jong, "Emperor Lothar," 229–35.

131. Hrabanus names Cassiodorus and Prosper as his two sources on the soul and Vegetius as his source on the military. By Prosper, he meant Julian Pomerius, whose *Vita contemplativa*

was extremely popular in the ninth century: Timmermann, "Sharers in the Contemplative Virtue." Hrabanus states that he included the chapters on the military in light of the recent incursions of barbarians: *TDA*, col. 1109C–D.

132. He indicates to Lothar that the work can easily be memorized: *TDA*, col. 1109B.

133. On Hrabanus's life and career, see Coon, *Dark Age Bodies*, 13–41.

134. Hrabanus, *TDA* 1, col. 1110D.

135. Hrabanus, *TDA* 1, col. 1110A–B. While Hrabanus links *spiritus* in humans with the breath, he never suggests a tripartite division into soul-spirit-body.

136. Hrabanus, *TDA* 1, cols. 1110C and 1111A.

137. Hrabanus, *TDA* 3, col. 1113A–C. Though the Bible describes God and the soul as speaking and moving, Hrabanus clarifies that this is a mere literary device for human comprehension.

138. See Hrabanus, *TDA* 1, col. 1111A.

139. Hrabanus, *TDA* 1, col. 1111A.

140. Hrabanus, *TDA* 4, col. 1114A; see also col. 1114B: "Et quid de hujuscemodi passionibus dicamus, cum frequentissime nimio potu et distentu ventris, sapientium animos obrui cernamus."

141. Hrabanus, *TDA* 4, col. 1114A, compares the soul to a fire shut into a small vessel and unable to escape. But a fire and vessel are corporeal bodies, so this metaphor cannot explain the soul's restriction.

142. This section closely follows Cassiodorus, *De anima* 10, ed. Halporn, 553–56.

143. Hrabanus, *TDA* 5, col. 1114B–C.

144. Hrabanus, *TDA* 5, col. 1114C–D (quoting Acts 7:49).

145. See also Ratramnus on the round and upright heads of the *cynocephali* (dog-headed people) as an important (though ultimately not essential) characteristic of humans: *Epistola de cynocephalis*, ed. Dümmler, 155; Matter, "Soul of the Dog-Man"; Wood, "Categorising the *cynocephali*."

146. Hrabanus underscores the body's symmetry and perfection (for example, the skull has six bones because six is a perfect number): *TDA* 11, col. 1119A–B.

147. Lv 17:14 and Dt 12:23.

148. Hrabanus, *TDA* 1, col. 1110B; Hincmar, *DAR* 1, col. 933A–B; Cassiodorus, *De anima* 3, ed. Halporn, 536–38.

149. Hrabanus, *TDA* 1, col. 1110B.

150. Although Hrabanus borrowed from Cassiodorus, he devoted more space to the issue of blood than his source. On Carolingian exegesis of Leviticus, see Firey, "Letter of the Law."

151. Hrabanus, *TDA* 2, col. 1112B–C (copying Cassiodorus but replacing "medendi artifices" with "naturarum investigatores"). On the consensus that forty days was when a fetus became a human being, see Elsakkers, "Vocabulary of Abortion," 386, 411.

152. Ratramnus, *De anima*, ed. Wilmart, 223; Hrabanus, *TDA* 1, cols. 1110C, 1110D, and 1111C.

153. Touati, "Raban Maur," 199, suggests that Hrabanus had read Vindicianus's *Gynaecia*, but this is not found in the one medical manuscript that Touati locates at Fulda (Paris, BnF lat. 6880, which includes Vindicianus's letter to Emperor Valentinian but not the *Gynaecia*).

154. On the persistence of Stoic beliefs in Gaul, Italy, and Spain, see Colish, *Stoic Tradition*, 239–302.

155. Gennadius of Marseille's *De ecclesiasticis dogmatibus* (ca. 470, commonly attributed to Augustine) was a particularly popular text and contained Stoic theories of the soul.

Lockett speculates that Gennadius was Candidus's source for the belief that only God is incorporeal. On Gennadius's influence and the category of "eclectic" Church Fathers, see Lockett, *Psychologies*, 200–227, 298–306. On Gregory's psychology of the soul as a response to the revival of Aristotelian theory in sixth-century Constantinople and Rome, see Dal Santo, *Debating*, 85–148.

156. On the six extant ninth-century manuscripts and the "traveling companions" of the *Visio*, see Contreni, "Building Mansions," 696–98.

157. On St. Petersburg, National Library, lat. O.v.I.5, see Curry, "Illustrated *Visio Baronti*"; Nees, "Illustrated Manuscript"; Contreni, "Building Mansions," 696–701; Nees, *Frankish Manuscripts*, cat. no. 59.

158. On the artistic and theological connections, see Nees, "Illustrated Manuscript," 112–28; Contreni, "Building Mansions," 696–706.

## Chapter 2

1. On Bernard of Septimania's career, see Depreux, *Prosopographie*, 137–39. On William's ambiguous status as a hostage, see Kosto, *Hostages*, 73–77. On what can be known about Dhuoda's life, see Le Jan, "Multiple Identities"; within a broader context of other laywomen, Garver, *Women*, 115–26, 144–59, 271–74.

2. For different perspectives on the form and function of the *Liber manualis*, see Jaffe, "Dhuoda's *Handbook*"; Cherewatuk, "*Speculum matris*"; Innes, "Keeping It in the Family," 17–23. On her sources, see Riché, *Manuel*, 33–37.

3. On the themes of duty and mutual assistance, see Nelson, "Dhuoda"; Olsen, "One Heart."

4. But see, recently, Polanichka, "Quasi per speculum," 7–16, which also addresses Dhuoda's interest in the natural world.

5. For a detailed study of Dhuoda's style, see Dronke, *Women Writers*, 36–54.

6. For a recent analysis, see Romig, *Perfect Man*, 34–66, 100–105, 158; Stone, *Morality*, discusses the manuals within a broader survey of moral literature. See also Savigni, "Laïcs dans l'ecclésiologie," 45–63; Sot, "Concordances"; Noble, "Secular Sancity." For a detailed study of the texts, sources, and manuscripts, see Sedlmeier, *Die laienparänetischen Schriften*.

7. On Eric, see Duval, "Paulin d'Aquilée." On Wido, see Smith, *Province and Empire*, 52–54, 58–59. On Matfrid, see Depreux, "Le comte Matfrid."

8. Jonas, *DIL* Preface, ed. Dubreucq, 1:122; Dhuoda, *LM* Prologue, ed. Riché, 80. This comes from Augustine's statement that scripture is a kind of mirror, in which a reader ought to be able to see the state of his/her soul: see Alcuin, *DVV* 5, col. 616C. On Augustine's use of *speculum*, see Bradley, "Backgrounds," 102–5.

9. On this genre, see Born, "*Specula principis*"; Anton, *Fürstenspiegel*; Rouche, "Miroirs des princes"; Dubreucq, "La littérature des *specula*." Cf. the argument that lay mirrors and mirrors for princes are fundamentally distinct: Sedlmeier, *Die laienparänetischen Schriften*, 24; Toubert, "La théorie du mariage," 237–41, 246–47.

10. Stone, *Morality*, 42. Hincmar's *De cavendis vitiis et virtutibus exercendis* (860s) is sometimes classed as a lay mirror, but since it was written for a king, it is not included here.

11. Given its author's unusual position, the *LM* has received far more attention from modern scholars, who have often emphasized the work's uniqueness and attributed it variously to Dhuoda's gender, her concerns as a mother, or her precarious political situation. On the changing representations of Dhuoda as author, see Stofferahn, "Many Faces."

12. Romig, *Perfect Man*, 34–66.

13. The three ecclesiastical authors state that the manuals were commissioned by their lay recipients. Some read such statements as a pretext (e.g., Rouche, "Miroirs des princes," 350–64), but see the convincing arguments of Noble, "Secular Sanctity," 24–31; Stone, "Rise and Fall," 365–67; Romig, *Perfect Man*, 42–43, 55–56.

14. Claussen, "Fathers of Power." On the honest advisor, see van Renswoude, *Free Speech*, 180–205.

15. Alcuin likely knew Paulinus's work because Eric of Friuli first requested a moral guide from Alcuin himself (see below). Jonas and Dhuoda both cite the *DVV*. Riché, *Manuel*, 384–85, finds correspondences to the *DIL* and *LE* in the *LM*; I find no compelling allusions to the *LE* but agree that there may be allusions to the *DIL* (see Riché, 312–13n1). Dubreucq, "La littérature des *specula*," 32, proposes that in writing her manual Dhuoda saw herself as fulfilling the duties of paternal religious instruction outlined by Jonas.

16. On mirrors and the common good, see Koziol, "Leadership."

17. On the two versions of the *LE*, the second of which was produced after Eric died in 799, see de Nicola, "Sancti Paulini," 189. Extant witnesses of the *DIL* fall into two groups, a shorter version with Matfrid's name that must date before 828 (when Matfrid was disgraced) and a longer version without it. Scholars date the first version 818–828 and the second 828–840, with many preferring a date closer to 829. See Dubreucq, *Instruction des laïcs*, 1:44–48 and 97–103; Sedlmeier, *Die laienparänetischen Schriften*, 200–208; Schröder, "Zur Überlieferung."

18. Jonas, *DIL* Preface, ed. Dubreucq, 1:124–26; Dhuoda, *LM* 1.1, ed. Riché, 96. On Dhuoda's intention to reach a court audience, see Nelson, "Organic Intellectuals," 11–13. On lay culture through Dhuoda's and Jonas's handbooks, see Sot, "Concordances."

19. Over 140 manuscripts of the *DVV* survive, with more than 35 witnesses from the ninth and tenth centuries: Szarmach, "Preliminary Handlist"; Szarmach, "Latin Tradition," 14–16. Hrabanus Maurus, Jonas of Orléans, and Halitgar of Cambrai all reused sections from the *DVV* in their own works. On the impact of Alcuin's text, see Newhauser, *Treatise on Vices*, 115–18.

20. Advisory literature for kings, for example, often borrowed from works addressed to a nonroyal audience, including texts reflecting on the monastic life as well as manuals for the lay nobility. Jonas's own royal mirror (the *De institutione regia*) borrowed from the *DIL*: Dubreucq, *Le métier de roi*, 35–49. On similarities between Smaragdus of Saint-Mihiel's advisory works for kings and for monks, see Kramer, *Rethinking Authority*, 123–68.

21. For similar approaches, see Romig, *Perfect Man*, 39–42; Stone, "Rise and Fall," 369–70; Smith, "Gender and Ideology," 62–67.

22. Jonas's *DIL* explicitly addressed topics appropriate to laywomen, but this is no reason to assume that the other manuals were not also read by women; they do not, after all, say anything about gendered activities like warfare. We know that one laywoman (Judith, daughter of Eberhard of Friuli) owned a copy of Alcuin's *DVV* (see Chapter 7), and Alcuin addressed a letter outlining similar moral points as in the *DVV* to *both* an elite nobleman and his wife (Ep. 69, ed. Dümmler, 112–13). On this letter, see Bullough, *Alcuin*, 370–71; Phelan, *Formation*, 143–44. On laywomen's familiarity with moral literature for men, see Garver, *Women*, 145.

23. For a similar comparison of subtler differences between Jonas's and Dhuoda's manuals, see Sot, "Concordances," esp. 360.

24. For example, the *DIL* is significantly longer than the other works. On the structure, sources, and transmission of each text, see Sedlmeier, *Die laienparänetischen Schriften*.

25. On the manuals teaching "qualities of mind," and on the *Admonitio generalis* of 789 similarly encouraging "states of mind" rather than "specific behaviors," see Romig, *Perfect Man*, 38, 63.

26. As Stone, *Morality*, 82–84, discusses, the manuals say almost nothing about military duties, although Wido supposedly requested guidance on this.

27. As Sedlmeier, *Die laienparänetischen Schriften*, 25–30, outlines, despite the absence of an extant dedicatory letter, a manuscript from the first half of the ninth century attributes the work to Paulinus, and the recipient (one *amicus suus in saeculo militans*) is assumed to have been Eric based on Alcuin's Ep. 98 (discussed below). A new edition of the *LE* by de Nicola is not widely available, so I have been able to consult only the first nine chapters in de Nicola, "Sancti Paulini," 196–209. On Paulinus's career, see Everett, "Paulinus."

28. Paulinus, *LE* 4–6, ed. de Nicola, 198–99. On the *interior homo* in Paulinus, see Deug-Su, "La *saecularis potestas*," 371–75, 398–99.

29. Paulinus's chief sources were Alcuin's letters, Julian Pomerius's *De vita contemplativa*, and the Pseudo-Basil *Admonitio ad filium spiritualem*. On these, and Paulinus's methods of adapting them, see Deug-Su, "*Liber exhortationis*."

30. Paulinus, *LE* 64, col. 274C: "quia caro est quae animam perdit." I do not find a clear distinction between Paulinus's use of *caro* versus *corpus*, as especially evident at *LE* 66, col. 281C.

31. Paulinus, *LE* 65, col. 278B.

32. The one mention of bodily resurrection is at *LE* 51, col. 254B.

33. Paulinus, *LE* 64, col. 277A.

34. See *LE* 8, 22, 37, 60, cols. 204B, 218A, 237A–238A, 268A–269A. Evagrius taught that there were eight chief demons that attacked the mind with their evil suggestions, but Brakke, *Demons*, 48–77, 240–46, argues that ascetic writing in the Latin West (especially John Cassian) internalized Evagrius's model of combat, to focus on the battle of the spirit against the flesh and not on demonic attacks directly against the soul.

35. See Paulinus, *LE* 64, col. 275B (quoting Rom 7:23).

36. See Paulinus, *LE* 64, col. 275A (drawing on Eph 6:12).

37. Paulinus, *LE* 64, col. 274C (referencing Mt 13:39).

38. Paulinus, *LE* 66, col. 279B: "Oratio animae ad Deum adversus mala carnis." The title is given by the editor but accurately summarizes the content that follows. According to de Nicola, "Sancti Paulini," 192, Paulinus did not himself divide the work into chapters. Cassiodorus's *De anima* also ended with a prayer to God: see Choy, "The Brother," 108.

39. Paulinus, *LE* 66, col. 281C.

40. Paulinus, *LE* 35, col. 233A (citing the Pseudo-Basil *Admonitio*, as noted by Deug-Su, "*Liber exhortationis*," 304).

41. For the parallels with the *Admonitio*, see Deug-Su, "*Liber exhortationis*," 293–98; Sedlmeier, *Die laienparänetischen Schriften*, 50–55. The *Admonitio*, once attributed to Basil of Caesarea, is now ascribed to Abbot Porcarius of Lérins (fl. 490). See the edition by Lehmann, "Die *Admonitio S. Basilii*," 200–246; and the attribution of authorship by de Vogüé, "Entre Basile et Benoît," 19–34. The oldest reference to the metaphor of the soul as a charioteer is from Plato's *Phaedrus*. Jerome also employed it in *Adversus Jovinianum* 2.10, col. 299B.

42. Paulinus, *LE* 35, cols. 233A–234A.

43. This was unlike Greek charioteers, who held the reins in their hands. Thanks to Nate Andrade for this observation.

44. Paulinus, *LE* 64, col. 280B.

45. Dhuoda, *LM* Incipit, ed. Riché, 68; trans. Neel, 2.

46. Dhuoda, *LM* 10.1, ed. Riché, 340. *Regula Benedicti* 7, ed. Venarde, 44–46, describes Jacob's ladder as the life of humility, with the sides representing the body and soul. This may have inspired Dhuoda, given her familiarity with the text. On her citations of the Rule, see Claussen, "Fathers of Power," 794–804; Riché, *Manuel*, 31, 34, 383–84.

47. Dhuoda, *LM* Praefatio and 4.2, ed. Riché, 86 and 208; trans. Neel, 6 and 46.

48. See, for example, *LM* 3.4–5, ed. Riché, 148–54. Dhuoda constantly compares the devotion and loyalty William owes to his lord and father to that he owes to God. On her conviction that the laity could perform both active and contemplative duties, see Claussen, "God and Man," 43–52.

49. Scholars note Dhuoda's "practical" tone: Nelson, "Dhuoda," 116; Jaffe, "Dhuoda's *Handbook*," 182. On spiritual discernment as key to William's role as royal counselor, see Mayeski, *Dhuoda*, 59, 118–19, 141–42.

50. Stone, *Morality*, 214–46, argues that wealth was not especially troubling to Carolingian moralists. See also Dronke, *Women Writers*, 44.

51. On these parallels (but also Dhuoda's insistence that the temporal not be mistaken for the eternal), see Polanichka, "Quasi per speculum," 1–9.

52. That is to say Dhuoda was not the exception among her contemporaries (in my opinion)—see the parallels between her work and Paschasius's attitude toward the body, as discussed below.

53. Dhuoda, *LM* 4.2, ed. Riché, 206.

54. Dhuoda, *LM* 4.2, ed. Riché, 206.

55. Dhuoda, *LM* 4.6, ed. Riché, 222. Nelson, "Monks, Secular Men," at 127, states that Dhuoda offered the "most frankly positive view of sexual activity to be found in a Frankish writer."

56. Dhuoda, *LM* 4.6, ed. Riché, 224: "Tamen si uenerint et *angelo* immittente *Sathanae*, mentem *colafizauerint* tuam." Cf. 2 Cor 12:7: "datus est mihi stimulus carnis meae angelus Satanae ut me colaphizet." Cf. Paulinus, *LE* 64, col. 275B: "ideo dicit Apostolus, Datus est mihi stimulus carnis meae; non dicit, animae meae, sed carnis meae angelus Satanae."

57. Dhuoda, *LM* 4.7, ed. Riché, 234.

58. Dhuoda, *LM* 4.7, ed. Riché, 232 (referencing Dt 34:7).

59. Dhuoda, *LM* 7, ed. Riché, 298–304. Nelson, "Dhuoda," 112–15, at 114 (where she also observes that this title is present in only one manuscript).

60. On her unusual "biological" authority, see Polanichka, "Maternity," 20–27.

61. Dhuoda, *LM* 7.1, ed. Riché, 298. On Dhuoda's Latin and use of Ovid's *Amores* here, see Nelson, "Dhuoda," 113–14; Dronke, *Women Writers*, 45–46.

62. On the two births, Dhuoda adapts Augustine, *In Iohannis Evangelium* 11.6, ed. Willems, 113–14. According to Heene, *Legacy of Paradise*, 155, Dhuoda's is the only Carolingian text to link spiritual and physical motherhood. On her use of exegesis to justify her pedagogical authority, see Mayeski, *Dhuoda*, esp. 65–92.

63. Paulinus, *LE* 64, cols. 276B–277A.

64. Paulinus, *LE* 64, col. 276B.

65. See Dhuoda's discussion of illness at *LM* 5.8, ed. Riché, 278–84, where she also notes that it might come as a loving chastisement, in which case William should neither forsake treatment nor become hopeless.

66. Similarly, Noble, "Secular Sanctity," 16, finds "considerable evolution in social thought" among lay manuals written in the 790s–820s.

67. Studies typically state that 30 witnesses of the *LE* survive, but de Nicola, "Sancti Paulini," 187, has found over 200 (almost all of which are attributed to Augustine, which likely accounted for its later popularity). Only one (Paris, BnF lat. 2996, *s*.IX$^{med}$) names Paulinus as the author.

68. On Paulinus as *praeceptor*, see Alcuin, Ep. 98, ed. Dümmler, 142. On their friendship, see Everett, "Paulinus," 119–29. On the question of citations (or lack thereof), see Bullough, *Alcuin*, 78–79, who observes that the *LE* shows signs of Alcuin sending copies of his own correspondence to Paulinus, who then reused quotations in his own admonitory work.

69. Alcuin, Ep. 98, ed. Dümmler, 142. On the dating, see Bullough, *Alcuin*, 446–48; on the significance, see Romig, *Perfect Man*, 42–43.

70. Alberi, "Sword Which You Hold," 117–31.

71. Alcuin, Ep. 249, ed. Dümmler, 402; Smith, *Province and Empire*, 52.

72. Romig, *Perfect Man*, esp. 39–43. See also Veronese, "Conjugality," 453, who argues that consensual politics required the support of the laity, and thus kings had to offer them a path to salvation without delay.

73. Wallach, "Alcuin on Virtues," 179, argues that Alcuin framed the work primarily as a lay equivalent to Gregory the Great's manual for clergy, the *Regula pastoralis*. Cf. Bullough, "Alcuin and Lay Virtue," esp. 84, who groups the *DVV* with Alcuin's admonitory letters to kings and laypeople and his *Disputatio de rhetorica* (from which the *DVV* borrows).

74. Alcuin, *DVV* 34, cols. 636D–637A. On Alcuin's use of Gregory's *Moralia in Iob* here, see Dubreucq "Autour du *De virtutibus*," 279–80.

75. Paulinus, *LE* 18 and 23, cols. 210B–C, 218B–219B, names various vices and their opposing virtues, but this is not a prominent theme of the work. Alcuin's sources and the extent to which he adapted them have been disputed: see Rochais, "Le *Liber de virtutibus*"; Wallach, "Alcuin on Virtues," 180–90; Sedlmeier, *Die laienparänetischen Schriften*, 129–49; Bullough, "Alcuin and Lay Virtue," 86–89.

76. Cassian and Gregory differed slightly on the number and order of the vices. From Gregory, Alcuin borrowed the secondary sins that derived from the eight chief sins; from Isidore, he took the idea of eight specific virtues that oppose the vices. On this, and for a chart comparing the lists of Cassian, Gregory, Alcuin, as well as Isidore, Jonas, and Hrabanus, see Dubreucq, "Autour du *De virtutibus*," at 276. On Christian virtue-and-vice literature, see Newhauser, *Treatise on Vices*, esp. 95–124; Bloomfield, *Seven Deadly Sins*, esp. 69–81.

77. On Carolingian manuscripts of the *Psychomachia*, see Woodruff, "Illustrated Manuscripts of Prudentius," 33–79.

78. Alcuin, (Preface to *DVV*) Ep. 305, ed. Dümmler, 464. I do not see a distinction between *anima/animus/mens* in the *DVV* (also true in the *LM*). Rosenwein, similarly, finds a "general equivalence" of *animus*, *anima*, *cor*, and *mens* in Alcuin's work: "Rereading *Askese und Laster*," 82.

79. Alcuin, *DVV* 16, col. 624D.

80. Alcuin, *DVV* 16, col. 625A.

81. Alcuin, *DVV* 16, col. 625A.

82. Alcuin, *DVV* 16, col. 624D.

83. Alcuin, *DVV* 18, col. 627B.

84. See Alcuin, *DVV* 16, col. 625A–B.

85. Paulinus, *LE* 48, col. 252A.

86. See, for example, *DVV* 3, col. 616A, where Alcuin uses similar language to discuss the two births of every Christian (*Nobilior est generatio spiritualis quam carnalis*) but only in order to contrast them, not to harmonize them, as Dhuoda did.

87. Alcuin, *DVV* 29, cols. 633D–634A.

88. Alcuin, *DVV* 29, col. 633D.

89. For the argument that the manuals sought to establish a *ministerium* for the laity, see Dubreucq, "La littérature des *specula*"; Noble, "Secular Sanctity"; Skinner, "Lay Sanctity," 30–33.

90. Alcuin, *DVV* 18, col. 627A.

91. Alcuin, *DVV* 27, cols. 632D–633A.

92. Cassian termed *gula* and *fornicatio* the natural vices and the other six the extranatural vices; Gregory listed these as carnal vices and the other five as spiritual vices. See Bloomfield, *Seven Deadly Sins*, 70, 73.

93. See Alcuin, *DVV* 27 and 28, cols. 633A and 633C.

94. See the discussion of *acedia* by Dubreucq, "Autour du *De virtutibus*," 277–78.

95. On emotions in Alcuin's text, see Rosenwein, *Generations of Feeling*, 67–85.

96. Jonas himself did not use the title *De institutione laicali* (Dubreucq, *Instruction des laïcs*, 43–44), but this has become conventional.

97. Jonas, *DIL* 3.6, ed. Dubreucq, 2:232–46, where he refers to Alcuin by name (at 244).

98. In the preface (ed. Dubreucq, 1:124–26), Jonas explains that he has divided the work into three books: Books 1 and 3 pertain to all the faithful, while Book 2 pertains to the laity (including laywomen). On the *DIL* as a handbook for *comes* in particular, see Veronese, "Conjugality," 447–53.

99. In 824, Matfrid led one of the armies against the Bretons, and in 827 he was responsible for a disastrous expedition in the Spanish March, which resulted in his disgrace in 828 (this date thus serves as the *terminus ante quem* of the first version of the *DIL*): Depreux, "Le comte Matfrid," 353–54; de Jong, *Penitential State*, 39–40, 148–53.

100. Similar passages are found in the Synod of 829, *Relatio episcoporum* of 829, *De institutione regia* of 831, and Council of Aachen 836; on Jonas's role in crafting these documents, see Debreucq, *Le métier de roi*, 34–42. On the two versions of the *DIL*, see above.

101. Veronese, "Conjugality," 444–49.

102. Jonas did not include Alcuin's section on the four cardinal virtues but only mentioned the eight pairs of virtues and vices.

103. Jonas, *DIL* 2.23, ed. Dubreucq, 2:96 (citing a sermon by Maximus of Turin, which Jonas attributes to Augustine).

104. Jonas emphasizes that human beings possess the image of God and animals do not: *DIL* 2.23, ed. Dubreucq, 2:100.

105. Jonas, *DIL* 2.8, ed. Dubreucq, 1:388.

106. He frequently introduces problems by describing interactions that he (purportedly) had with lay members of his flock. On Jonas's role as a bishop, see Dubreucq, *Instruction des laïcs*, 33–43; Dubreucq, *Le métier du roi*, 9–26; Delaruelle, "Jonas d'Orléans," 129–43.

107. Jonas, *DIL* 1.20, ed. Dubreucq, 1:312.

108. Jonas, *DIL* 2.1, ed. Dubreucq, 1:318–20. Cf. Augustine, *De bono coniugali* 9.9, ed. Zycha, 199–201, who holds out as the third and best option to have no need to use these necessary things.

109. Jonas, *DIL* 2.1, ed. Dubreucq, 1:322 (citing Isidore's *De ecclesiasticis officiis*).

110. Scholars have seen Jonas's work as a crucial step in defining the laity by the state of marriage, but as Romig notes, Jonas states in the preface that Matfrid had asked for guidance on the married life—so the *DIL*'s emphasis may reflect its patron's as much as its author's concerns: *Perfect Man*, 191n150. On Carolingian moralists' constitution of an *ordo coniugatorum*, see Toubert, "La théorie du mariage"; cf. Chélini, *L'aube*, 79–83, who believes that instead of offering the laity its own *ordo*, these authors subjected nobles to a monastic ideal that they could never fully fulfill.

111. Things to be sought for their own sake include wisdom, friendship, and health: Jonas, *DIL* 2.1, ed. Dubreucq, 1:318. On Augustine's understanding of how marriage limited the disordering power of lust, see Cavadini, "Reconsidering Augustine."

112. See Jonas, *DIL* 2.1, ed. Dubreucq, 1:314–30, at 316 and 324.

113. On these rules, which referenced both Old Testament purity laws and Christian liturgical cycles, see Chélini, *L'aube*, 199–205.

114. Jonas, *DIL* 2.6, ed. Dubreucq, 1:368.

115. On Jonas's belabored concern with regulating marital sex (especially compared to the other lay mirrors), see Stone, *Morality*, 285–89, 298–302.

116. Jonas, *DIL* 2.6, ed. Dubreucq, 1:374 (citing Augustine's *De bono coniugali*).

117. Here we see how Jonas's agenda drove the process of compilation: he selected those passages from authorities that accorded with his overarching themes.

118. Jonas, *DIL* 1.10, ed. Dubreucq, 1:208. On Jonas as one of Pomerius's "most attentive readers," see Timmermann, "Sharers in the Contemplative Virtue," 34–39.

119. Jonas, *DIL* 3.6, ed. Dubreucq, 2:232.

120. Jonas, *DIL* 3.6, ed. Dubreucq, 2:232.

121. Jonas, *DIL* 1.10, ed. Dubreucq, 1:214 (citing Pomerius's *De vita contemplativa*).

122. See, for example, *DIL* 1.10, ed. Dubreucq, 1:208.

123. For example, Jonas only once alludes to Gal 5:17 (a passage that appears in both the *LE* and *LM*) and slightly alters the quotation, which diminishes the sense of direct conflict between body and soul. See *DIL* 3.16, ed. Dubreucq, 2:330: "et uitia quibus *caro aduersus spiritum concupiscit*."

124. The last six chapters treat of burial, the resurrected body, the day of judgment, and eternal rewards and punishments. Thus, there is a thematic progression throughout the *DIL* from baptism to the final judgment.

125. Jonas, *DIL* 3.16, ed. Dubreucq, 2:320–34 (relying heavily on Augustine's *Enchiridion*).

126. Smaragdus, *Expositio*, Prologus 2, ed. Spannagel and Engelbert, 10. On Smaragdus, see Ponesse, "Smaragdus of St Mihiel"; Coon, *Dark Age Bodies*, 101–13.

127. Smaragdus, *Expositio*, Prologus 3, ed. Spannagel and Engelbert, 13.

128. These two passages are cited five times.

129. Smaragdus, *Expositio* 7.9, ed. Spannagel and Engelbert, 165–66; trans. Barry, 271.

130. Hildemar's commentary is derived from oral lectures to his students. On Hildemar (also known as Hildemar of Corbie), see de Jong, "Growing Up"; Coon, *Dark Age Bodies*, 63–67, 103–8.

131. The issue of baths offers a keen point of comparison: while canons from 816 allowed only biannual bath times, Smaragdus encouraged the use of baths for the infirm, and Hildemar broadened accessibility even more by allowing baths for those laboring. See Ponesse, "Smaragdus of St Mihiel," 389; Hildemar, *Expositio regulae* 36, ed. Mittermüller, 407–9; Smarag-

dus, *Expositio* 36.8, ed. Spannagel and Engelbert, 250. On the dangers of bathing, see Coon, *Dark Age Bodies*, 125.

132. Hildemar, *Expositio regulae* 4, ed. Mittermüller, 148. On Hildemar's and Smaragdus's approaches to bodily regulation within the cloister, see Coon, *Dark-Age Bodies*, 63–68, 102–33.

133. Hildemar, *Expositio regulae* 4, ed. Mittermüller, 149.

134. See Smaragdus, *Expositio* Prologus 21, ed. Spannagel and Engelbert, 35; Hildemar, *Expositio regulae*, Prologus 21, ed. Mittermüller, 46.

135. See Savigni, "Esegesi medievale."

136. Unlike earlier exegetes, who had claimed that "earthly Adam" represented the body of the devil, opposed to the body of Christ, Angelomus underscored the humility of this *Adam terrenus*: Savigni "Esegesi medievale," 606.

137. See Savigni, "Esegesi medievale," 605–7. Note that "spiritalis effectus" is similar to the vocabulary used by Alcuin in the *DVV*. On the dating of Angelomus's exegesis, see Laistner, "Some Early Medieval Commentaries," 28.

138. Boucaud, "*Factus est homo*." Irenaeus's views were themselves a reaction against Gnostic antagonism toward the body.

139. Savigni, "Esegesi medievale," 600; Appleby, "Beautiful on the Cross," 14.

140. Appleby, "Beautiful on the Cross," sees this as a long-standing reaction against Spanish Adoptionism and its claim that Christ's humanity was "adoptive."

141. Paschasius, *De corpore et sanguine Domini* 19, ed. Paulus, 101; discussed by Appleby, "Beautiful on the Cross," 14.

142. See Boucaud, "*Factus est homo*," 147–49; Appleby, "Beautiful on the Cross," 12–14.

143. See the detailed analysis of the Iconoclasm Controversy by Noble, *Images*.

144. On this work, see Freeman, "Carolingian Orthodoxy."

145. See the comment in the *Libri Carolini* that "God is to be sought not in visible things, not in manufactured things, but in the heart," as cited and translated by Chazelle, "Matter, Spirit, and Image," 176. Noble, *Images*, 223, claims that Theodulf's insistence on the manufactured quality of images is his most repeated point.

146. The *Libri Carolini* acknowledged that God had designated a limited number of material objects as conduits of the spiritual (the Eucharist, liturgical objects, the cross, saints' relics, scripture, and the Ark): Chazelle, "Images, Scripture, the Church."

147. Unlike any material image, the soul was a true image of God because it possessed some qualities of his nature. See Chazelle, "Matter, Spirit, and Image," 171–72.

148. Nobles, *Images*, 268, notes that the *Libri Carolini* is never referenced in the *Libellus* produced in 825.

149. *Concilium Parisiense* (825), ed. Werminghoff, Conc. 2.2, 512. On this colloquy and its use of Pseudo-Dionysius, see Moore, *Sacred Kingdom*, 252.

150. On this colloquy, see Noble, *Images*, 263–85.

151. Alcuin, Ep. 305, ed. Dümmler, 464.

152. Paulinus, *LE* 4, ed. de Nicola, "Sancti Paulini," 199 (citing Alcuin, Ep. 115); Jonas, *DIL* 1.17, ed. Dubreucq, 1:264 (citing Bede's *Homiliarum evangelii libri II*).

153. Romig, *Perfect Man*, 56–59.

154. Alcuin, *DVV* 7, col. 618B.

155. *Capitulare missorum generale* (802) 3, ed. Boretius, Capit.1, 92. Recent assessments of this oath include Davis, *Charlemagne's Practice*, 348–61; Heydemann, "People of God," 113–19; Esders, *Sacramentum fidelitatis*, 530–98.

156. Koziol observes that, as compared to earlier oaths, the oath of 802 was new because it focused on a "positive injunction to behave" rather than a prohibition of disloyalty: "Leadership," 191–92. With particular regard for the *DIL*, Delaruelle, "Jonas d'Orléans," 142–43, asserts that there was an increasing turn toward individualism in the Christian spirituality of the eighth and ninth centuries.

157. On Charlemagne's determination, especially after 800, to ensure that his subjects (including women) disciplined their bodies and minds, see Nelson, "England and the Continent," 13.

158. *Admonitio ad omnes regni ordines* (823–25) 3, ed. Boretius, Capit. 1, 303. On the *admonitio*, see Guillot, "Une *ordinatio* méconnue."

159. See Savigni, "Laïcs dans l'ecclésiologie," 45–63, who argues that Paulinus and Alcuin offered the laity the chance to be "interior monks" while Jonas and Dhuoda were more interested in establishing a separate *ordo* or *ministerium* for the laity.

160. Compare, too, Dhuoda's harmonious model of governance to how Nithard describes the contemporaneous rule of Charles the Bald: his exercise of royal power was not hierarchical or severe but consensual and horizontal, grounded in mutual assistance between himself and his men. Nithard, *Historiarum libri* 1.1 and 3.5, ed. Lauer, 4 and 102–6.

## Chapter 3

1. See Davis, *Charlemagne's Practice*, 252–59, 372–77; Hartmann, *Die Synoden*, 128–40; Kramer, *Rethinking Authority*, 59–91.

2. Patzold, *Episcopus*, 72–83, regards events starting in 810 as the impetus for the synods; the *ARF*, ed. Pertz and Kurze, 129, record problems already in 809.

3. *Concilium Cabillonense* (813) 45, ed. Werminghoff, Conc. 2.1, 282. On this, see Moore, *Sacred Kingdom*, 281; Geary, *Living with the Dead*, 182.

4. *Concilium Cabillonense* (813) 32 and 33, ed. Werminghoff, Conc. 2.1, 279–80.

5. On this council and its penitential ideology, see Firey, *Contrite Heart*, 195–205. On the different approaches taken by the five regional councils, see Kramer, *Rethinking Authority*, 77–89.

6. On the bodily cavity as a "site of otherness within the self," see Holmes, *Symptom and Subject*, esp. 15–16, 275.

7. For Gregory the Great, relic miracles proved that the soul lived on after death: *Dialogi* 4.6, de Vogüé, 3:38–40. See Dal Santo, *Debating*, 86–116.

8. Alcuin, *DRA* 1, ed. Curry, 39.

9. Alcuin, *Disputatio puerorum* 34–35, ed. Rabin and Felsen, 28 (drawing on Isidore, *Etymologiae* 11.1.16). Rabin and Felsen, 10–14, question Alcuin's authorship, suggesting instead an origin in the Regensburg-Salzburg region.

10. Hrabanus, *DRN* 2.1 and 6.1, cols. 31D, 139A, 142A–D.

11. Bede, *De natura rerum* 3, ed. Jones, 194; trans. Wallis, 75.

12. Bede *De natura rerum* 4, ed. Jones, 195–96. On the early medieval reception of Bede's scientific works, see Kendall and Wallis, *On the Nature of Things*, 33–42.

13. Isidore, *De natura rerum* 9.1, ed. Fontaine, 207.

14. Isidore, *Etymologiae* 4.5.3; trans. Barney, 109. Hrabanus copied everything Isidore included regarding the four humors: *DRN* 18.5, cols. 500B–501B. On the humors, see Chapter 6. On Hrabanus's interest in medicine, see Touati, "Raban Maur."

15. Coon, *Dark Age Bodies*, 238–39, associates the instability of the elements with the gendered body: the monastic, male body was stabilized through discipline, while the effeminate body manifested the violent fluctuations of the cosmos.

16. Alcuin, *Disputatio puerorum* 31, ed. Rabin and Felsen, 28.

17. Alcuin, *Disputatio puerorum* 21–22, ed. Rabin and Felsen, 26.

18. On this theme, see also Gregory, *Dialogi* 4.5, ed. de Vogüé, 3:36–40.

19. Hrabanus, *TDA* 2, col. 1112B–D.

20. Hrabanus, *TDA* 11, col. 1119A.

21. Hrabanus, *TDA* 11, col. 1119B.

22. Oliver and Mahoney, "Episcopal Anatomies," read Hrabanus's exegesis of the body as shaped by the Iconoclasm Controversy.

23. Hrabanus, *DRN* 6.1, col. 167B–D.

24. Hrabanus, *DRN* 6.1, col. 163A. On his other sources, see Heyse, *Hrabanus Maurus' Enzyklopädie*. On distinctions from Isidore, see Phelan, "New Insights," 80–85; Touati, "Raban Maur," 192–200.

25. Head-to-toe ordering was found in late antique remedy collections like Alexander of Tralles's *Therapeutica*: see Slaveva-Griffin, "Byzantine Medical Encyclopedias," 968, 976.

26. Both are edited by Rose, *Theodori Prisciani*, 426–83, and discussed in *BTML*, 154. Shared passages in these two works led Beccaria ("Sulle tracce I," 39–56) to argue that they derive from a single anatomical work by Vindicianus. Cf. Cilliers, "Medical Writings," 1018–19; Vázquez Buján, "Vindiciano," 25–46, who argues that the *Gynaecia* was by Vindicianus, but the *Epitome* was a later compilation (based on the *Gynaecia* and a text extant only in Paris, BnF, lat. 7027, *De natura generis humani*). An edition and translation of the *Gynaecia* according to one twelfth-century manuscript is offered by Cilliers, "Vindicianus's *Gynaecia*." Little is known about Vindicianus apart from the fact that he held the position of proconsul in Africa at the time of Theodosius I, was the teacher of the medical writer Theodorus Priscianus, and likely knew Saint Augustine: Cilliers, "Contribution."

27. The *Gynaecia* is transmitted in manuscripts associated with the monasteries of Saint-Denis (Paris, BnF lat. 11219) and Corbie (St. Petersburg, National Library, F.v.VI.3); Beneventan manuscripts include Montecassino, Archivio dell'Abbazia 97 and Glasgow, UL Hunter 404. On extant witnesses, see Cilliers, "Vindicianus's *Gynaecia*," 155–56.

28. Vindicianus, *Epitome altera* 1, ed. Rose, 467 (punctuation mine).

29. Vindicianus, *Epitome altera* 1, ed. Rose, 467 (on *alape* in this list, see *adipe* in Cilliers, "Vindicianus's *Gynaecia*," 168).

30. Vindicianus, *Gynaecia* 2, ed. Rose, 428–31.

31. Vindicianus, *Epitome altera* 2–16, ed. Rose, 467–71.

32. Translation based on witnesses III and V in Vindicianus, *Gynaecia* 11, ed. Rose, 439. See also *Epitome altera* 18, ed. Rose, 474; Cilliers, "Vindicianus's *Gynaecia*," 190–91.

33. Vindicianus, *Gynaecia* 12, ed. Rose, 440–41; trans. Cilliers, "Vindicianus's *Gynaecia*," 193.

34. See Vindicianus, *Gynaecia* 12–13, ed. Rose, 440–43; Cilliers, "Vindicianus's *Gynaecia*," 192–93.

35. The five-figure series (showing the bones, arteries, veins, nerves, and muscles) probably originated in late antique Alexandria but was not available in Latin texts until the twelfth century: Wallis, *Reader*, 238–39. Illustrations depicting the fetus in utero, which accompanied

the Latin gynecological text by Muscio, survive in Brussels, BR 3701-15: Hanson and Green, "Soranus of Ephesus," 1047, 1058, 1072.

36. Von Staden, "Physis and Technē," 23–24.

37. It was also sometimes translated as *qualitas*. On *virtus* and *dynamis* in early medieval medical texts, see MacKinney, "*Dynamidia*"; Dendle, "Plants," 56–57; Miller, "*Dynamis* and *Physis*."

38. Isidore, *Etymologiae* 4.10.2; trans. Barney, 114.

39. MacKinney, "*Dynamidia*," 403, argues for two distinct applications of *dynamidia*, according to a text's roots in Hippocratic writings (dietetic material) or Galenic writings (pharmaceutical material).

40. MacKinney, "*Dynamidia*," 403, citing Chartres, BM 62, f. 54r: "Vera haec est virtutis demonstratio omnium medicamentorum qui ad artis medicinae pertinet."

41. MacKinney, "*Dynamidia*," 412.

42. See Probst, "Isidors Schrift," 36. Cf. MacKinney's rejection of this theory: "*Dynamidia*," 401–2.

43. On early medieval beliefs that plants, stones, and animals might possess a hidden divine potency that could be tapped through following a recipe, see Dendle, "Plants," 52–56.

44. MacKinney, "*Dynamidia*," 414, speculates that *virtus* was more common than *dynamidia* because of the latter's Greek origin, but Carolingian medical codices often drew attention to the Greek term for a disease or herb with the recurrent phrase "quod Greci vocant." In Montecassino, Archivio dell'Abbazia 97 (*s*.X$^{in}$) Greek terms are highlighted by being written in a majuscule script and are sometimes overlined. See Everett's discussion of Greek vocabulary in *Alphabet of Galen*, 103–6.

45. On the *Herbarius* of Pseudo-Apuleius (300s) and the five-part *materia medica* corpus, see Howald and Sigerist, eds., *Antonii Musae*; van Arsdall, *Medieval Herbal Remedies*, 68–80; Collins, *Medieval Herbals*, 165–79.

46. *Herbarius* 12, ed. Sigerist and Howald, 45. On the illustration of this scene in Florence, Biblioteca Medicea Laurenziana, Ms. Plut. 73.41 (Beneventan script, *s*.IX$^{1}$), see Collins, *Medieval Herbals*, 171, 180–81.

47. Paris, BnF lat. 6862 (*s*.IX$^{2/4}$) ff. 6r–63v: with Antonius Musa's *De herba vetonica* and the *Herbarius* interpolated with information from Pseudo-Dioscorides's *Ex herbis femininis*. On the manuscript's date and origin, see Collins, *Medieval Herbals*, 184–88, who proposes Tours or Metz as a site of production; Hubert et al., *L'Empire carolingien*, 349, who suggest Hautvillers; Wickersheimer, *Manuscrits latins*, 67–70; *Katalog* 3.4417; *Codici* 24. One of the most striking elements of the manuscript is its illustration of Scolapius gathering betony (f. 18v), which Collins (p. 188) argues is a Carolingian addition not found in an earlier archetype.

48. Paris, BnF lat. 6862, ff. 6r–8v.

49. Paris, BnF lat. 6862, f. 42v.

50. Paris, BnF lat. 6862, f. 20r: "Incipit epistola Antoni Muse de herba vetonica quantas virtutes habet." This is the first herb in the compendium and the longest entry.

51. For the invocation, see *De herba vettonica*, ed. Howald and Sigerist, *Antonii Musae*, 11. For the prayer, see Paris, BnF lat. 6862, f. 19r (right margin).

52. St. Gall, SB 762 (*s*. IX$^{1/4}$), pp. 25–216, with a table of contents at 2–20. *Katalog* 3.5848 suggests Saint-Germain-des-Prés or Auxerre as the origin; see also *Codici* 137. According to MacKinney ("*Dynamidia*," 405n24), *virtus* appears thirty-four times in Book 1; it also appears in the incipits to Books 1, 3, and 4 (at pp. 25, 138, and 187), and in the *Epistula Anthimi*

(pp. 217–60), which follows Book 4. Books 1, 2, and 4 (known as the *Dynamidia Hippocratis*, ed. Rose, *Anecdota Graeca*, 2:123–56) and the *Epistula Anthimi* all bear some relationship to a Latin translation of the Hippocratic *De victus ratione*: MacKinney, "*Dynamidia*," 404–8; *BTML*, 73–74.

53. *Dynamidia Hippocratis*, ed. Rose, *Anecdota Graeca*, 2:136.

54. *Dynamidia Hippocratis*, ed. Rose, *Anecdota Graeca*, 2:151.

55. *De quattuor elementis corporis* was (with one exception) always transmitted with the *Epistula de ratione ventris*; both are edited by Scherer, "*Epistula de ratione ventris*," 73–80. See also a text entitled *Epistola Yppocratis de quatuor humoribus*, in Paris, BnF lat. 11219, f. 18v (*s*.IX$^{med}$).

56. On the increasing use of *vitium* over *morbus* or *aegritudo* from the third century onward, see Migliorini, "Alcune denominazioni," 99–100. Everett, *Alphabet of Galen*, 90, translates *vitium* as "natural defect" and notes its use fourteen times in the text (vs. *aegritudo* once and *morbus* never).

57. On *receptaria*, see Sigerist, *Studien und Texte*; Jörimann, *Frühmittelalterliche Rezeptarien.*

58. For a detailed discussion of each term, see Migliorini, "Alcune denominazioni," 93–132.

59. Stoll, *LAB*, 485, translates *vitium* as "das Gebrechen, der Fehler, das Leiden." For a comparable discussion of "evil" as both physiological malady and malevolent force in English medical writings, see Tormey, "Treating the Condition of 'Evil.'"

60. *Tereoperica*, ed. López Figueroa, "Estudio," 154–55.

61. Quintus Serenus, *Liber medicinalis*, ed. Vollmer, with chapter headings seemingly original to the work (Vollmer, xxiii). The text is typically attributed to the third or fourth century; for more on it, see Chapter 4.

62. Sigerist, *Studien und Texte*, 78. On the possible attribution of this recipe to Archbishop Theodore of Canterbury, see Lapidge, "School of Theodore," 50. See also the antidote ascribed to Vindicianus, which "purges all vices of the body," ed. Rose, *Theodori Prisciani*, 256.

63. Anthimus, *DOC* 14, 58, 79, ed. Liechtenhan, 9, 23, 29.

64. Caelius Aurelianus, *Chronicae passiones*, Praefatio, ed. and trans. Drabkin, *On Acute Diseases*, 440–41. Muscio's *Gynaecia* and Celsus's *De medicina* also employed the term *vitia.*

65. *Teroperica*, ed. López Figueroa, "Estudio," 166. Cf. Isidore, *Etymologiae* 4.13.5. See Glaze, "Master-Student," 490–94, for how the *Tereoperica* draws on Agnellus of Ravenna's commentary on Galen's *De sectis.*

66. Dendle, "Plants," at 57, argues that Galenic balance was not prominent in the early Middle Ages and that Old English medicine understood illness as an "external and invasive force, often zoomorphized." Humoral balance is discussed further in Chapter 7.

67. Alcuin, *DVV* 34, cols. 636D–637A. Here, the virtues refer to the four classical, cardinal virtues of temperance, justice, prudence, fortitude. On Alcuin's influence over ideas of the virtues, see Bejczy, *Cardinal Virtues*, 28–67; Mähl, *Quadriga virtutum*, 83–160.

68. See Alcuin, *DVV* 30, 32, 33, 34, cols. 634B, 635A, 635C, 636A. While Cassian and Gregory had established an authoritative set of capital sins, they did not supply a simplistic schema of paired virtue-vice, as Alcuin did: O'Sullivan, *Early Medieval Glosses*, 4. See also Newhauser "Preaching the Contrary Virtues," 135–39, 143–46.

69. See Langum, *Medicine and the Seven Deadly Sins*, 13, 29–34; Straw, *Gregory the Great*, 41–46.

70. This is summarized by Isidore, *Etymologiae* 4.9.5–7.

71. See Arbesmann, "Christus medicus," 1–2, 9.

72. Firey, *Contrite Heart*, 159–95, at 167, argues that there was a "revolution in moral theology," grounded in the virtues and vices, which occurred first in the Rhineland and then spread to other areas of the empire.

73. See McNeill, "Medicine for Sin."

74. Councils in 813 and 829 expressed concern about the diversity of penitential texts and their uncertain authorship: Meens, *Penance*, 113–18, 130–39.

75. Halitgar, *Paenitentiale Pseudo-Romanum*, Prologue, ed. Schmitz, *Die Bussbücher*, 291. On the date, compilation, and sources of this penitential, which constituted Book 6 within a larger work and which Halitgar claimed he took from the archive of a Roman church, see Meens, "Historiography," 74–82; Kottje, *Die Bussbücher*, 144–48, 157–67; 185–90.

76. Hildemar, *Expositio regulae* 58, ed. Mittermüller, 541.

77. Alcuin intended the letter to circulate beyond the monastery of Tours; he sent it to Bishop Arn of Salzburg in 802: see Driscoll, "*Ad pueros sancti Martini*," 37–41.

78. Alcuin, *Ad pueros sancti Martini* 2, ed. Driscoll, 50.

79. Alcuin, *Ad pueros sancti Martini* 3–4, ed. Driscoll, 52–55. See Firey, *Contrite Heart*, 97–98, on Pomerius as the source for medical metaphors of confession.

80. Firey, "Blushing Before the Judge," 176.

81. Booker, "By the Body Betrayed."

82. See Booker, "By the Body Betrayed," on Charlemagne, Ep. 85, ed. Dümmler, 128: "timor vel erubiscentia in facie foris ostendit, quod homo intus in corde non retinet."

83. *Concilium Aquisgranense* (836) 15, ed. Werminghoff, Conc. 2.2, 709 (quoting Gregory's *Regula pastoralis*).

84. In 833, as part of his public penance, the bishops wrote out all of Louis's sins, so that he might see and thus recognize his iniquity: Booker, *Past Convictions*, 166–75.

85. The conscience was also compared to a witness or an accuser: Firey, "Blushing Before the Judge," 181–90.

86. On the dangers of external appearance *not* according with inner reality, see Booker, "Hypocrisy."

87. Alcuin, *DVV* 32, col. 635A.

88. See Alcuin, *DVV* 27, col. 633A, where he states that, if the roots of the eight vices are cut, the branches of other evils will be easier to cut away.

89. *Epistola primitus legenda de disciplina artis medicinae*, Paris, BnF lat. 11219, f. 13r: "et pulsum tangendo discas quod intus sit vitium." A similar statement is also found in St. Gall, SB 751, and Karlsruhe, BLB 120.

90. On the classical Greek tradition, see Ferngren and Amundsen, "Virtue and Health/Medicine," 3–22.

91. On how Anthony remained "unaffected," see Rubenson, "Anthony and Pythagoras," 197–204.

92. See Brown, *Body and Society*, 213–40.

93. See Nithard, *Historiarum libri* 4.5, ed. Lauer, 138–40, on his father's body being found intact "absque aromatibus" twenty-nine years after his death. Polanichka and Cilley, "Very Personal History," 193–95, argue that this anecdote was rebutting claims about Nithard's parents' illegitimate sexual union. For other examples of preserved bodies (starting with Jerome's *Vita Hilarionis*), see Angenendt, "*Corpus incorruptum*," 320–32. Kitchen, "Gregory of Tours,"

416–23, suggests that the preserved body was, for Gregory, a sign of Christian order standing against the disordered society portrayed in his *Histories*.

94. Heydemann, "Relics and Texts," 191–95. On this text, see Head, *Hagiography*, 42–49; Angenendt, "*Corpus incorruptum*," 329–30.

95. Jonas, *Vita secunda S. Huberti* 25, col. 816A–B.

96. Jonas, *Vita secunda S. Huberti* 25, col. 816B. His description of the face as dewy could signal retention of heat and moisture, which decreased in the elderly according to Galenic theory.

97. Jonas, *Translatio S. Huberti* 33, col. 818D.

98. *Annales Bertiniani* 877, ed. Grat, 216–17; *Annales Fuldenses* 877, ed. Kurze and Pertz, 90. On Charles's death as that of a tyrant, modeled on the death of Antiochus IV in 2 Mc 9:8–28, see Nelson, "La mort," 61–65.

99. The investigators also saw a dragon fly out of the coffin: Hincmar, *Quierzy (Nov. 858)* 7, ed. Hartmann, Conc. 3, 415. The vision is not part of the original *Vita Eucherii* but only appears in later versions, which drew on Hincmar's account: Dutton, *Politics of Dreaming*, 174.

100. Preservation was not a secure signifier of sanctity, since many saints' bodies survived only as dust and bones; but even these were understood to be whole, with the saint fully present in every fragment: see Bynum, *Resurrection*, esp. 81–86, 104–8.

101. The author of the *Life of Pachomius* deliberately counterposed his protagonist to the *Life of Anthony*: see Crislip, *Thorns in the Flesh*, 109–37.

102. See Ferngren and Amundsen, "Virtue and Medicine," 7, 46–47. Perkins, *Suffering Self*, 1–13, finds a common emphasis on "the body in pain" across Christian, Stoic, and romance texts of the second century.

103. See Crislip, *Thorns in the Flesh*, esp. 5–13, 22–35.

104. For a list of references to health in Alcuin's letters, see Edelstein, *Eruditio und sapientia*, 256–59; on aging, see Dutton, *Charlemagne's Mustache*, 153–56.

105. Though, in a letter to Benedict of Aniane, Alcuin thanks him for the herbal medicines he sent: Ep. 56, ed. Dümmler, 100.

106. See Alcuin, Ep. 121 and 226, ed. Dümmler, 178 and 370.

107. Alcuin, Ep. 146, ed. Dümmler, 236.

108. Alcuin, Ep. 161, ed. Dümmler, 259.

109. See Dutton, *Politics of Dreaming*, 60–80; Carozzi, *Le voyage de l'âme*, 369–75; Carozzi, "Les carolingiens dans l'au-delà," 367–76.

110. Einhard, Ep. 2 (ca. 825), ed. Hampe, 109; trans. Dutton, *Charlemagne's Courtier*, 144.

111. Lupus, Ep. 20, ed. Dümmler, 26–27; trans. Regenos, 21.

112. See Dhuoda, *LM* 10.4, ed. Riché, 348–52. Similarly: Alcuin, Ep. 226, ed. Dümmler, 370.

113. On Symeon the Elder, see Harvey, "Sense of a Stylite."

114. Venantius Fortunatus, *De vita S. Radegundis* 26, ed. Krusch, 373. On the different emphases of the two extant lives of Radegund, see Wehlau, "Literal and Symbolic."

115. Brown, *Rise of Western Christendom*, 248–57.

116. Cf. Diem, "Carolingians and the *Regula Benedicti*," 260–61, who believes that the Benedictine Rule, as interpreted by the Carolingians, was a *Regula Columbani* "in disguise."

117. See *Capitulare Francofurtense* (794) 42, ed. Werminghoff, Conc. 2.1, 170; Fouracre, "Origins of the Carolingian Attempt," 162.

118. On Ardo's agenda, see Kramer, *Rethinking Authority*, 169–213; Savigni, "L'immagine del santo fondatore"; Coon, *Dark Age Bodies*, 49–59.

119. Ardo, *Vita S. Benedicti Anianensis* 2, ed. Waitz, 201–2; trans. Cabaniss, 67. On Benedict's austere practices, see Williams, "Working for Reform," 19–42.

120. Ardo states that Benedict preferred to follow the harsher rules of Pachomius and Basil: *Vita Benedicti* 2, ed. Waitz, 202.

121. On this transformation (accompanied by a name change from Witiza to Benedict), see Lifshitz, *Name of the Saint*, 57–68.

122. Ardo, *Vita Benedicti* 21, ed. Waitz, 208; trans Cabaniss, 83 (with slight modifications).

123. See Crislip, *Thorns in the Flesh*, 94–96.

124. Rudolf, *Vita Leobae* 7 and 11, ed. Waitz, 124–26.

125. Rudolf, *Vita Leobae* 11, ed. Waitz, 126.

126. A contrast to fourth-century ascetic writings (e.g., Palladius's *Life of Evagrius* vs. Evagrius's own prescriptions): Crislip, *Thorns in the Flesh*, 97–100.

127. Smaragdus, *Expositio* 36.4, ed. Spannagel and Engelbert, 249 (citing Isidore's *Regula monachorum*).

128. Hildemar, *Expositio regulae* 36, ed. Mittermüller, 413.

129. Cf. Basil, *Regulae fusius tractatae* 55, PG 31, cols. 399D–400A, which indicates that, if sickness is sent as a punishment, it is wrong to seek medical treatment.

130. On the Carolingians' intensifying concern with any disjuncture between interior and exterior, see Booker, "Hypocrisy."

131. The most obvious exceptions were when someone deliberately insulted a saint. For a statistical analysis, see Kroll and Bachrach, "Sin and the Etiology." Pilsworth, "Medicine and Hagiography," 262, notes that when the *Vita Ambrosii* was rewritten in the ninth century the new version deemphasized the links between sin and illness.

132. The apocryphal Latin *Vita Adae et Evae* explicitly linked the first sin and bodily illness (chs. 30–36): see the electronic edition of the different versions of this text (ca. 200–600 C.E.) by Anderson and Stone at http://www2.iath.virginia.edu/anderson/vita/vita.html (accessed July 2021).

133. Dutton, *Politics of Dreaming*, 85–91, at 88 (noting a change of author in the year 820). On the problems of interpretation, see also Palmer, "Climate of Crisis," esp. 16–17; Ashley, "Power of Symbols."

134. *ARF*, ed. Pertz and Kurze, 153–54: drawing connections between moisture in the air and the outbreak of disease, this entry also points to an awareness of Hippocratic theory (as discussed further in Chapter 6).

135. See Dutton, "Observations," 167–80.

136. See Hen, "*Annals of Metz*," 179–83, who argues that the natural disasters of 805–808 prompted the *Divisio regni* of 806. Around the same time (805–806), Charlemagne issued preemptive instructions that in future cases of famine, pestilence, and other ills, the people should not wait for an edict but entreat God's mercy immediately: *Capitulare missorum in Theodonis villa datum secundum* 4, ed. Boretius, Capit. 1, 122–23.

137. Charlemagne, *Ad Ghaerbaldum episcopum epistola*, ed. Boretius, Capit. 1, 245. On the evidence for colder weather, famine, and epidemic disease from 805–807 (and increased subsistence crises across the realm from 790–815), see Newfield, "Contours of Disease," 172–73, 314–16, 346, 429–32.

138. Charlemagne, *Ad Ghaerbaldum episcopum epistola*, ed. Boretius, Capit. 1, 245–46 (emphasis mine).

139. *Annales Bertiniani*, ed. Grat et al., 156. The sinfulness of the king could cause disorder in the natural world, as expressed in the Irish *De duodecim abusivis saeculi*: see Meens, "Politics, Mirrors of Princes."

140. Geary, *Living with the Dead*, 177–93.

141. On the diffusion of Gregory's *Miracula*, see Bourgain, "Works of Gregory of Tours," 143–45.

142. Gregory of Tours, *De virtutibus S. Martini* 4, Preface, ed. Krusch, 199; trans. Van Dam, *Saints*, 285.

143. Bachrach and Kroll, "Sin and the Etiology," 405–6; Kitchen, "Gregory of Tours," 397–40. On the sick as external to the community, see Van Dam, *Saints*, 86–94, 109–13.

144. On *translationes*, see Geary, *Furta sacra*, 45–48, 118–20; Appleby, "Hagiography and Ideology," 3, 93–142; Smith, "Old Saints"; Heinzelmann, *Translationsberichte*, esp. 94–99.

145. According to Appleby, "Hagiography and Ideology," 95–96, the work was composed in stages over 828–834. Cf. Dutton, *Charlemagne's Courtier*, xxiv, which offers 830–831 as the earliest date.

146. Dutton, *Politics of Dreaming*, 91–99.

147. Einhard, *Translatio* 3.13, ed. Waitz, 252–53, claims that Louis ignored the martyrs' advice.

148. Einhard, *Translatio* 3.14, ed. Waitz, 253–54. On Wiggo's critique, see Booker, *Past Convictions*, 232–33.

149. At Einhard, *Translatio* 4.14, ed. Waitz, 262. On Einhard's perception of his own sinfulness, see Smith, "Sinner and the Saints." On miraculous cures (vs. medical cures) as appropriate for those weak in faith, see Bede, *Expositio actuum apostolorum* 28.8, ed. Laistner, 96.

150. On the theme of reincorporation, see Van Dam, *Saints*, 89–94.

151. There are five chief conditions, which apply to both men and women and which focus on long-term disability, not illness: *caecus, surdus et mutus, paralysis, nervorum contractio*, and *spasmon/tremulosa* (some translate into modern categories, but others do not). On *medici* using the Greek term *spasmon*, see *Translatio* 4.14, ed. Waitz, 261–62. On impairment and illness, see Metzler, *Disability in Medieval Europe.*

152. Most of the brief entries are in Book 4 (with fifty-two of the seventy-two miracles), which Einhard says was composed from little books sent to him from the places to which his relics traveled.

153. There is no mention of discharges from the bowels, which were associated with demonic possession following the example of the heretic Arius (d. 336). On St. Martin curing through defecation, see Rousselle, *Croire et guérir*, 116, 126–28. On demons in the bowels, see Caciola, *Discerning Spirits*, 203–5. On Gregory's use of bodily fluids in the *De virtutibus S. Martini*, see Nugent, "Bodily Effluvia," 51–56.

154. Einhard, *Translatio* 3.2, ed. Waitz, 249. On vomit's association with sin: 2 Pt 2:22.

155. Einhard, *Translatio* 3.6, ed. Waitz, 250.

156. Sometimes these actions occur in a vision, sometimes they are visible to spectators: compare *Translatio* 3.9 and 4.2, ed. Waitz, 251 and 256. For similar examples of saints using violent force to heal, see the seventh-century Byzantine text, the *Miracles of St. Artemios*. Penitential literature often emphasized the pain of the doctor's cures.

157. On humoral purgation, see Duden, *Woman Beneath the Skin*, 104–78.

158. Amalarius, *Liber officialis* 3, Preface, ed. Knibbs, 2:2.

159. A clear exception is when outsiders attempt to harm the saints, as when the Normans enter a church and are immediately struck by disease: *Translatio S. Germani Parisiensis* 15, ed. de Smedt, 81.

160. With possession, almost all victims are women (but see the case of a male cleric in Rudolf, *Miracula sanctorum* 5, ed. Waitz, 334, and another example in Appleby, "Hagiography and Ideology," 189).

161. Appleby, "Hagiography and Ideology," 187–92. On Hrabanus's efforts (as abbot of Fulda) to translate relics to churches owned by the monastery, and on Rudolf's documentation of these efforts, see Raaijmakers, *Community of Fulda*, 214–35. Einhard's *Translatio* mentions three exorcisms, but these are not described like the healing of disabilities.

162. Rudolf, *Miracula sanctorum* 12, ed. Waitz, 338. A black fly exits: *Miracula sanctorum* 11, ed. Waitz, 337 (recalling Gregory the Great's *Vita Benedicti*). A possessed woman is slapped by a saint, and fluid (*sanies*) runs from her mouth: Jonas, *Vita secunda S. Huberti* 7, col. 811A.

163. Caciola, *Discerning Spirits*, 129–75, finds a connection between the porousness and coldness of women's bodies and their susceptibility to demonic possession.

164. Einhard, *Translatio* 1.10, ed. Waitz, 243.

165. On healing as release from blockages, see Brown, *Ransom of the Soul*, 175–76; Van Dam, *Saints*, 111–14.

166. See, for example, Rudolf, *Miracula sanctorum* 2, 4, 5, 10, 12, ed. Waitz, 330–31, 333–34, 336, 338.

167. Dhuoda, *LM* 5.8, ed. Riché, 278–84, at 280; trans. Neel, 72.

## Chapter 4

1. Bamberg, Staatsbibliothek, Msc. med. 1: currently 75 ff., but Stoll, *LAB*, 14–15, estimates that missing folios account for 36 percent of the original remedies.

2. Sometimes termed the *defensio artis medicinae* (there is no title in the manuscript). First discussed by Sudhoff, "Eine Verteidigung." See also two essay collections from the 1990s: *Das Lorscher Arzneibuch: Klostermedizin in der Karolingerzeit*; Keil and Schnitzer, *Das Lorscher Arzneibuch und die frühmittelalterliche Medizin*; and recent assessment by Fischer, "Das *Lorscher Arzneibuch*." English translation by Wallis, *Reader*, 84–93.

3. *LAB*, f. 1r, ed. Stoll, 48.

4. See Keil, "Einleitung"; Keil, "Klostermedizin." Cf. Fischer, "Das *Lorscher Arzneibuch*."

5. Some material from this chapter has previously appeared in Leja, "The Sacred Art: Medicine in the Carolingian Renaissance," *Viator* 47 (2016): 1–34.

6. On baptism, see Phelan, *Formation*; Wood, *Missionary Life*, esp. 79–99; Cramer, *Baptism and Change*, esp. 185–220; Reimitz, "Conversion and Control."

7. We have to assume that various types of surgeries were being performed after battle, even if we have little evidence about what these treatments were.

8. See the Introduction.

9. Extant medical manuscripts with Visigothic elements include: Glasgow, UL Hunter 96 (*s.*VIII$^{ex}$/IX$^{in}$); Paris, BnF nouv. acq. lat. 203 (*s.*VIII$^{ex}$/IX$^{in}$); Paris, BnF lat. 10233 (*s.*VII$^{ex}$).

10. Studies on the relationship between early Christianity and classical medicine tend to focus exclusively on the Greek East and conclude that most of the patristics held a generally positive attitude toward Hippocratic and Galenic teachings: see Amundsen, *Medicine, Society, and Faith*; Temkin, *Hippocrates*; Ferngren, *Medicine & Health*. The Fathers' use of medical metaphors is treated in Chapter 5.

11. Nemesius's *De natura hominis* was not translated into Latin until the eleventh century (by Bishop Alfanus of Salerno). Basil treats medicine in Question 55 of his *Longer Rules*, but Rufinus's Latin adaptation depended upon an earlier recension of the text (known as the *Shorter Rules*) and did not include anything on the medical art.

12. On the Carolingians' reception of the Fathers, see Otten, "Texture of Tradition"; Alibert, "La transmission des textes patristiques." Beside Origen's statement (in his *Homilies on Numbers*) that *medicinae scientia* must come from God, the canon Martin Hiberniensis of Laon (819–875) made a marginal notation indicating its significance: Contreni, *Cathedral School*, 116; Contreni, "Masters and Medicine," 346n50. Yet, Origen himself held an ambiguous attitude toward Greek medicine, praising it as a gift from God but indicating that perfect Christians use prayer, not medicine: Ferngren, *Medicine & Health*, 27–28.

13. On Jerome, see Pease, "Medical Allusions." Augustine speaks approvingly of the North African medical writer Vindicianus in *Confessionum libri* 4.3, 7.6, ed. Verheijen, 42, 97–98. Bede included snippets of Hippocratic material in *De natura rerum* (ch. 37) and *DTR* (chs. 30 and 35) but without any discussion of medicine as a distinct field of study.

14. The apologist recommends Gregory's *Homiliae in Hiezechihelem*, *Homiliae in Evangelia*, and *Dialogi* and notes that Gregory himself sought medical treatment (*Dialogi* 4.57). He seems familiar with Bede's *De schematibus et tropis* and *Expositio Apocalypseos* (on the latter, see Chapter 6). From Isidore, he uses the *Etymologiae*, *Liber differentiarum*, and *Sententiae*: Fischer, "Vernachlässigte Quellen," 167–69. He may cite Jerome's *Commentaria in Esaiam*, or this could be an indirect citation via Isidore. Fischer (personal correspondence) has suggested that the opening lines of the apology draw from Jerome's preface to Job in the Vulgate.

15. Book 4 of the *Etymologiae* is devoted to medicine. Brown, *Rise of Western Christendom*, 364–68, describes the *Etymologiae* as a work of emancipation from the Roman past. On Isidore as a medical authority, see Ferraces Rodríguez, "Isidoro de Sevilla," 33–37.

16. On this analogy (stretching back to Plato and Democritus), see Holmes, *Symptom and Subject*, 204–11.

17. Cassiodorus, *Institutiones* 1.31, ed. Mynors, 78–79, discussed in the Introduction.

18. Despite quoting the *Institutiones*, the apology never names Cassiodorus. The apology may reference the Benedictine Rule (ch. 53) within its interpolated quotation of the *Institutiones*: *LAB*, f. 4v, ed. Stoll, 62. Benedict's Rule addressed how the monks should serve the infirm, not what they should read (discussed in Chapter 5).

19. See Bischoff, *Abtei Lorsch*, 31–33, where the script is described as the older Lorsch style; cf. *Katalog* 1.223, which dates it to the beginning of the ninth century; Stoll, *LAB*, 13, gives 795. On the cultural and educational agenda at Lorsch, see the essays in Becker et al., *Karolingische Klöster* (esp. Licht at 145–62 that the older Lorsch style be redated).

20. Stoll, "Ein Arbeitsbericht," 30. The manuscript was owned by Otto III, then Henry II, then given to the cathedral of Bamberg; see Platte, "Der Weg des Arzneibuchs."

21. On the layout, see Stoll, "Ein Arbeitsbericht," 33–38.

22. Bischoff, *Abtei Lorsch*, 32. For Abbot Richbod as the author, see Keil, "Klostermedizin," 23; for a rebuttal, see Fischer, "Das *Lorscher Arzneibuch*," 180–84; Berschin, "Lateinische Kultur," 3–6. On Hrabanus as a possible author, see Touati, "Raban Maur," 201.

23. Given that Lorsch was a male monastery, I use the male pronoun.

24. Berschin, "Lateinische Kultur," 5, argues that the apology was only copied, not composed, at Lorsch, pointing to the apologist's unusual spelling of *Baedano presbytero*; this spelling, however, appears in a computus compilation ascribed to Lorsch (Vatican, BAV

Pal. lat. 1449, f. 16r, *s.*IX[1]). Fischer, "Medizinische Handschriften in der Karolingerzeit: Einblicke und Einsichten" (unpublished paper), suggests a northern Italian composition for the exemplar.

25. All of the works listed above by Gregory, Cassiodorus, Isidore, and Bede are found in the Lorsch library catalogues A or B (dated 830–840): Häse, *MBKL*, A56/57, A65, B166, B167, B168, B124, B 178/79, B180/81, B183, B200, B204; the *Epistula Anthimi* (*LAB*, ff. 72r–75r) is listed in a catalogue dated to 860: Häse, *MBKL*, Ca419.

26. Bede was ordained in 702. The apology states that Bede called Gregory the Great an *orator*, and the only time he alludes to this is in *De schematibus et tropis* 1.12, ed. Kendall, 149. On the dating of this text to 710, see Franklin, "Date of Composition."

27. On Bede's reputation, see the essays in DeGregorio, *Companion to Bede*, Part III.

28. No evidence survives on these critics or detractors, but see Alcuin, Ep. 148, ed. Dümmler, 239, for the observation that many are so cowardly that they do not study the things established by God in nature and rebuke those who do.

29. Though the Lorsch apology is clearly not addressed to Charlemagne, note that Alcuin refers to Charlemagne ordering a defense of a work that he composed on the ruler's orders: Ep. 172, ed. Dümmler, 284.

30. Manuscripts dated VIII$^{ex}$/IX$^{in}$ and discussed in this book: Paris, BnF lat. 11218 and nouv. acq. lat. 203; Glasgow, UL Hunter 96; Einsiedeln, SB 304; St. Gall, SB 877; St. Petersburg, National Library, lat. F.v.VI.3; and Modena, Archivio Capitolare O.I.11.

31. For reappraisals of the long-held stereotype that debate was stifled in the early Middle Ages, see the special issue edited by de Jong and van Renswoude, *EME* 25 (2017); Cameron, *Dialoguing in Late Antiquity*; van Renswoude, *Free Speech*.

32. Van Renswoude, "Art of Disputation."

33. Cf. Isidore, *Etymologiae* 4.9.1: "medicinae curatio spernenda non est."

34. Jerome, *Tractatuum in psalmos series altera*, Ps 96, ed. Morin, in *S. Hieronymi presbyteri opera*, 444.

35. On biblical interpretation according to literal and spiritual levels, see Cavadini, "From Letter to Spirit"; Chazelle and Edwards, *Study of the Bible*.

36. *LAB*, f. 3v, ed. Stoll, 56–58 (referencing Ex 15:23–25 and 2 Kgs 2:19–22).

37. See Hrabanus, *Enarrationum in epistolas beati Pauli* 7.14, cols. 1574D–1575D. On patristic exegesis of this passage, see Burns Jr., *Romans*, 334–38.

38. *LAB*, f. 2r and 2v, ed. Stoll, 50 and 54.

39. *LAB*, f. 1v, ed. Stoll, 50. A similar reading is performed on Is 1:6 and Jer 8:22.

40. On medicine as *utillima ars*, see Cassiodorus, *Variae* 6.19, ed. Fridh, 248.

41. *LAB*, ff. 1r and 3v, ed. Stoll, 48, 58. On the usefulness of creation for food and medicine (with reference to Dioscorides and Pliny), see Jerome, *Adversus Jovinianum* 2.5–6, cols. 303A–307C.

42. *LAB*, f. 3v, ed. Stoll, 58 (citing Jn 9:1–7: note that Jesus states the man's blindness is *not* due to sin).

43. Sir 38:1–15. On this biblical book (ca. 195–175 B.C.E.), see Schmidt, *Wisdom, Cosmos, and Cultus*.

44. Sir 38:4, at *LAB*, f. 4r, ed. Stoll, 58.

45. *LAB*, f. 4r, ed. Stoll, 58.

46. *Epistola Solomonis*, in Brussels, BR 3701-15 (*s.*IX$^{2/3}$), f. 7r. This codex consists of two units, the first of which (ff. 1–33) contains thirty-three medical treatises, almost all titled

*epistolae* (including both versions of the *Disputatio Platonis et Aristotelis* from Chapter 1). On the dating and contents, see *Katalog* 1.708; *Codici* 6; Wiedemann, "Untersuchungen," 94–100.

47. See Hrabanus, Ep. 21 (ca. 835–840), ed. Dümmler, 427–28. On its status as the first commentary, see Paxton, "Curing Bodies," 242n40.

48. Hrabanus, *Commentaria in Ecclesiasticum* 8.13, col. 1030D.

49. Hrabanus, *Commentaria in Ecclesiasticum* 8.13, col. 1030B–C: "Unde non debemus ea spernere, quae noverimus ad utilitatem nostrum et sanitatem creatorem nostrum nobis procreasse, sed cum gratiarum actione ea percipere, et ad usus nostros convertere." Cf. *LAB*, ff. 3r–4r, ed. Stoll, 56 and 58: "Sed non ideo humana refutanda medicina, sed cum gratiarum actione in labore utenda" and "nullus terrenam debet spernere medicinam."

50. Hrabanus, *DRN* 18.5, col. 501C. On the *DRN*, see Phelan, "New Insights," 80–85.

51. On his aims, Hrabanus states at *DRN* 18.5, col. 501C: "Setting aside those matters that the writers of secular literature have covered concerning disease and the art of medicine, let it suffice to relate those matters here which we read about in the divine books." He does not want to cover knowledge found in Isidore but wishes to provide a spiritual companion to the *Etymologiae*. Cf. Paxton, "Curing Bodies," 249–50, on Hrabanus's desire to suppress the reading of classical medicine.

52. Unlike the *Etymologiae*, Hrabanus's *DRN* treated medicine under Bk. 18, "Weights and Measures." This may reflect ninth-century medical manuscripts, which often included Isidore's chapter on weights and measures (found as Bk. 16 in the *Etymologiae*, while medicine was Bk. 4).

53. The terms *utile/utilitas* or *spernere* never appear in Sirach but do in Hrabanus and the *LAB*.

54. On this notary, see Bischoff, *Manuscripts and Libraries*, 61; Bullough, "*Aula Renovata*," 138, 157n50. Two witnesses of the verses survive, one of which was copied at Saint-Gall in the later ninth century: Zurich, Zentralbibliothek C. 78, f. 57v; see *Codici* 141.

55. The first attestation of the *Liber medicinalis* is by Marcellus of Bordeaux around 400.

56. The two families of manuscripts of the *Liber medicinalis* both descend from the copy produced for Charlemagne, according to Rouse, "Quintus Serenus," 381–85.

57. Jacobus, *Versus ad Carolum*, ed. Dümmler, 97–98.

58. See also the *Capitulare de villis* (ca. 800) 70, ed. Boretius, Capit. 1, 90–91, which lists herbs to be cultivated on royal estates.

59. *LAB*, f. 5r, ed. Stoll, 64. Walafrid dedicated his poem to Abbot Grimald of Saint-Gall: *De cultura hortorum* 27, ed. Berschin, 94.

60. On Walafrid's view of the cosmos, see Dendle, "Plants," 47–49; on his herbal knowledge, see Stoffler, *Der Hortulus*, 44–119.

61. Cf. Verbaal, "Eros im Kräutergarten," who claims Walafrid's primary interest was adolescent sexuality, not plants. There is every likelihood the poem contains multiple layers. On Walafrid's use of the *Liber medicinalis*, see Vollmer, *Quinti Sereni*, vi; Stoffler, *Der Hortulus*, 16–19.

62. On the *utilis/inutilis* king, see Peters, *Shadow King*, 47–72; Booker, *Past Convictions*, 216–18. On use vs. enjoyment, see Augustine, *De doctrina christiana* 1.7–10, ed. Green, 9–11.

63. Magic was primarily defined by its association with demons (including the pagan gods), but there was little consensus on how to categorize particular practices and beliefs. For a nuanced analysis, see Kieckhefer, "Specific Rationality"; Palmer, "Defining Paganism"; Markus, "From Caesarius"; Jolly, *Popular Religion*. Cf. Flint, *Rise of Magic*, which treats "magic" as a static category opposed to the rational.

64. Tatian (d. ca. 180) condemned medications as magical arts encouraged by demons: Amundsen, *Medicine, Society, and Faith*, 158–69; Temkin, *Hippocrates*, 119–23. Stoll, "Ein Arbeitsbericht," 45–52, reads the apology as a response to Tatian's beliefs.

65. Prognostics are discussed in Chapter 6.

66. This occurs in the *De herba vettonica*, *Curae herbarum*, and *Precatio omnium herbarum*; see McEnerney, "*Precatio terrae*," 182–87; Collins, *Medieval Herbals*, 156, 225n63; Ferraces Rodríguez, "Problemas de edición," 65.

67. On the (perceived) persistence of divinatory practices and natural magic, see Filotas, *Pagan Survivals*, 145–52, 223–43.

68. Augustine, *De civitate Dei* 5.2–7, ed. Dombart and Kalb, 129–35; *Expositio epistulae ad Galatas* 35.1–3, ed. Divjak, 103.

69. Augustine, *De doctrina christiana* 2.110, ed. Green, 65.

70. Augustine, *De doctrina christiana* 2.111, ed. Green, 65. On Augustine's attitude to nature, see Jolly, *Popular Religion*, 73–92.

71. For a recent corrective, see Petit, "Galen, Pharmacology."

72. Palmer, "Defining Paganism"; Koziol, "Truth and Its Consequences."

73. Known as the *Indiculus superstitionum et paganiarum*, ed. Boretius, Capit. 1, 222–23, the list has been associated with Boniface and the reforming councils held in 743–744; see Dierkens, "Superstitions, christianisme et paganisme."

74. Bede, *DTR* 28, ed. Jones, 364–66. Vulture medicine has typically been cast as pagan superstition, but note that Jerome specifically draws attention to the medical benefits of the vulture in *Adversus Jovinianum* 2.6, col. 306A.

75. On Christians gathering twigs from trees that Christ planted and stone chips from Golgotha, see Smith, "Portable Christianity," 148–49.

76. Boniface was primarily a reformer and only secondarily a missionary: Wood, *Missionary Life*, 57–78.

77. The designation of Saxons as pagans was a political tool shaped by the wars: Rembold, *Conquest and Christianization*, 190–205.

78. See Riché, "La magie"; Meens, "Magic"; Hen, "Early Medieval West"; Filotas, *Pagan Survivals*.

79. *Admonitio generalis* 64, ed. Mordek et al., 216; *Capitulare missorum generale* (802) 25, ed. Boretius, Capit. 1, 96. See also Theodulf of Orléans, *Zweites Kapitular* 10.19, ed. Brommer, Capit. episc. 1, 178: "bibere maleficium vel inmundam rem causa medicinae."

80. *Concilium Parisiense* (829) 69, ed. Werminghoff, Conc. 2.2, 669. Alcuin also railed against the carrying of amulets: Ep. 290, ed. Dümmler, 448.

81. For example, Halitgar, *Paenitentiale Pseudo-Romanum*, nos. 31–40, ed. Schmitz, *Die Bussbücher*, 296.

82. As with the *DRN*, Hrabanus relied heavily on the *Etymologiae* (here, Bk. 8.9): *De magicis artibus*, cols. 1095–1110. On his sources, see Flint, *Rise of Magic*, 54–56.

83. Paschasius, *Epitaphium Arsenii* 2.8–9, ed. Dümmler, 68–72; Hincmar, *De divortio Lotharii*, ed. Böhringer, 205–17; Ward, "Agobard of Lyons"; Rider, *Magic and Impotence*, 31–42.

84. Meens, "Magic," 286; Palmer, "Defining Paganism," 408, 423. Cf. Flint, *Rise of Magic*, 59–69.

85. On local efforts to eradicate superstitious beliefs, see Agobard, *De grandine et tonitruis*, ed. van Acker, 3–15; Dutton, *Charlemagne's Mustache*, 169–88.

86. Thorndike, *History of Magic*, 1:584.

87. Paris, BnF lat. 9332, f. 251v, ed. MacKinney, "Unpublished Treatise," 494–96. On the assimilation of pagan charms and Christian liturgy, see Jolly, *Popular Religion*, esp. 114–23.

88. Paris, BnF lat. 6862 (*s*.IX$^{2/4}$), f. 15r: "Contra pustella: Apollo medicus, adiuro te per trecentos sexaginta et quinque dies quos habet annus versus ut extollas tumores, dolores de corpore humano, dico, praedico . . . maledicta pustella."

89. Paris, BnF lat. 6862, f. 12v: "Pretantatio vel plagas et de qualibet causa factus fuerit vulnus. Incantatio sic: sicut Dominus noster IHS XPS in cruce pendens lancea perforatus latere est et neque doluit, neque tumuit, neque fistulam fecit, sic et tu plaga neque doleas, neque tumeas, neque fistulam facias." See Wickersheimer, *Manuscrits latins*, 70. See, similarly, the marginal note in Paris, BnF lat. 6882A, f. 8r (*s*.IX$^{1}$).

90. St. Gall, SB 44, pp. 324, 339, 354, 357. On this manuscript, see Chapter 7.

91. The *Dicta Aristotelis* in St. Gall, SB 44 is edited by Jörimann, *Frühmittelalterliche Rezeptarien*, 10–37. On the *Problemata Aristotelis*, see *BTML*, 40–41.

92. Montecassino, Archivio dell'Abbazia 69, p. 545 (in mixed capitalis and uncial, with a decorated initial). On the manuscript, see *Codici* 94; Lowe, *Beneventan Script*, 2:63; *Katalog* 2.2805. Lowe, *Scriptura Beneventana*, pl. 22, suggests that it was one of two medical codices commissioned by Abbot Bertharius (856–884).

93. Glasgow, UL Hunter 96, f. 48r. The codex is written in a minuscule with Visigothic elements; see *Katalog* 1.1396; *CLA* 2:156. St. Gall, SB 877, p. 33: on this composite manuscript (with medical texts pp. 33–59), see *Codici* 138; von Euw, *Die St. Galler Buchkunst*, 356–57; Bischoff, *Manuscripts and Libraries*, 114.

94. London, BL Arundel 166, f. 71v. In the tenth century, the prefatory letters from Marcellus's *De medicamentis* were added to the original core of this manuscript, ff. 14–90 (*s*.IX$^{1/3}$): see *Katalog* 2.2412; *Codici* 83, suggests an origin of southern Germany.

95. Certain texts and remedies are also attributed to Christian figures (e.g., Ezra, Moses, and Solomon).

96. Montecassino, Archivio dell'Abbazia 69, p. 544. See also Einsiedeln, SB 304 (*s*.VIII$^{ex}$/IX$^{in}$), p. 1: "In nomine dei summi" heads a list of "obscure" vocabulary.

97. The original *vademecum* (*s*.IX$^{in}$), now found in St. Gall, SB 217 (pp. 251–74 and 335–42) and St. Gall, SB Fragmentum 1396 (pp. 9–13, 15, 16, 19, 20–22), was written in northern Italy and may have been joined there to a *materia medica* compilation in a similar hand (St. Gall, SB 217, pp. 275–334); both ended up at Saint-Gall where they were combined with Gregory's *Regula pastoralis*: Köpp, *Vademecum*, 12–14; *Codici* 131; Bischoff, "Italienische Handschriften," 177–78, 190; Niederer, *Der St. Galler Botanicus*, 51–62.

98. St. Gall, SB 217, p. 251.

99. St. Gall, SB 217, p. 252: "In nomine D<omi>ni n<ost>ri IHU XPI incipit s<an>c<t>am ars medicine." Cf. Köpp, *Vademecum*, 25 and 106, who construes the abbreviations as "incipit scientiam ars medicine." The phrase "s<an>c<t>am artem medicinae" appears in Paris, BnF lat. 11219, f. 13v.

100. See a contemporaneous book of medical cures, which included a "recipe" for protection against the devil and feverish chills by repetitively invoking the cross, blood, resurrection, and ascension of our lord Jesus Christ: St. Gall, SB 759, p. 91 (*s*.IX$^{in}$, Brittany). On the manuscript, *Codici* 135; *Katalog* 3.5846; Bischoff, "Ursprung und Geschichte eines Kreuzsegens," in *MS* 2:275–84, at 281.

101. Paris, BnF lat. 9332 (*s*.IX^in), likely produced at Fleury or in the Loire area, was at Chartres by the eleventh century: *Codici* 31; MacKinney, *Early Medieval Medicine*, 197n218; *La médecine médiévale*, no. 8; Collins, *Medieval Herbals*, 149; Nees, *Gundohinus Gospels*, 61–64.

102. Paris, BnF lat. 9332, f. 140r. This manuscript is the first witness to the Latin translation of Alexander's *Therapeutica*, which condensed the original twelve books into three and was probably completed in Rome or Ravenna: see Langslow, *Latin Alexander*, 18, 35–36, 49–50.

103. Paris, BnF lat. 9332, f. 140r: "Alexander sapiens medicus exposuit unc libellum artis medicinae."

104. Paris, BnF lat. 9332, f. 140r: "Scancta [*sic*] crux psalva nos quia per te Christus de suo sacrosancto sanguinae redimet nos." See Bischoff, "Kreuz und Buch im Frühmittelalter und in den ersten Jahrhunderten der spanischen Reconquista," in *MS*, 2:284–303, at 291.

105. See Langslow, *Latin Alexander*, 8; Thorndike, *History of Magic*, 1:575–84; Wallis, *Reader*, 25–26. A recipe following the *Therapeutics* included Christian elements like the Lord's prayer: see Burridge, "Incense," 245–46.

106. Kitzinger, *Cross*, 51–55, 67 (also noting the cross-initials throughout the *Therapeutics*).

107. Paris, BnF lat. 9332, f. 140v: "In nomine domini nostri Iesu Christi incipit Alexandri Hiatrosofiste Therapeutcon liber primus." The title *iatrosophist* (late fourth century) typically referred to physician-philosophers who taught medicine.

108. Montecassino, Archivio dell'Abbazia 97, p. 109, at the start of the *Liber Aurelii de acutis passionibus*. The *Liber Aurelii* and the *Liber Esculapii*, on acute and chronic diseases respectively, were loose Latin translations of Soranus of Ephesus's work and traveled together in the early Middle Ages.

109. On the *digitus medicinalis*, see Isidore, *Etymologiae* 11.1.71.

110. Alba Iulia, Biblioteca Batthyáneum MS R II 1, p. 36. See also Erlangen, Universitätsbibliothek MS 2000 (fragment, *s*.IX^med).

111. Munich, Bayerische Staatsbibliothek Clm 14000, f. 97v.

112. On the manuscript, see *Codici* 95; Lowe, *Beneventan Script*, 1:19, 134, 178, 200, 224, 295; Lowe, *Scriptura Beneventana*, pl. 36. Everett, *Alphabet of Galen*, 125–27.

113. Montecassino, Archivio dell'Abbazia 97, p. 199.

114. Bischoff notes that it is the only folded manuscript he has seen that contains an illustration: "Über gefaltete Handschriften, vornehmlich hagiographischen Inhalts," in *MS*, 1:95–100, at 99.

115. On instrumental value, see Kitzinger, *Cross*, 11–12; on apotropaic uses, see Nees, *Gundohinus Gospels*, 204–10; on economy of healing, see Jones, "Image," 23.

116. *LAB*, f. 2r, ed. Stoll, 52.

117. *LAB*, f. 1v, ed. Stoll, 50 (*passione* was corrected by another hand to *passionum*, which still does not reflect the Latin of the source, Isidore, *Sententiae* 3.3.4, ed. Cazier, 201: "ex intemperantiae passione"). See also the similarities with an anonymous Pauline commentary: PL 68, col. 534C–D.

118. *LAB*, f. 1v, ed. Stoll, 50.

119. *LAB*, f. 2r, ed. Stoll, 50.

120. *LAB*, f. 3r, ed. Stoll, 54 (quoting Isidore, *Sententiae* 3.3.7).

121. *LAB*, f. 3r, ed. Stoll, 54 (quoting Heb 12:6, Prv 3:12).

122. *LAB*, f. 3r–v, ed. Stoll, 56.

123. For Carolingian exegesis on Paul's letters, see Levy, "Commentaries."

124. Paris, BnF lat. 11219 (*s*.IX$^{med}$), f. 12r: "Per omnes curas adhibenda sunt dei medicamenta, quia divina potentia dignata est revivificare corpora mortificata." The treatise is also found in Brussels, BR 3701-15, f. 7r (for similarities between these two manuscripts, see Chapter 5). This line also appears in the preface to the *Teraupetica*, transmitted in 11219 (at f. 104r) and London, BL Arundel 166 (at f. 14r). Cf. the reading of Ferraces Rogríguez, "Un recetario medico inexplorado," 30, 35–39, based on the *Teraupetica*'s use of Theodorus Priscianus's *Euporista*.

125. Paris, BnF lat. 11219, f. 12r: "Et numquid non praesciunt [Brussels, BR 3701-15, f. 7r: non prescivit] ipse dolores nostros quos patimur et genera infirmitatum. Quod et credo quia cum corpora nostra plasmavit tunc et egritudines varias ad nos regendos ordinavit. Pro peccatis enim nostris se ipsum tradidit. Et intantum nos dilexit ut omnes mundi species et pulchritudines ad humanos usus crearet." See also Wiedemann, "Untersuchungen," 143–44.

126. *LAB*, f. 4r, ed. Stoll, 60.

127. This exempts the doctor from blame if a cure is not effected (see Sir 38:9–11).

128. *LAB*, f. 4r, ed. Stoll, 60.

129. *LAB*, f. 1v, ed. Stoll, 50.

130. *LAB*, f. 1v, ed. Stoll, 50 (quoting Isidore, *Liber differentiarum* 2.38, ed. Andrés Sanz, 99).

131. The schemata between two of Alcuin's works (PL 101, col. 947) are found in two extant manuscripts: Matter, "Question-and-Answer," 650. Hrabanus, *DRN* 15.1, col. 413D. Walafrid's citation includes interpolations: St. Gall, SB 878, p. 332. Ermenrich, *Lettre à Grimald* (ca. 854), ed. Goullet, 68. On Abbot Richbod (784–804), a student of Alcuin, as the link between him and the *LAB*, see Glaze, "Perforated Wall," 84–87. On Richbod's friendship with Alcuin, see Bullough, *Alcuin*, 371–72, 400.

132. Isidore, *Liber differentiarum* 2.38, ed. Andrés Sanz, 96–100. On the Insular connections (especially the same division of *physica* in the seventh-century Irish text known as the *Anonymous ad Cuimnanum*), see Bischoff, "Eine verschollene Einteilung der Wissenschaften," in *MS*, 1:273–88.

133. Earlier Roman encyclopedists like Varro had recognized nine arts, but Martianus Capella, Augustine, Boethius, and Cassiodorus followed a sevenfold scheme (as did Isidore at *Etymologiae* 1.2). See Wagner, "Seven Liberal Arts"; Shanzer, "Augustine's Disciplines"; Stahl, *Martianus Capella*, vol. 1. On Isidore's recognition of medicine as a liberal, not manual, art, see Montero Cartelle, "La medicina."

134. On the reception of the *De nuptiis*, see Teeuwen and O'Sullivan, *Carolingian Scholarship*.

135. Whitney, *Paradise Restored*, 57–73, 62–63. See also Contreni, "John Scottus."

136. Wallis, "Is there a 'Carolingian Medicine'?" (unpublished paper), cites Paris, BnF lat. 13955 (*s*.IX$^{3/4}$) as an example of a liberal arts compendium that included medicine and architecture; Glaze, "Perforated Wall," 91, cites two examples of liberal arts handbooks that included medicine, as listed in the Reichenau library catalogues. See also Bern, Burgerbibliothek 363 (*s*.IX$^{3/4}$), which includes Dioscorides's *De materia medica* alongside works on grammar, rhetoric, and dialectic (and a Virgilian commentary with marginal notes of "de medicina" at, for example, ff. 5v, 27v, 31r, 31v, 34v, 35v, 52r, 52v, 57r).

137. *LAB*, f. 1v, ed. Stoll, 48.

138. Bücker, "Christianizing the Arts"; Luhtala, "Early Medieval Divisions."

139. Alberi, "Better Paths."

140. Alcuin, *Carm.* XXVI, lines 12–17, ed. Dümmler, 245; trans. Godman, *Poetry*, 118–19.

141. Isidore, *Etymologiae* 4.3. For adaptations, see *Epistola Ysogogus* in Paris, BnF lat. 11219, f. 20r; *Epistola quantis annis latuit medicina* and *De inventoribus medicinae et artem eius*, in Brussels, BR 3701-15, ff. 5v–6r. These may not have drawn on Isidore but on a common source: Ferraces Rodríguez, "Isidoro de Sevilla," 22–33; Fischer, "Neue oder vernachlässigte Quellen," 169–72; Fischer, "De epistulis." Another history treats the life of Hippocrates and different ancient medical sects: *LAB*, f. 6r, ed. Stoll, 66; St. Gall, SB 751, p. 355–56. See also the history that begins with Chiron in Glasgow, UL Hunter 96, f. 48r; Sigerist, "*Lecciones Heliodori*," 148–49; Laux, "*Ars medicinae*," 418–19.

142. Lozovsky, "Perceptions of the Past," 129–30.

143. Hibernicus Exul, *De artibus liberalibus* c. 8, ed. Dümmler, 410. Kassel, Universitätsbibliothek 2° Ms. phys. et hist. nat. 10 (*s*.IX$^{2}$), ff. 1r, 39r, 39v. Collins, *Medieval Herbals*, 189–91, compares these portraits to productions at Charles the Bald's court, arguing against the claim that they are copies of a southern Italian model. On the manuscript, see Broszinski, *Kasseler Handschriftenschätze*, 82–88; *Codici* 58. On the image of *Scolapius medicus mag<ister>*, with the suggestion that the flowers reference *Christus medicus* iconography as well medicinal substances used in the transmitted remedies, see Fricke and Holler, "Rosenrot," 113–14.

144. Kassel, Universitätsbibliothek 2° Ms. phys. et hist. nat. 10, ff. 1v–2r.

145. For the Carolingians, see the *Chronicon universale* (Apollo at 3958, Hippocrates at 4783), ed. Claszen, "*Chronicon Moissiacense*," 2:17, 32 (borrowing from Isidore's *Chronica Hispalensis* and Bede's *Chronicon maiora*). On the *Chronicon universale*, see Reimitz, *History*, 345–51.

146. Cf. *Epistola Paraxagore*, a history lacking Christian themes in Brussels, BR 3701-15, f. 10r–v; Schubring, "*Epistula Paraxagorae*."

147. Paris, BnF lat. 11218, ff. 6r–10v. If taken as περιοδευτικῶν (*periodeutikon*), the title may refer to "of medical treatments." Boscherini, *Parole*, 71–111, construes the title as *peri dieteson* and offers a discussion and edition, identifying Seneca's *Epistola* 95, the prologue to Celsus's *De medicina*, Pliny's *Historia naturalis*, and Tertullian's *De anima* as possible sources to the first section of the text. On the manuscript, see Chapter 5.

148. Paris, BnF lat. 11218, ff. 6r–v.

149. Paris, BnF lat. 11219, ff. 43r–45r. For an edition, discussion of sources, and transmission history, see Glaze, "Master-Student," here 490.

150. *Epistola peri hereseon*, ed. Glaze, "Master-Student," 490 and 494.

151. *Epistola Luce aevvangeliste*, in Paris, BnF lat. 4883 (*s*.IX$^{ex}$), f. 3r. Edited by Andrés Sanz, "Isidoro de Sevilla," 62–63; Rose, *Theodori Prisciani*, 463. On the manuscript, see *Katalog* 3.4343; *Codici* 21; Wickersheimer, *Manuscrits latins*, 63–64. The first few lines of the letter and the anatomical text that follows it survive in Munich, Bayerische Staatsbibliothek, clm. 5257 (*s*.XI–XII) and Vatican, BAV, Pal. lat. 1098 (*s*.XV). Given its reference to Isidore, this framework cannot predate the seventh century (as Andrés Sanz notes), so 4883 likely reflects a ninth-century augmentation of an earlier, shorter text. Wickersheimer, "Les écrits médicaux," 614, rightly opposes a suggestion that the letter must reflect a Greek original.

152. *Epistola Luce aevvangeliste*, in Paris, BnF lat. 4883, f. 3r: "Constat Hypocratem medicum per tempora sua pagana scripsisse volumina et ideo ibi aliqua esse obscura quaedam vero genetalia. . . . Et ideo nos qui artis medicine curam exercemus et Christiani sunt et libros Hypocratis habemus, quod ille dixit utile probatum tenemus, quod vero ille aut minus aut obscure dixit nos aelucidando transcribimus ut melius legentis intellegat. Quod ibi aliquid

addamus ex libris sancti Isydori aut sancti Augustini aut sancti Gregorii aut Luce evvangeliste, quia toti isti de arte medicine plura dictaverunt. Credentis nobis ad futurum domini nostri Iesu Christi auxilium ut tanto melius proficiat artis nostre operatio quanto ab eo qui est omnipotens medicus libri nostri corrigantur omnem carentes mendatium." The temporal structure of the letter is strange, with Luke appearing as both author and subject.

153. See Lupus of Ferrières's collation of classical texts: Brown, "Introduction," 43–44; Noble, "Lupus of Ferrières," 246–50.

154. See Nees, *Tainted Mantle*, 65–68, 111–30. Cf. Teeuwen, "Seduced by Pagan Poets," 74, who suggests that angst increased over the ninth century as non-Christian texts were copied and studied by a greater range of students.

155. *LAB*, f. 1r, ed. Stoll, 48: "quasi aurum . . . in sterquilinio repperitur." Fischer, "Medizinische Handschriften in der Karolingerzeit: Einblicke und Einsichten" (unpublished paper), suggests Cassiodorus or Origen as the source for this Virgilian phrase, but see Alcuin, Ep. 207, ed. Dümmler, 345, who, unusually, also uses *sterquilinio*, not *stercore*. On the phrase "aurum colligere de stercore," see Folliet, "La fortune du dit de Virgile."

156. http://www.unesco.org/new/en/communication-and-information/memory-of-the-world/register/full-list-of-registered-heritage/registered-heritage-page-5/lorsch-pharmacopoeia-the-bamberg-state-library-mscmed1/ (accessed July 2021).

157. On the transformation of bitter water as a medical art, compare Hrabanus, *Commentaria in Ecclesiasticum* 8.13, col. 1031A and *LAB*, f. 3v (n36 above). On not spurning medicine, compare Hrabanus and *LAB* (n49 above). On the interpretation of Rom 13:14, compare Hildemar, *Expositio* 36, ed. Mittermüller, 415–16: "*Carnis curam ne feceritis in concupiscentiis*. Vido modo, cum dicit *in concupiscentiis*, intelligitur, concessisse in necessitatibus curam carnis esse habendam," with *LAB*, f. 3r–v, ed. Stoll, 56: "Licet Paulus diceret: Carnis curam ne feceritis, quia statim adiecit: in desideriis. Quod enim in desiderio prohibuit, in necessitate nimirum concessit."

158. On Charlemagne's duty to provide "sanitas corporum" to his subjects, see the royal blessing discussed by Nelson, "Kingship and Empire," 217–18. On links between Charlemagne's court and Lorsch, consider also the scribe Rado (d. 808), who worked in both the royal chancery and Lorsch's scriptorium and was known to Alcuin: Becker et al., *Karolingische Klöster*, 74–79, 149–52, 284.

159. Sedulius Scottus, *Carm.* XXXI, lines 4 and 11, ed. Traube, 197–98; trans. Doyle, *On Christian Rulers*, 132.

## Chapter 5

1. *ARF* (817), ed. Pertz and Kurze, 146. Cf. Astronomer, *Vita Hludowici* 28, ed. Tremp, 372–74.

2. *Annales Bertiniani* (870), ed. Grat et al., 175.

3. On illness and accidents in the lives of Carolingian kings, see Hack, *Alter*, 123–46, 231–53; Winter, "Corps, maladie et pouvoir."

4. Alcuin, *Carm.* XXVI, lines 12–17, ed. Dümmler, 245.

5. Einhard, *Vita Karoli* 22, ed. Holder-Egger, 27; trans. Dutton, *Charlemagne's Courtier*, 30.

6. Eigil, *Vita Sturmi* 25, ed. Engelbert, 161. Alcuin knew Wintar: Ep. 8, ed. Dümmler, 34.

7. *Annales Fuldenses* (869), ed. Kurze and Pertz, 69.

8. For an overview, see Siraisi, *Medieval & Early Renaissance Medicine*.

9. The Roman term *archiater* still appears in Merovingian sources. On this title and its use, see Nutton, "*Archiatri*"; MacKinney, *Early Medieval Medicine*, 47–49, 67–69.

10. We know the names of only two royal physicians: Wintar, under Charlemagne, and Zedechias, under Charles the Bald.

11. On Merovingian doctors, see Finot, "Les médecins"; Jones, *Social Mobility*, 250–82; Hack, *Alter*, 339–42; MacKinney, *Early Medieval Medicine*, 60–80. On the Ostrogoths and Lombards, see Pilsworth, *Healthcare*, 177–215. On Visigothic Spain, see Amundsen, "Visigothic Medical Legislation," at 565, which concludes that there was a "non-clerical, non-monastic, professional medical class."

12. Heiric of Auxerre, *Miracula S. Germani* 86, col. 1248B. Wintar is referred to as *medicus domini regis* in Eigil, *Vita Sturmi* 25, ed. Engelbert, 161. A charter of King Zwentibold of Lotharingia (896) grants land to one *clericus* Everhelmus, designated a *regalis medicus* in the later *Gesta episcoporum Tullensium*: Hack, *Alter*, 352–53. Contreni, "Masters and Medicine," 335–36, finds in an 845 charter from Charles the Bald one Johannes *medicus* with ties to the court (and speculates this was Eriugena).

13. Payment due a *medicus* for treatment is found in *Pactus legis Salicae* 29.18, ed. Eckhardt, 117 (but not in the *Lex Salica Karolina*). The *medicus* determines the severity of a wound in the *Lex Alamannorum* 57.5–7, ed. Lehmann, 117; *Lex Baiwariorum* 5.3, ed. von Schwind, 339. On doctors in the law codes, see Oliver, *Body Legal*, 76–79, 88–89, 157–58. A *medicus* must be sought for a blow in Halitgar, *Paenitentiale Pseudo-Romanum*, no. 51, ed. Schmitz, *Die Bussbücher*, 297.

14. Cassiodorus, *Institutiones* 1.31, ed. Mynors, 78–79. *LAB*, f. 4v, ed. Stoll, 60, changes Cassiodorus's phrase to "the sick" (*aegrotantes*).

15. *Regula Benedicti* 36, ed. Venarde, 130.

16. This does not mean all extant texts *necessarily* reflect monastic writing; see the wariness expressed by Davis, *Charlemagne's Practice*, 188; Brown et al., *Documentary Culture*. On the catalogues, see the Introduction.

17. For more on the plan, see Chapter 7. The best way to navigate it is through the digital reproduction at http://www.stgallplan.org/en/plan_notes.html (accessed July 2021).

18. For the list of goods to be purchased at Cambrai market (likely for Corbie): *Polyptyque de l'abbé Irminon*, ed. Guérard, 2:336. For Fontenelle's annual supply of honey and spices for the sick (and a little house, supplied with plenty of meat, poultry, and eggs): *Gesta abbatum Fontanellensium*, ed. Lohier and Laporte, 122–23. For more examples, see McCormick, *Origins*, 708–16.

19. These are Geilo/Teilo and Sigibertus/Sigipreth, the latter of whom Zettler suggests succeeded the former as the Reichenau *medicus* in the 840s. See *Das Verbrüderungsbuch*, ed. Autenrieth et al., 218; Zettler, "Exkurs I," 265–69.

20. Adalhard, *Consuetudines Corbeienses*, ed. Semmler, in *Initia consuetudinis*, 367; discussed by C. W. Jones in Horn and Born, *Plan of St. Gall*, 3:93–123.

21. On Adalric of Saint-Vaast (abbot from 742) as *probatissimus medicus*, see Ulmarus of Saint-Vaast, *Miracula S. Vedasti* 9, ed. Holder-Egger, 401. On Dido of Saint-Pierre-le-Vif (abbot 847–869), see below. On Decorosus, a *medicus* and *monachus*, sent as an envoy for Charlemagne in 791, and on Gisulfus, *abbas et medicus*, as an envoy of Queen Angilberga (wife of Emperor Louis II), see Hack, *Alter*, 353. Walafrid mentions a brother *medicinali scientia instructus* who performs a phlebotomy on himself: *Vita S. Galli* 2.36, ed. Krusch, 333. Two tenth-century examples that may be indicative of ninth-century conditions are one Kerolt (described as *medicus, monachus atque presbyter*) and the famous monk-physician Notker, both from Saint-Gall: see Zettler, "Exkurs I," 271–72. The monk Richer (ca. 950–1000) studied

medicine under teachers at Reims and Chartres and references the bishop of Amiens's learning: MacKinney, "Tenth-Century Medicine"; Lake, *Richer*, 187–88, 259–69.

22. The capitulary of Thionville from 805 includes a heading "De medicinalia arte," but the phrase "ut infantes hanc discere mittantur" is found only in the edition by Baluze: *Capitulare missorum in Theodonis villa datum primum* 7, ed. Boretius, Capit. 1, 121. The meaning is unclear and cannot be taken to indicate that all clerics were to learn medicine: Paxton, "Curing Bodies," 234–35; cf. MacKinney, *Early Medieval Medicine*, 95.

23. Hack, *Alter*, 351–53.

24. Pilsworth, *Healthcare*, 187–215. On *medici* as a respected, largely literate group in northern Italy, see Pilsworth, "Could You Just Sign."

25. Contreni, "Masters and Medicine," 333–39.

26. Bishop Wigbert of Hildesheim (880–908) is described as *medicinae artis peritissimus* in the *Chronicon Hildesheimense* 6, ed. Pertz, 851. On Chartres and Reims, see MacKinney, *Early Medieval Medicine*, 106–51, and "Tenth-Century Medicine"; Contreni, "Masters and Medicine," 338.

27. Cf. Pilsworth, *Healthcare*, 210, that *monachi* could not be titled *medici* based on the charter evidence.

28. The term *medica* appears twice but refers to saints: Fortunatus, *De vita S. Radegundis* 1.29, ed. Krusch, 374; Wolfhard of Herrieden, *Miracula S. Walburgae* 2.7, ed. Holder-Egger, 547. Einhard criticizes foolish women who use herbs and incantations: *Translatio* 3.16, ed. Waitz, 254.

29. See Chapter 7. Hildemar, *Expositio regulae* 36, ed. Mittermüller, 407, states that an attendant for the sick must be a monk, not a canon or layman.

30. Einhard, *Translatio* 3.20, ed. Waitz, 255.

31. *Ex miraculis S. Quintini* 11, ed. Holder-Egger, 267. See also the eleventh-century story about Notker the monk (d. 975) examining the Duke of Bavaria's urine: Wallis, "Signs and Senses," 278.

32. Ardo, *Vita Benedicti* 11, ed. Waitz, 205. Lupus, Ep. 72, ed. Dümmler, 68–69, praises Abbot Dido of St. Pierre-le-Vif's knowledge of healing and asks him to assume care for brothers unsuccessfully healed by *medici* who came to the monastery (noted in MacKinney, *Early Medieval Medicine*, 92).

33. See *Formulae Augienses* Coll. C 10 and 22, ed. Zeumer, 369, 374.

34. On clerical *medici* in monasteries, see Pilsworth, *Healthcare*, 210–14.

35. On early medieval deontological writings, see MacKinney, "Medical Ethics"; Hirschfeld, "Deontologische Texte"; Galvão-Sobrinho, "Hippocratic Ideals"; Fischer, "*Isagoge* of Pseudo-Soranus." There are similarities with the *Physician, Decorum, Precepts*, and *Oath* from the Hippocratic Corpus, but no Latin translations of these survive from the early medieval West. On correspondences (especially when it pertains to the *medicus*'s deportment, clothing, and bodily grooming) among the Latin texts, an Arabic treatise, and a Greek original extant in two fourteenth-century manuscripts, see Deichgräber, *Medicus gratiosus*, 83–107. On Hippocratic ethics, see Edelstein, *Ancient Medicine*, 87–110; Nutton, *Ancient Medicine*, 87–102; Jouanna, *Greek Medicine*, 261–85.

36. Markus, "From Caesarius," 169.

37. The texts have consistently been associated with Greek medicine in imperial centers: on their origins, Hirschfeld, "Deontologische Texte," 354–57, favors Oribasius's environs, MacKinney, "Medical Ethics," 7, sixth-century Ravenna.

38. The content, title, and framework of the texts differ in the extant witnesses. Some survive as prefaces, some in letter *corpora*, some in ensembles (that were themselves reconfigured) like the *Sapientia artis medicinae*, the *Ars medicinae*, and the *Isagoge* of Pseudo-Soranus. On these tangled transmission histories, see Fischer, "*Isagoge* of Pseudo-Soranus"; Baader, "Die Anfänge"; Wiedemann, "Untersuchungen," 5–81; Laux, "*Ars medicinae*"; Wlaschky, "*Sapientia artis medicinae*."

39. St. Gall, SB 751 (*s*.IX$^{med}$), p. 358, ed. Hirschfeld, "Deontologische Texte," 363. On various dates proposed for the manuscript (*s*.IX$^{1/4}$–IX$^{2}$) and its origins in northern Italy (before arriving at Saint-Gall), see Bischoff, *Manuscripts and Libraries*, 129–30; *Codici* 133; *Katalog* 3.5844. Paris, BnF lat. 11219, f. 12v has a different version of this text. See also Brussels, BR 3701-15, f. 12r: "Quid est perfectus medicus? Sapiens, memoriosus, litteris eruditus."

40. The first, *De sacramento dando vel qualiter legat*, in Paris, BnF lat. 11219, f. 13v–14r (f. 14 is badly mutilated), as reconstructed from the (now mostly destroyed) Chartres, BM 62 (*s*.X) by MacKinney, "Medical Ethics," 15. The second, St. Gall, SB 751, p. 355, ed. Hirschfeld, "Deontologische Texte," 367. See also the "preface" to the Pseudo-Soranus *Quaestiones medicinales*, ed. Rose, *Anecdota Graeca*, 2:244–45 (with the preface being a separate text rather than an introduction to the *Quaestiones*, as argued by Fischer, *Sorani*, 17).

41. Isidore and the preface to Pseudo-Soranus, *Quaestiones medicinales* may have drawn on a common source: Fischer, "Neue oder vernachlässigte Quellen," 154–55.

42. Isidore, *Etymologiae* 4.13.1–4.

43. *Etymologiae* 4.13 (alone or as part of Bk. IV) appears in: Glasgow, UL Hunter 404, ff. 3r–11v (*s*.X); Berlin, Staatsbibliothek, Phillipps 1790, ff. 36r–v (*s*.IX$^{med}$); St. Gall, SB 752, pp. 161–78 (*s*.IX$^{ex}$); London, BL Add. 8928, ff. 1v–5v (*s*.X); Montecassino, Archivio dell'Abbazia 97, pp. 13–20 (*s*.X$^{in}$).

44. Paris, BnF lat. 11218, f. 7r: "Qui disciplina et dei timorem habuerit leccione ingenio racione vitae temporis cursum, pulsus venarum, aetatis, personas hominum, volatilium, piscium, herbarum, arborum vel saxorum [saxosum] et omnia que arte vel manu fieri possunt cognitor."

45. Cassiodorus also underscored a doctor's need to read assiduously: *Variae* 6.19, ed. Fridh, 249.

46. On Augustine's "mechanical arts" (grouped under the divine disciplines), see Klingshirn, "Divination and the Disciplines," 128–35.

47. Augustine, *De doctrina christiana* 2.115, ed. Green, 66.

48. On the *De doctrina*, see Amos, "Augustine and the Education."

49. See *De doctrina*, Bk. 4. On monastic interest in the Roman orator, see Coon, "Somatic Styles," esp. 66–67.

50. Paris, BnF lat. 11219, f. 12r: "Interea moneo te medice sicut et ego monitus sum a magistro, lege semper, desidiosus noli esse. Susceptos infirmos require, de eorum cura cogita, pudicitiam sectare, castitatem ama, secretum domus serva. Si aliquid nosti in infirmis tace, de aliis detrahere noli." Also in Brussels, BR 3701-15, f. 7r; Glasgow, UL Hunter 404, f. 27v, where it is titled *Ammonitio Theodori medici*. Wiedemann, "Untersuchungen," 136, counts fourteen medieval witnesses.

51. Practical matters addressed include age of training, clothing and mannerisms, payment, and pulse-taking. See, for example, *Quomodo debes visitare infirmum* in Montecassino, Archivio dell'Abbazia 97, p. 4.

52. *Qualis esse debeat medicus*: Paris, BnF lat. 11219, f. 13v; St. Gall, SB 751, p. 358. Compare with Pseudo-Soranus *Quaestiones medicinales*, ed. Rose, *Anecdota Graeca*, 2:245.

53. See other characteristics in *Epistola Arsenii*; *De his qui inchoant*; *Epistola primitus legenda de disciplina artis medicinae* (discussed at *BTML*, 42, 75; Kibre, *Hippocrates Latinus*, 179–81).

54. St. Gall, SB 751, p. 356: "Gravitas enim multa animae significat."

55. *Epistola Arsenii* in Brussels, BR 3701-15, f. 5v: "Oportet inprimis probare natura." Contrast ancient deontological treatises, where ethical precepts *instilled* good conduct: Galvão-Sobrinho, "Hippocratic Ideals," 447–50.

56. St. Gall, SB 751, p. 355, ed. Hirschfeld, "Deontologische Texte," 364–65. See also MacKinney, "Medical Ethics," 15.

57. Paris, BnF lat. 11218, f. 8v: "Verumtamen medicine per multus transiit sed paucus sapientis invenit."

58. MacKinney, "Medical Ethics," 3, 30.

59. *Epistola Arsenii*, ed. Hirschfeld, "Deontologische Texte," 361.

60. Jerome, Ep. 52, "Ad Nepotianum presbyterum," ed. Hilberg, *Epistulae*, 1:438–39.

61. See de Jong, *Penitential State*, 113–15, 151–52; Margalhan-Ferrat, "Le concept de *ministerium*"; Patzold, *Episcopus*, 135–84; Kramer, *Rethinking Authority*, 59–96; Booker, *Past Convictions*, 140–46, 165–81.

62. *Capitulare Francofurtense* 14, ed. Werminghoff, Conc. 2.1, 168; *Regula Benedicti* 31, ed. and trans. Venarde, 116–17.

63. See McKitterick, *Charlemagne*, 268–70; Esders, "Faithful Believers"; Esders, "Rechtliche Grundlagen."

64. See *LAB*, f. 6r; Paris, BnF lat. 11219, ff. 13v–14r (likely, before mutilation); St. Gall, SB 751, pp. 355–56. See also Chartres, BM 62, f. 1r–v (*s*.X) and the eleventh- and twelfth-century manuscripts with section III in Laux, "*Ars medicinae*," 419–21 and with letters J and K in MacKinney, "Medical Ethics," 15–16.

65. Paris, BnF lat. 11219, f. 13v: "Coniurare etiam debet qui medicinalem artem et naturae scientiam vult inchoare." On the original Hippocratic Oath, see von Staden, "In a Pure and Holy Way," 406–8.

66. Cf. Galvão-Sobrinho, "Hippocratic Ideals," 445. Cassiodorus refers to doctors taking oaths in the manner of priests (*sacerdotii genere sacramenta*): *Variae* 6.19, ed. Fridh, 249.

67. French, *Medicine Before Science*, esp. 1–4.

68. See García-Ballester et al., *Practical Medicine*; Green, *Making Women's Medicine*; McVaugh, *Rational Surgery*.

69. On methods of categorization, see Pomata, *Contracting a Cure*, 120–40.

70. Filotas, *Pagan Survivals*, 219 and 223, finds fifty different terms for "magic practitioner."

71. See Nutton, *Ancient Medicine*, 164–70. Contrast Galen: Mattern, *Rhetoric of Healing*, 14–27.

72. Locating change by the fifth century: Jones, *Social Mobility*, 252–60; Nutton, "From Galen to Alexander," 12–15.

73. Pliny the Elder, *Historia naturalis* 29.8 (framed by a critique of foreign Greek practices). On Roman denunciations of Greek physicians, see von Staden, "Liminal Perils."

74. On the *Historia naturalis*, see Eastwood, *Ordering the Heavens*, 19–20; Borst, *Buch der Naturgeschichte*. On the adaptations of Pliny (often attributed to Plinius Secundus Iunior), see Önnerfors, ed., *Plinii Secundi Iunioris*; Önnerfors, ed., *Physica Plinii*; Hunt, trans., *Medicina Plinii*. The preface of the *Medicina Plinii* was also found in Marcellus's *De medicamentis*.

75. *Medicina Plinii* 1, ed. and trans. Hunt, 14–15 (and Broderson's Introduction, 4). On the preface, see Segoloni, "Il prologus"; Doody, "Authority and Authorship." See also the preface to Pseudo-Apuleius, *Herbarius*, ed. Howald and Sigerst, 15.

76. A physician is executed for the death of a queen in Gregory of Tours, *Historiae* 5.35, ed. Krusch and Levison, 241–42.

77. *Annales Bertiniani* (877), ed. Grat et al., 216–17.

78. For evidence of Jewish doctors, see Gregory of Tours, *Historiae* 5.6, ed. Krusch and Levison, 203; *Formulae Salzburgenses* 38 (ascribed to Arn of Salzburg), ed. Zeumer, 448, as cited by Blumenkranz, *Juifs et chrétiens*, 21–22; Skinner, *Health and Medicine*, 81–82 (on southern Italy). Correcting a mistake about Charlemagne's doctor: Hack, *Alter*, 353–57. There is insufficient evidence to draw generalizations about the number of Jewish practitioners (cf. Bachrach, *Jewish Policy*, 71–72, 138).

79. Jewish doctors may have fared reasonably well under Charlemagne's and Louis's relatively favorable policies toward Jews. Jewish scholars friendly with Carolingian intellectuals and Jewish merchants who crossed the Mediterranean may have been instrumental in furthering medical knowledge and procuring ingredients in the eighth and ninth centuries. On Jewish-Christian relations and trading activity, see Bachrach, *Jewish Policy*, 66–105; Elukin, *Living Together*, 43–58; McCormick, *Origins*, 647–49, 667–78, 766.

80. Regino of Prüm, *Chronicon* (877), ed. Kurze, 113 (noted in Hack, *Alter*, 348).

81. Cf. Lk 8:43–48 and Mt 9:20–22, which do not mention doctors.

82. On Gregory's own illness, see *De virtutibus S. Martini* 2.1, ed. Krusch, 159. On Gregory and medicine, see Van Dam, *Saints*, 82–93; James, "Sense of Wonder." Einhard, *Translatio* 4.1 and 4.6, ed. Waitz, 256, 257.

83. Flint, "Early Medieval *medicus*." See also Van Dam, *Leadership and Community*, 256–76; Jones, *Social Mobility*, 260–65. Cf. Pilsworth, *Healthcare*, 115–19, who finds few incompetent *medici* in northern Italian hagiography.

84. On the medical marketplace, see Horden, "Sickness and Healing," 416–20.

85. Dutton, *Politics of Dreaming*, 91.

86. See *ARF* (826), ed. Pertz and Kurze, 171–72; Einhard, *Translatio* 2.8–9, ed. Waitz, 247.

87. Smith, "Old Saints," 320–24, with table at 335–39.

88. See Geary, *Furta Sacra*, 23, 34–37.

89. For criticism of other relics, see Einhard, *Translatio* 3.5, 3.15, Preface 4, 4.14, ed. Waitz, 249, 254, 256, 261–62.

90. Paxton, *Christianizing Death*, 128–30. See also Poschmann, *Penance*, 234–49.

91. Gerbald of Liège, *Erstes Kapitular* 21, ed. Brommer, Capit. episc. 1, 21.

92. *Concilium Cabillonense* 48, ed. Werminghoff, Conc. 2.1, 283. For further Carolingian mandates, see Poschmann, *Penance*, 242–43.

93. Jonas, *DIL* 3.14, ed. Dubreucq, 2:296–302.

94. Paxton, *Christianizing Death*, 149–53.

95. For Benedict's emphasis on the temporal healing of the body (vs. Irish focus on spiritual purification), see Paxton, *Christianizing Death*, 148–61.

96. Alcuin, *Carm.* XXVI, line 15, ed. Dümmler, 245; trans. Godman, *Poetry*, 118–19. *LAB*, f. 4v–5r, ed. Stoll, 60–62. Similarly, the treatise *Qualis esse debeat medicus* states that physicians must care for the rich and poor equally, only accepting payment if it is offered: Hirschfeld, "Deontological Texts," 363; MacKinney, "Medical Ethics," 12.

97. Burridge, "Incense," argues for a similar overlap between "religion" and "medicine" in examining the multipurpose uses of incense.

98. Mk 2:17, Lk 5:31, Mt 9:12; see also Lk 4:23.

99. See Mk 2:1–12.

100. Temkin, *Hippocrates*, 17.

101. Asclepius was worshipped at 670 shrines across the Roman Mediterranean by the second century: Ferngren, *Medicine & Health Care*, 67.

102. Temkin, *Hippocrates*, 79–85, 97, 118–19, 181–89. Cf. Ferngren, *Medicine & Health Care*, 26–41, 64–85.

103. Augustine, *De civitate Dei* 3.17, 8.26, ed. Dombart and Kalb, 83–85, 246–47. On condemnations of Asclepius in late antique Christian writers, see Patterson, "*Adversus paganos*." cf. Reid, "First Dispensation," 225–26.

104. Augustine, *De civitate Dei* 22.8, ed. Dombart and Kalb, 815–27.

105. Arbesmann, "Christus medicus." See also Bochet, "Maladie de l'âme"; Blanchard, "Christ médecin"; Reid, "First Dispensation," 163–221.

106. Pease, "Medical Allusions."

107. On Gregory's medical metaphors, see Straw, *Gregory the Great*, 99, 142–43, 153, 204–5. Pomerius's *De vita contemplativa* may have inspired Gregory: Timmerman, "Sharers in the Contemplative Virtue," 2–3, 24–28.

108. Gregory, *Regula pastoralis* 3.36, ed. Rommel, 2:518.

109. *Concilium Cabillonense* (813) 34, ed. Werminghoff, Conc. 2.1, 280; *Concilium Aquisgranense* (816) 23, 134, ed. Werminghoff, Conc. 2.1, 344, 410; *Concilium Aquisgranense* (836) 15, ed. Werminghoff, Conc. 2.2, 709.

110. *Regula Benedicti* 27, 28, ed. and trans. Venarde, 106–11 (with slight modifications). On Benedict's medical terminology, see Molland, "*Ut sapiens medicus*."

111. Noble, "Monastic Ideal"; Diem, "Carolingians and the *Regula Benedicti*"; Kramer, *Rethinking Authority*, 53–93, 176–84.

112. Booker, *Past Convictions*, 155–56; de Jong, *Penitential State*, esp. 113–22, 126–28, 203–4.

113. *Libellus Trecensis* and *Libellus Parisinus*, ed. Wilmart, *Precum libelli*, 13, 42; Alcuin, *Ad pueros sancti Martini* 3, 4–6, ed. Driscoll, 52–56; Firey, "Blushing Before the Judge"; Choy, "The Brother," 102–3.

114. Jerome, *Commentarium ad Philemon* 23–24, ed. Bucchi, in *Commentarii in epistulas Pauli*, 105.

115. *Concilium Cabillonense* (813) 34, ed. Werminghoff, Conc. 2.1, 280.

116. Hrabanus, *Commentaria in Ecclesiasticum* 8.13, col. 1030C.

117. *Interea moneo te*, in Paris, BnF lat. 11219, f. 12r: "gratia dei tecum et in usu medicinae, et susceptis tuis salus a deo veniat qui solus est medicus. Feliciter. Amen."

118. *Epistola Luce aevvangeliste*, in Paris, BnF lat. 4883, f. 3r.

119. *Epistola de homine et voce*, in Brussels, BR 3701-15, f. 5r: "Lucas dicit ibi laudatur medicus ubi operatur dominus. Hypocratis quoque ait tantum proficit medicus quantum permittit dominus" (the full text is edited by Fischer, "*De coelo uita*," 215–16). The *Epistola Luce aevvangeliste* in Paris, BnF lat. 4883, f. 3r includes a variant: "omnis administratio et omnis medicina a deo procedit et ibi laudabitur medicus ubi voluerit dominus."

120. Cf. Augustine on the physician's ineffectiveness because he is trying to cure a body that he did not create: *Enarrationes in Psalmos* 102.5, ed. Dekkers and Fraipont, CCSL 40, 1455.

121. *LAB* f. 3v, ed. Stoll, 56–58.

122. Paris, BnF lat. 11218 (*s*.VIII$^{ex}$/IX$^{in}$), possibly produced in Burgundy, held at the abbey of Saint-Bénigne of Dijon by the seventeenth century: see *Katalog* 3.4669; *Codici* 34; Wickersheimer, "Une vie des saints Côme et Damien," 41. It is a small, easily portable codex, which was produced by rearranging and expanding an earlier compilation, as indicated by scattered quire signatures. The various hands are early Caroline minuscule, including those that copied space-filling recipes, so the rearrangement was likely complete by the early ninth century.

123. Paris, BnF lat. 11218, f. 2r: "Incipit passio sanctorum Quosme et Damiani medicorum" (mixed capitalis and uncial). This version of the *passio* corresponds most closely to BHL 1970; trans. Wallis, *Reader*, 62–66. On ninth-century witnesses, see Cross, "Cosmas and Damian," 15–18.

124. *Passio*, in Paris, BnF lat. 11218, f. 2r: "Docti autem sunt famuli dei ad revelacione spiritus sancti, in multa sciencia artis medicinae et curabant secundum scriptura divina."

125. Cf. Anastasius Bibliothecarius's Latin translation (Rome, 870s) of Sophronius of Jerusalem, *Miracula SS. Cyri et Ioannis*, m. 22 and m. 30 (where Cyrus and John are called co-martyrs and co-physicians to Cosmas and Damian), ed. Mai, *Spicilegium Romanum III*, 239–40 and 317 (PG 87.3, cols. 3486B–C, 3519C). On Sophronius's response to a Hippocratic, rationalist skepticism of the saints, see Dal Santo, *Debating*, 174–82.

126. Paris, BnF lat. 11218, f. 2r: "Quicumque autem aegrotantur et haec passio super eum lecta fuerit, dominus misertus erit ei."

127. Paris, BnF lat. 11218, ff. 6r–10v. On this text, see Boscherini, "Malattia e corruzione," 71–111.

128. Paris, BnF lat. 11218, ff. 7v and 8r: "O tu sapiens si fragilitas humana delinquit cur sapienciam laceras [*corr. a* lazeras]? . . . O tu aeger qui te in inmundicia credis et alterius malo, non solum placandum deum postulacionem poteris, nec tuum advocatum medicum qui inmundicia plenus est auditur."

129. Paris 11218, f 8r: "Suscepti eorum manifeste hac celere adplecantur morte."

130. Paris 11218, f. 7v: "VITA MEDICI [canonical capitalis] castitas fidis subrietas faciunt permanere sapientes in sapiencia."

131. Paris 11218, f. 8v: "in quibus fidis non vacellit sed ars pura et consciencia non ficta."

132. Paris 11218, f. 8r: "Melius est cum imperito sancto vivere vel cum eius parva arte quamvis imperita portare, quam cum perfecto et omni iniquitate et inmundicia plenum adhibere." A similar statement is attributed to Erasistratus and found in the Pseudo-Soranus *Quaestiones medicinales* and *Isagoge*.

133. Paris 11218, f. 9r: "Tu quid est corpus quod videre potes curas, numquid in hanimam quam non vides tenere potes?"

134. On the transformative power of hagiography, see Rapp, "Holy Texts," 222.

135. *Ad demonium remedium* in Paris, BnF lat. 11218, f. 69r.

136. *Isidori Hispalensis versus* 16–24, ed. Sánchez Martín, 227–33, who gives the *LAB* as the earliest witness with the medical verses. See also Sudhoff, "Die Verse Isidors." The Lorsch library catalogue of 830–840 (Häse, *MBKL*, B171) includes the verses: "Breviarium eiusdem [Isidore] super divinae historiae libros et versus, qui scripti sunt in armaria eius, ab ipso conpositi."

137. See the end of *Epistula quantis annis latuit medicina* in Brussels, BR 3701-15, f. 6r, as noted by Fischer, "De epistulis," 265.

138. *LAB*, f. 5r. Cf. Vatican, BAV, Pal. lat. 276, f. 40v (*s*.IX$^{1}$), where red ink is used for the names of Church Fathers but not for the physicians; Milan, BA C.74 sup., f. 141r, where all verse

titles are condensed into the margin (the Isidore verses were added by a later ninth-century Italian hand: *Katalog* 2.2630).

139. Gregory of Tours, *Historiae* 10.31, ed. Krusch and Levison, 535.

140. Under the title to the *passio* in Paris, BnF lat. 11218, the feast day is noted as "v kalendas octobris." On the cult of Cosmas and Damian, see Harrold, "Saintly Doctors," 26–80.

141. On their depictions in Rome and Ravenna, see Knipp, "Chapel of Physicians"; Harrold, "Saintly Doctors," 88–110. On connections with Constantinople, see Maskarinec, *City of Saints*, 32–37.

142. On the iconography of the boxes, see Harrold, "Saintly Doctors," 91–92, 107; Nordhagen, *Frescoes of John VII*, 55–66.

143. See, respectively, Knipp, "Chapel of Physicians," 11–12; Harrold, "Saintly Doctors," 119; Paxton, *Christianizing Death*, 70.

144. Gregory of Tours, *Liber in gloria martyrum* 97, ed. Krusch, 103–4; trans. Van Dam, *Glory of the Martyrs*, 91.

145. Paris, BnF lat. 11219: see *Codici* 35; Wiedemann, "Untersuchungen," 100–102; Wickersheimer, "Un manuscrit médical," 173–89; Vázquez Buján, "Codicologie et histoire"; Vezin, "Le point d'interrogation," 184, 191–92; López Figueroa, "Estudio," 101–6.

146. *Liber epistolarum* at ff. 12r–41v. Compare with Brussels, BR 3701-15, ff. 1r–14v (*s.*IX$^{2/3}$), a unit that lacks a section heading but contains a set of numbered treatises, most of which are titled *epistula* (extant are letters 9–26 and 38–50, with pages missing at the beginning and after f. 8). The Paris and Brussels manuscripts share eleven letters in common, seven of which are exclusive to these two manuscripts, but they did not rely on the same exemplar: Wiedemann, "Untersuchungen," 57–81.

147. *Epistola quod per omnes curas adhibenda sint medicamenta* in Paris, BnF lat. 11219, ff. 12r–12v: " Digna enim est professio talem medicum vocare, qui praestat animi sanitates et corporis salubritates, quare enim non postulemus illum qui animam et corpus suo imperio formavit . . . Sic enim constituit operatores quos docuit gratia sua ut exerceant se spiritalibus usibus. Cum diligentia curent corpora et animas recuperent. Sed multi sunt qui studia videntur inpendere corporis requirunt auxilium, et animam affligunt neglecto. Sed quia animam et corpus procurat salvare, ab omnipotente deo factus inmortalis pristinam merebitur accipere sanitatem et de reatu eius securitatem." Cf. Brussels, BR 3701-15, f. 7r, and Wiedemann's collation of the two texts, "Untersuchungen," 143–44.

148. See also Alcuin, Ep. 213, ed. Dümmler, 356–57; trans. MacKinney, *Early Medieval Medicine*, 86: "they [*medici*] do not presume to say that they are the creators [*creatores*] of herbs or of any other kinds of drugs from the composition of which the health of sick men is regained, but they say they are only the servants [*ministros*] in collecting and combining them into one body."

149. On the earliest witness to this reform rite, see Paxton, *Christianizing Death*, 148–53. An edition from the Rodradus Sacramentary (ca. 850, Corbie) is found as no. 433, ed. Deshusses, *Le sacramentaire grégorien*, 3:145–46.

150. See Paxton, *Christianizing Death*, 153–55, who delineates the Roman and Visigothic precedents.

151. *Sacramentaire grégorien* nos. 4022 and 4026, ed. Deshusses, 3:134–35.

152. *Sacramentaire grégorien* nos. 3990 and 4026, ed. Deshusses, 3:128 and 135.

153. *Tereoperica* (Paris 11219, f. 42r), ed. López Figueroa, "Estudio," 153: "Ex tunc et nunc et usque in eternum confitebimur cum dei auxilio esse manifestum certantis studium fructuosum opus ad omnes egritudines mitigandas et cum dei gratia curandas corporum uexatas."

154. *De his qui inchoant*, in Paris, BnF lat. 11219, f. 13v: (attributed to Erasistratus) "Si autem unum e duobus defuerit melius est virum esse bonum absque doctrina quam cum arte sancta mores habere malos et inprobum esse." See also the *Epistola pepiodeotecon* on the importance of both skill and morality.

155. *Epistola Arsenii ad Nepotianum* in Paris, BnF lat. 11219, ff. 14r–15r (f. 14 is damaged). It survives in two other ninth-century manuscripts: Brussels, BR 3701-15, and St. Gall, SB 751. Saint Arsenius (d. ca. 455) was the pseudonym chosen by Paschasius Radbertus for his hero, Wala, in the *Epitaphium Arsenii*.

156. *Epistola Arsenii*, Paris, BnF lat. 11219, f. 15r: "Quid est medicus? Lenis auxiliator vivificans corpus, refrenans dolores, desiccans humores, dieta invitat, febres effugat . . ."

157. *Epistola Arsenii*, Paris, BnF lat. 11219, ff. 14v–15r: "sicut lucerna quae domum inluminat omnes videre facit excluso tenebrae incessu, ita sic laeta medici astutia omnes tristitias in gaudium convertit et tota membra egrotantis confortat et animum recreat."

158. See also a question and answer text, *Liber interrogationis Yppocratic medici*, in Paris, BnF lat. 11219, f. 26v: "Sanitas, quod appellatur? Modis duobus: unum in quo anime intellegimus sanitatem, alium quo corporis praeceptum."

159. *Epistola Arsenii*, Paris, BnF lat. 11219, f. 15r: "docens praesentia, denuntians futura, aeterna manifestat."

160. Isidore, *Etymologiae*, 4.10.2; trans. Barney, 114.

161. Cassiodorus, *Variae* 6.19, ed. Fridh, 249; Wallis, "Signs and Senses," 277.

162. On saints' visions of death, see Wallis, "Signs and Senses," 278; Kreiner, "Autopsies and Philosophies," 116–20.

163. Alcuin, *Vita Willibrordi* 30, ed. Levison, 137; trans. Talbot, in *Soldiers of Christ*, ed. Head and Noble, 210.

164. *LAB*, f. 4r, ed. Stoll, 58. A string of biblical citations interpolated into the quotation from Cassiodorus's *Institutiones* also cements this point.

165. *LAB*, f. 4r, ed. Stoll, 58–60.

166. See also *De ratione medicine* in Glasgow, UL Hunter 404, f. 25r: "Et qui non timet dominum quere medicum et non inveniet eum."

167. Flint, "Early Medieval *medicus*," 143.

168. That the doctor and priest might be one and the same is suggested by manuscripts like the handbook produced at Lorsch for secular clergy, Vatican, BAV Pal. lat. 485 (*s*.IX$^{3/4}$), which includes Benedict of Aniane's reform rite for the sick alongside medical texts like bloodletting prognostics and monthly regimens; on the manuscript, see Paxton, "*Bonus liber.*"

169. See Margalhan-Ferrat, "Concept de *ministerium*"; Savigni, "Laïcs dans l'ecclésiologie," 45–63; Moore, *Sacred Kingdom*, 336–42.

170. In his figural poem of Christ's body, Hrabanus drew attention to the term for the fourth finger on Christ's right hand (called the *medicus* for its use in applying ointments), implicitly linking the divine and human physician; see Coon, *Dark Age Bodies*, 218.

## Chapter 6

1. On astronomical phenomena that year, see Ashley, "What Did Louis the Pious See."

2. Astronomer, *Vita Hludowici* 3.58, ed. Tremp, 518–24.

3. Astronomer, *Vita Hludowici* 3.62, ed. Tremp, 540. More astronomical omens accompany Louis's death.

4. But see Booker, *Past Convictions*, 293n129, on the Astronomer's interest in medicine (and possible identity as Walafrid).

5. On astronomy's importance within medicine in the late Middle Ages, see French, "Astrology in Medical Practice."

6. On practical vs. theoretical medicine, see Riddle, "Theory and Practice."

7. In an otherwise nuanced summary, Horden, "Medieval Medicine," 51, states that the early Middle Ages "presents too fragmented and confusing a picture for historians to find much sense in it. . . . The theory, Galenic or other, has been drained out of the surviving medical texts. . . . Instead, all is mutability." The Hippocratic Corpus, too, presents numerous inconsistencies and contradictions; these do not render it incoherent but merely reflective of ongoing debate.

8. Usually found as some variation on *Epistula Ypocratis ad regem Antiochum/Antigonum/Antigonem* (sometimes *et Antonium*). Beccaria, *I codici*, 463, lists twenty-four copies in pre-Salernitan manuscripts; Opsomer and Halleux, "La lettre d'Hippocrate," 345–46, list fifteen from the ninth century.

9. And in world chronicles like that in Bede's *DTR*.

10. For example, Paris, BnF lat. 11218.

11. The Greek text is from Diocles of Carystus to one Antigonus: on the author, recipient, and transmission of the letter (it survives in Paul of Aegina's work), see van der Eijk, *Diocles of Carystus*, 2:352–60. On the Latin letter's complex transmission history, which includes multiple recensions and translations (probably themselves based on different Greek versions) and intersects with the history of the *Epistula ad Maecenatem* (which derived from the same source), see Opsomer and Halleux, "La lettre d'Hippocrate"; Fischer, "Diokles von Karystos," 345–51; *BTML*, 96–100. Marcellus contains the earliest Latin witness in *De medicamentis*, ed. Niedermann, 1:18–24.

12. Bede, *DTR* 30, ed. Jones, 372–74; this version has similarities to Paul of Aegina's Greek text: Fischer, "Diokles von Karystos," 351. On the *DTR*'s reception, see Westgard, "Bede and the Continent," 206–10.

13. Here, the version in Uppsala, Universitetsbiblioteket C. 664 (*s*.IX$^{1}$) and St. Gall, SB 44 (*s*.IX$^{2}$), edited by Nelson, "Zur pseudohippokratischen *Epistula*," 203–17, at 213. Cf. Marcellus, *De medicamentis*, ed. Niedermann, 1:18; Stadler's edition (based on a manuscript from ca. 1300), "Epistola Pseudohippocratis," 21.

14. *Epistula ad Antiochum*, ed. Nelson, 213.

15. *Epistula ad Antiochum*, ed. Nelson, 214.

16. *Epistula ad Antiochum*, ed. Nelson, 214.

17. Sometimes compilers extended the *Epistula ad Antiochum* to cover other organs: see St. Gall, SB 44, pp. 217–18.

18. *Tereoperica*, ed. López Figueroa, "Estudio," 179–81. On the text, see López Figueroa, "From Cassius Felix," 383–401.

19. Alcuin, *DVV* 30, col. 634B–C.

20. On favoring practical information, see Phelen, "New Insights," 72, who argues that Hrabanus's *De institutione clericorum* "ignored most of Augustine's meta-argument while lifting out concrete advice."

21. But contrast the concern about inconsistencies among different penitentials: Meens, *Penance*, 114–18.

22. Here, the version in Nelson, "Zur pseudohippokratischen *Epistula*." Marcellus divides the year into five and names more "humors" (*umor, fleuma, fel, acres biles, sanguis*); Bede divides the year into quarters (circa ninety days) but does not assign only one humor to each (cf. *DTR* 35, ed. Jones, 392–93). On Bede's agenda, see Wallis, *Reckoning of Time*, 312–21.

23. *Epistula ad Antiochum*, ed. Nelson, 215. The versions edited by Stadler and Nelson never advocate sex, but those in Bede and Marcellus do. On similar excisions for reasons of Christian morality in the Latin *Diseases of Women I*, see Mazzini, "Christianesimo e scienza pagana," 75–77.

24. On the theory of contraries, see Kaye, *History of Balance*, 141–47.

25. St. Gall, SB 878, pp. 327–31; St. Gall SB 265, pp. 93–97 (*s*.IX$^{2/3}$); on the latter, see *Codici* 132; *Katalog* 3.5707.

26. On the letter's translation of Greek (Hippocratic) teachings for a Latin audience, see Zurli, "L'epistola a Pentadio," 458–62; Jouanna, *Greek Medicine*, 357–59, doubts Vindicianus's authorship; cf. Stok, "Fonte e datazione." Jouanna, "Théorie des quatre humeurs," argues that the text is a translation of a Greek original (attributed to Hippocrates), different versions of which also appear in the *Epistula ad Maecenatem* (group C) and Pseudo-Soranus *Isagoge*.

27. Vindicianus, *Epistula ad Pentadium*, ed. Rose, *Theodori Prisciani*, 485–86.

28. The organs are the liver, spleen, head, heart, and bladder: Vindicianus, *Epistula ad Pentadium*, ed. Rose, 486.

29. Vindicianus, *Epistula ad Pentadium*, ed. Rose, 487 (on *respiratio* here, see Jouanna, *Greek Medicine*, 350n44).

30. Vindicianus, *Epistula ad Pentadium*, ed. Rose, 486–87.

31. Vindicianus, *Epistula ad Pentadium*, ed. Rose, 488–89. On the temperaments, see Jouanna, "Théorie des quatre humeurs"; Klibansky et al., *Saturn and Melancholy*, 12–15, 55–66.

32. On the gradual systematization of fourfold humoral thinking, see Schöner, *Das Viererschema*, 92–103.

33. Vindicianus mentions that heat rules the upper parts of body and cold the lower, but this division is not correlated with gender. Soranus of Ephesus (who rejected the humors and qualities) dominated early medieval Latin gynecological material: Green, "Transmission," 25–34, 172–73, 315–17. On "complexion" in later medieval thought, see Cadden, *Meanings of Sex Difference*; Siraisi, *Medieval & Early Renaissance Medicine*, 101–6.

34. Vindicianus, *Epistula ad Pentadium*, ed. Rose, 490.

35. Vindicianus, *Epistula ad Pentadium*, ed. Rose, 489–90.

36. Schöner, *Viererschema*; Stewart, *Galen's Theory*, 1–26; Temkin, *Galenism*; King, "Female Fluids," 23–33; Siegel, *Galen's System*, 196–241.

37. By equating blood with a perfect mixture of the four elements (rather than with air, as later), Galen resisted a complete fourfold systematization: Jouanna, *Greek Medicine*, 335–59.

38. The latest date for the Latin translation is the early eighth century, when a version of the text appears in Bede's *DTR* 35, ed. Jones, 392–93: Jouanna, "Théorie des quatre humeurs," 167–68.

39. Paris, BnF lat. 11219 (see Chapter 5); inconsistencies remain at f. 15v: "quadrifida corporis elementa hoc est fel sanguis et humor," where a later hand has written "flegma" above the line. Not all texts in Carolingian manuscripts speak exclusively of the same four humors, but the scheme clearly dominated. On such inconsistencies in ancient texts, see King, "Female Fluids," 30.

40. *De arte prolixa* (which begins a commentary on the *Aphorisms*) in London, BL Arundel 166 (*s*.IX$^{1/3}$), ff. 82v–83r: "In principio creavit deus celum et terram. Extra autem homo factus est et pro quo omnia facta sunt. Igitur ex iiii elementis dicitur constare mundus ex igni, aqua, terra, vento et aere." On the text and manuscript, see Kibre, *Hippocrates Latinus*, 29–34, 153; *Katalog* 2.2412; *Codici* 83. At f. 88v, one finds a copy (lacking a title) of the *Epistula ad Antiochum*.

41. Compare with Isidore, *Etymologiae* 4.5.7 and the *Liber Aurelii*, ed. Daremberg, "*De acutis passionibus*," 479.

42. Wlaschky, "*Sapientia artis medicinae*," 103–13, at 104 (based on St. Gall, SB 44, pp. 187–91; Glasgow, UL Hunter 96, ff. 53r–54v; St. Gall, SB 751, pp. 446–47, 453–55, where it is entitled *Epistula prima Ypogratis*). See also Paris, BnF lat. 11219, noted above.

43. Wlaschky, "*Sapientia artis medicinae*," 111–13.

44. On the First Bible of Charles the Bald (produced 845 at Tours), see Dutton and Kessler, *Poetry and Paintings*, esp. 62–65, 89, 94. On intersections between *Maiestas Domini* illuminations and scientific diagrams, see Kühnel, *End of Time*.

45. Dhuoda, *LM* 1.5, ed. Riché, 104–6; trans. Neel, 10 (referencing Isidore, *Liber numerorum* 5, PL 83, cols. 183B–184A).

46. Barcelona, Biblioteca di Catalunya 569 (*s*.XIV). On this codex, see Riché, *Manuel*, 45–50; Vernet, "Un nouveau manuscrit."

47. Chandler, "Barcelona BC 569."

48. Here, named the *Expositio computus de divisionibus temporum* (Barcelona 569, ff. 24r–56v) and attributed to Bede but drawn from the *Sententiae in laude compoti*: see Chandler, "Barcelona BC 569," 273; Cordoliani, "Une encyclopédie carolingienne," 237–43.

49. On *computus*, calculation, and numerology as one of Dhuoda's four main concerns, see Garver, *Women*, 153–58.

50. On the poetic (vs. practical) nature of computus, see Wallis, "Images of Order."

51. Wallis, *Reckoning of Time*, 264–66; McCluskey, "Natural Knowledge"; Borst, *Ordering of Time*, 33–41; Kühnel, *End of Time*, 87–101.

52. Bede *DTR* 71, ed. Jones, 544; trans. Wallis, 249 (discussed at lxxi).

53. Bede, *DTR* 70, ed. Jones, 540.

54. Ramírez-Weaver, *Saving Science*, 5–11, 29–37, at 69.

55. See Borst, *Der Streit*; Borst, *Die karolingische Kalenderreform*. Cf. Palmer, "Calculating Time." *Admonitio generalis* 70, ed. Mordek, 224; *Capitulare missorum in Theodonis villa datum primum* 6, ed. Boretius, Capit. 1, 121; *Quae a presbyteris discenda sint* 8, ed. Boretius, Capit. 1, 235.

56. Wallis, "Bede and Science."

57. Eastwood, *Ordering the Heavens*; Ramírez-Weaver, *Saving Science*; Stevens, *Cycles of Time*; Dutton, *Charlemagne's Mustache*, 93–127.

58. On Corbie's translation of the *Aratus Latinus* (first ca. 735 and then revised ca. 790), see Le Bourdellès, *L'Aratus Latinus*, 251–63; Ramírez-Weaver, *Saving Science*, 50, 74–75, 169–75.

59. Einhard, *Vita Karoli* 25, ed. Holder-Egger, 30; trans. Dutton, *Charlemagne's Courtier*, 32.

60. Lohrmann, "Alcuins Korrespondenz"; Dutton, *Charlemagne's Mustache*, 98–102; Kühnel, *End of Time*, 102–10.

61. Ramírez-Weaver, *Saving Science*, 145–56; Eastwood, *Ordering the Heavens*, 27–28, 373–425.

62. Eastwood, *Ordering the Heavens*, esp. 3–15, 180–89; Ramírez-Weaver, *Saving Science*, esp. 195–225; McCluskey, *Astronomies and Cultures*, 114–64.

63. *Capitulare missorum in Theodonis villa datum primum* 6–7, ed. Boretius, Capit. 1, 121. On the expansion of computus, see Wallis, "Medicine in Medieval Calendar Manuscripts."

64. On dividing the solar cycle into four calendar "seasons," see Eastwood, *Ordering the Heavens*, 128–39, 276–82, 333–72. Wallis, *Reckoning of Time*, 319–21, notes that Bede's discourse on the number four is found at the midpoint of the *DTR* (which included the letters to Antiochus and Pentadius).

65. Only fragments of a Latin translation of the Hippocratic *On the Nature of Man* survive from the early medieval West (e.g., Paris, BnF lat. 7027): Mazzini, "*De natura humana.*"

66. Coon, *Dark Age Bodies*, 21–23, 217–46. See also Kitzinger, *Cross*, 27–39; Chazelle, *Crucified God*, 99–118.

67. The quadripartite divisions in Hrabanus resemble those in Pentadius. On the cross in early medieval scientific diagrams, see Kühnel, "Carolingian Diagrams."

68. Hrabanus, *In honorem sanctae crucis* C7, ed. Perrin, 71. For Jerome's rumination on the sacredness of the number four, see Darby, "Codex Amiatinus," 367–68.

69. Alcuin, Ep. 145, ed. Dümmler, 233; cited by Dutton, *Charlemagne's Mustache*, 98.

70. On Charlemagne's wisdom in discerning these patterns, see Alcuin, Ep. 148, ed. Dümmler, 238–39. Ramírez-Weaver, *Saving Science*, 27, on astronomy as seizing the "Adamic mantle" of dominion over the cosmos.

71. Lupus, Ep. 30, ed. Dümmler, 37; trans. Regenos, 96.

72. Such diagrams (*rotae*) were composed by Isidore himself: Obrist, "Le diagramme isidorien"; Kühnel, "Carolingian Diagrams," 363–68.

73. On prognostics, see Liuzza, *Anglo-Saxon Prognostics*; Chardonnens, *Anglo-Saxon Prognostics*; van Rhijn, "Pastoral Care," and forthcoming research from her project "Prognostic Thinking (750–1000): Texts, Manuscripts, Global Connections." Chardonnens, 8, defines a prognostic as: "A codified means of predicting events in the life-time of an individual or identifiable group of individuals, using observation of signs and times, or mantic divination." Liuzza, 59–77, argues for a discrete "prognostic" genre by the eleventh century.

74. See also Galen's *De diebus decretoriis* (*On critical days*).

75. Some migrated from a medical to a computistical context. On circulation, see Liuzza, *Anglo-Saxon Prognostics*, 71; Chardonnens, *Anglo-Saxon Prognostics*, 142–57.

76. Chardonnens, *Anglo-Saxon Prognostics*, 8–15, sorts prognostics into descriptive, proscriptive, or prescriptive.

77. See also weather prediction, as in Juste and Chiu, "*De tonitruis* attributed to Bede," 110–24.

78. On Egyptian Days, see Chardonnens, *Anglo-Saxon Prognostics*, 271–80, 330–58; Steele, "*Dies Aegyptiaci.*"

79. St. Gall, SB 752 (*s.*IX$^{ex}$), at 82 (*Medicina Plinii* at pp. 6–80). On such diagrams, see Wickersheimer, "Figures médico-astrologiques." On the manuscript, see *Codici* 134.

80. St. Gall, SB 752, p. 82, ed. Sigerist, "Sphere," 294. The Sphere of Apuleius originally derived from a Greek model: Chardonnens, *Anglo-Saxon Prognostics*, 182–83.

81. St. Gall, SB 751 (*s.*IX$^{med}$), pp. 165–67.

82. The translated text purportedly came from unearthed ivory tablets written by Democritus and then buried: see Sudhoff, "Die pseudohippokratische Krankheitsprognostik," 86, 89–104; Sigerist, "Die *Prognostica Democriti*," 157–59.

83. A partial translation of the *Prognostica* is found in St. Gall, SB 44; no complete Latin translation survives before the late ninth century; see Sigerist, "Fragment," 87–90; Paxton, "*Signa Mortifera*," 632–34.

84. St. Gall, SB 751, p. 166: "[*post corr.*] Si sub lingua papula apparuerit sicut est peduculum porcinum et labacrum labare desideraverit in initia passionis ipsius morietur." *Lunaria* often give an exact number of days within which recovery/death will occur.

85. Unlike other manuscripts, St. Gall, SB 751, compares the pustule not to a lentil but to a louse.

86. On *lunaria*, see Weißer, *Krankheitslunar.*

87. St. Gall, SB 751, p. 176: "Luna xviii, tarde convalescit." *Lunaria* freely mix present and future tense, but I stick with the latter. The codex contains several *lunaria*: Weißer, *Krankheitslunar*, 57–58.

88. On this remedy, see Pseudo-Bede, *De minutione sanguinis*, ed. Giles, 350.

89. St. Gall, SB 751, pp. 376–77. Dates listed varied, but the basic idea was that one could not undertake certain tasks because God had cursed these days.

90. See Laux, "*Ars medicinae*," 432. St. Gall, SB 751, pp. 175–76, contains a *lunare* for bloodletting immediately followed by two *lunaria* for illness.

91. With the example of a Montecassino manuscript, see Wallis, "Signs and Senses."

92. Van Rhijn, "Pastoral Care," esp. 275–78; cf. Flint, *Rise of Magic*, 88–142; Chardonnens, *Anglo-Saxon Prognostics*, 103–6, 131–38.

93. The same manuscript might hold prescriptions against prognosticating and prognostic texts: van Rhijn, "Pastoral Care," 284–88, 294–97.

94. Gerbald of Liège, *Zweites Kapitular* 10, ed. Brommer, Capit. episc. 1, 29; Hrabanus, *De magicis artibus*, cols. 1095A–1109A; Augustine, *Enchiridion de fide, spe et caritate* 21.79 ed. Evans, 93; Augustine, *Expositio epistolae ad Galatas* 34–35, ed. Divjak, 102–4.

95. See Wallis, "Signs and Senses," on both diagnosis and prognosis as fortunetelling.

96. Augustine, Ep. 55, 12–15, ed. Goldbacher, *Epistulae II*, 182–86.

97. Gerbald of Liège, above. Consider, too, that Democritus was named as a magician in Isidore, *Etymologiae* 8.9.2. On hesitancy with astrological predictions, see Dutton, *Charlemagne's Mustache*, 108–11.

98. Dutton, *Charlemagne's Mustache*, 103.

99. Bede, *DTR* 28, ed. Jones, 364–66; Pseudo-Bede, *De minutione sanguinis*, ed. Giles, 350.

100. As Wallis observes with computus manuscripts: "Images of Order," 57–62.

101. Wallis, "Medicine in Medieval Calendar Manuscripts," 116–17; McCluskey, *Astronomies and Cultures*, 97–113.

102. Van Rhijn, "Pastoral Care," 296–97.

103. See Vatican, BAV Pal. lat. 485; Vatican, BAV Pal. lat. 1449; El Escorial, Real Biblioteca di San Lorenzo, L III 8. On these, van Rhijn, "Pastoral Care," 291–96; Paxton, "*Bonus liber.*"

104. Liuzza, *Anglo-Saxon Prognostics*, 60.

105. Berlin, Staatsbibliothek, Phillipps 1790, f. 39v. Consisting of various units by different hands, the manuscript has been dated from the early to the later ninth century: *Katalog* 1.429; *Codici* 50. On its prognostics, see van Rhijn, "Pastoral Care," 289–91. Each of the six parts of nature is associated with a part of the person (e.g., the ocean as blood). *Vita Adae et Evae* (here, ch. 55.1), electronic edition by Anderson and Stone at http://www2.iath.virginia.edu/anderson/vita/vita.html (accessed July 2021).

106. Canon 6, ed. Hartmann, "Unbekannte Kanones," 44–45; noted by Filotas, *Pagan Survivals*, 139.

107. On the regulation of excretion, see Tuten, "*Necessitas naturae.*"

108. For an attempt to merge liturgical and medical time, see the text in Tironian notes ascribed to one *Marcus medicus*, which links the two solstices and two equinoxes to events in Christ's life and to the four humors with their four qualities: Bern, Burgerbibliothek 109, f. 136v (*s*.IX$^{3/4}$). For the intriguing suggestion that Marcus was an Irish monk at Saint-Médard de Soissons, who was known to Heiric of Auxerre, the possible author of the Tironian excerpts and marginalia in Bern 109, see Contreni, "What Was Emperor Augustus," 385–86.

109. Paxton, "*Signa Mortifera*."

110. On Paris, BnF lat. 11218, f. 100v: Paxton, "*Signa Mortifera*," 646, who notes a unique reference to the dissolution of the body and soul here.

111. On the Carolingians' lack of concern with variety (even in the case of baptismal treatises), see Keefe, *Water and the Word*, esp. 38, 132.

112. *Lunaria* functioned by determining the day on which the sufferer *decumbit* (lies down or falls sick); given the difficulty (even with modern technology) of determining when an illness "begins," we can surely envision a malleable method of "reading" a prognostic, so as to inspire hope in the patient.

113. This is assuming twenty-four Egyptian Days, but there were also sets of three and twelve. Phlebotomy was also forbidden during the Dog Days (the hottest days of summer, associated with the appearance of Sirius, usually from mid-July to early September).

114. Dietary texts are often found alongside prognostics but are not usually predictive. On the development of the dietary calendar as isolated text in the early Middle Ages, see Pucci Donati, *Dieta*, 73–111.

115. Groenke, "Monatskalendarien," identifies four versions in ninth-century manuscripts; cf. Fischer, "Gesund durchs Jahr."

116. Groenke's Calendar VII is the exception, running from May through April. Wallis, "Medicine in Medieval Calendars Manuscripts," 112–15, argues for a shift from seasonal to monthly calendars between Late Antiquity and the early Middle Ages; cf. Chardonnens, *Anglo-Saxon Prognostics*, 471–73.

117. Vatican, BAV Pal. lat. 1088 (*s*.IX$^{med}$), f. 60v: "Ad cibum et potionem quos per singulos menses usitare oportet" (on the manuscript, possibly produced around Lyon, see *Codici* 103; *Katalog* 3.6574). London, BL Arundel 166, f. 67v: "Ratio per quisque mense quod observare debemus." Paris, BnF lat. 11218, f. 56v: "Hic est virtus de duodicem mensibus quod observandum est propter sanitatis corporum quale observacione debeant habere."

118. Byzantine calendars mentioned bathing and anointing, but Latin ones focused on bloodletting and purging: Groenke, "Monatskalendarien," 273–76.

119. *LAB*, f. 8r, ed. Stoll, 76. See, Groenke, "Monatskalendarien," 158. On spices mentioned, see McCormick, *Origins*, 711–16.

120. Groenke, "Monatskalendarien," 136–38.

121. For example, in June drink cold water: Groenke, "Monatskalendarien," 104–6.

122. This is especially true in Calendar I: see Groenke, "Monatskalendarien," 98, 102, 106, 108.

123. Discussed further in the Conclusion.

124. It should be noted, however, that the cost of substances like cinnamon, pepper, and cloves would have precluded their use by any but the wealthy.

125. On this understanding of nature, see McCluskey, "Natural Knowledge," 290–92.

126. Dendle, "Plants," 49.

127. Dutton, *Charlemagne's Mustache*, 103.

128. On Eriugena's belief that nature was "habitually uncustomary," see Kreiner, *Legions of Pigs*, 67. On scholastic perceptions of nature, see Bartlett, *The Natural*, 1–17.

129. Conceptualizing medical treatments as luxurious may seem counterintuitive, but this refers to how they could soothe, energize, and pamper the body (e.g., on bathing and *luxuria*: Coon, *Dark Age Bodies*, 125, 201).

130. Pseudo-Bede, *De minutione sanguinis*, ed. Giles, 349: "Omni tempore, die ac nocte si necessitas urget, in acutis passionibus, oportet phlebotomiam adhibere." On extant witnesses, see Voigts and McVaugh, "Latin Technical Phlebotomy," 2. It survives in Brussels, BR 3701-15, f. 11v, and London, BL Arundel 166, f. 67r. Laon, BM 426 bis, f. 118r (*s*.IX$^{ex}$) contains a modified version (without *necessitas*).

131. *LAB*, f. 3r–v, ed. Stoll, 56.

132. *LAB*, f. 2v, ed. Stoll, 52.

133. *LAB*, f. 4r, ed. Stoll, 58.

134. Hildemar, *Expositio regulae*, 36, ed. Mittermüller, 415–16. For the Latin parallels, see Chapter 4.

135. Mk 2:26–27. See also 4 Mc 5:13.

136. Bede, *In Marcum* 1.2.27, ed. Hurst, 464.

137. Bede, *Expositio Apocalypseos* 1.9, ed. Gryson, 317; trans. Wallis, *Commentary on Revelation*, 152–53. Bede's source (and possible the Lorsch author's too) was Primasius's sixth-century commentary.

138. See, for example, *Paenitentiale Theodori, Discipulus Umbrensium* 6.2, 7.6, ed. Finsterwalder, *Die Canones*, 297, 299; *Paenitentiale Excarpsus Cummeani* 3.14, 7.5, 13.20, 13.32, ed. Schmitz, *Die Bussbücher*, 606, 621, 633, 635; Halitgar, *Paenitentiale Pseudo-Romanum*, nos. 24, 44, 89, ed. Schmitz, *Die Bussbücher*, 295, 297, 299. On these penitentials, see Meens, *Penance*, 58, 90–96, 108–10, 130–39.

139. *Capitulatio de partibus Saxoniae* 4, ed. Boretius, Capit. 1, 68. See also *Admonitio generalis* (789) 48, ed. Mordek et al., 204: "Omnibus. Item in eodem, ut ecclesiastica ieiunia sine necessitate rationabili non solvantur."

140. The language of *necessitas* and *periculum* may be drawn from a letter by Pope Leo I on the provision of penance, which was cited by the Council of Metz in 859: *Metz* 10, ed. Hartmann, Conc. 3, 442: "qui in tempore necessitatis et in periculi urgentis instantia praesidium poenitentiae et mox reconciliationis implorant, nec satisfactio interdicenda est." See Roumy, "L'origine et la diffusion."

141. Heito, *Capitula ecclesiastica* 7, ed. Boretius, Capit. 1, 363.

142. See Roumy, "L'origine et la diffusion," 303–4.

143. On the legal notion of a state of exception (with brief reference to the role of necessity), see Agamben, *State of Exception*, esp. 24–26.

144. See Oribasius, *Synopsis* 1.11, ed. Mørland, in *Oribasius Latinus*, 49; ed. Bussemaker and Daremberg, in *Oeuvres*, 5:813 (drawing on Galen, *De curandi ratione per venae sectionem*). Thanks to Cloudy Fischer for the link between Oribasius and Pseudo-Bede.

145. In addition to the abovementioned pseudo-Bede *De minutione sanguinis*, see St. Gall, SB 217, p. 255, ed. Köpp, *Vademecum*, 27: "Omni tempore, diae et nocte, si necessitas fuaerit, fleuotomandus est."

146. "*Sapientia artis medicinae*," ed. Wlaschky, 106.

147. Unique to Brussels, BR 3701-15, f. 12r: "Redimitur anima per detractionem sanguis veniente occurrere morbo, necessitas tempus non expectat." Edited and discussed by Wiedemann, "Untersuchungen," 148–49, 189–203. Compare *Quid per singulos menses flevotomia*, in Paris, BnF lat. 11219, f. 35v: "Reliquis mensibus nisi fortis necessitas exierit, non est tempus flevotomia. Nam si necessitas fuerit, nec diem nec tempus nec horam flevotomi non expectat praeces."

148. Cf. Bourbon, "Necessity and Timeliness," which argues that in the Hippocratic gynecological treatises necessity stands for the unavoidability of a sequence of pathological reactions.

149. Though likely practiced prior to its first documentation in 816: Yearl, "Time of Bloodletting," 114–21.

150. *Synodi primae Aquisgranensis decreta authentica* 10, ed. Semmler, in *Initia consuetudinis*, 459–60. The Murbach statutes (816) elaborated on the type of food to be given after bloodletting, and the statutes of Corbie (prior to 826) noted that reading was to be carried out for those being let: Adalhard, *Consuetudines Corbeienses* 33 and *Statuta Murbacensia* 12, ed. Semmler, in *Initia consuetudinis*, 413, 445–46.

151. On the later development, see Yearl, "Bloodletting as Recreation."

152. See Nightingale, *Once Out of Nature*, 47–48, 188–96.

153. See also the dietary text by Anthimus (discussed in Chapter 7), in which certain types of meat are forbidden except "si necessitas exegerit": *DOC* Prologus, ed. Liechtenhan, 2.

154. Smaragdus, *Expositio* 36.9, ed. Spannagel and Engelbert, 250 (citing Augustine's *Regula ad servos Dei*).

155. *Epistula Arsenii ad Nepotianum*, in Paris, BnF lat. 11219, f. 15r: "intrinseca sentitor, dicitur salutaris praeceptor vel liberator artifex oportunus, quis ad necessitatem praeliator."

156. St. Gall, SB 751, p. 339: "intrinsecus sentitur dicitur medicus salutaris praeceptor vel liberator artifex oportunus qui a necessitate liberat." See the variation in Brussels, BR 3701-15, f. 5v: "intrinseca sentitur dicitur medicus salutaris praeceptor vel liberator artifex oportunus qui ad necessitatem subveniat."

157. Ps 106:19 and Bar 6:36. See also the Old Gelasian Sacramentary, *Liber Sacramentorum Romanae ecclesiae* no. 1382, ed. Mohlberg et al., 201: "Exaudi, domine, praeces nostras . . . ita te fontem pietatis agnoscimus, a quo et a peccatis nostris nos ablue et a necessitatibus liberari confidemus."

158. On Walafrid's career, see Booker, "New Prologue," 83–86; Stevens, "Walahfrid Strabo"; Fees, "War Walahfrid Strabo" (who argues that Walafrid was *not* Charles's tutor).

159. St. Gall, SB 878 (with medical texts interspersed from pp. 327–93). Bischoff argues for texts copied by Walafrid himself (at different points in his life) and by at least ten other scribes: "Eine Sammelhandschrift Walahfrid Strabos (Cod. Sangall. 878)," in *MS*, 2:34–51. Cf. Schmidt, "Karolingische Autographen."

160. On Walafrid's interest in natural science and computus, see Stevens, "Computus-Handschriften"; Corradini, "Rhetoric of Crisis," 313–21.

161. There are two versions of the *Epistula ad Antiochum* at pp. 327–31 and 374–76 (this from Bede's *DTR*); the first bears the same (atypical) title to Paris, BnF lat. 11219, f. 41r (*Epistola Ypocratis ad Antiocum et Antonium*), but the text itself is not similar.

162. For the liberal arts, see Alcuin's *Disputatio de vera philosophia*, copied at pp. 322–23, 340–44.

163. St. Gall, SB 878, p. 332: "Medicorum scientia mortalibus utilissima est . . . Scientia curationum quae pigmentorum herbarumque vim et lignorum sucos atque paene omnium rerum naturas ad temperamentum corporis vel salutem sollicite perquirit."

164. The use of this definition (as discussed in Chapter 4) suggests ties to Alcuin, whose *De vera philosophia*, letter on Lenten fasting (pp. 335–39), and name (p. 277) appear in the *vademecum*. Note that Alcuin's own *Disputatio Pippini* 10–64, ed. Orchard, 181–90, moves from discussing the body to the natural world.

165. From this perspective, Walafrid's *De cultura hortorum*, was the perfect pairing to the *vademecum* because there he *did* offer remedies (focusing on ailments causing pain of the head, chest, stomach, and bladder—the exact four bodily divisions in the *Epistula ad Antiochum*).

## Chapter 7

Epigraph: St. Gall, SB 878, p. 335: "Sensus corporis equi, anima auriga / Corpus puer, anima pedagogus / Animae imperio, corporis servitio magis utimur / Luxoriora res vinum et contumeliosa ebrietas, omnis quicumque his miscetur non erit sapiens / Sapientiae operam dare non possumus si mensae abundantiam cogitemus." For the first three lines, see Sallust, *Bellum Catilinae* 1.2, trans. Ramsey and Rolfe, 20–21. For the fourth line, see Prv 20:1.

1. These five aphorisms appear in the same order in Jerome, *Adversus Jovinianum* 2.10–11, cols. 312C–314B, alongside many of the themes discussed in this chapter (dietary regimens, moderation, the danger of plethora).

2. See Agnellus of Ravenna, *Lectures* 1, ed. Westerink, 2: "[Ars medicinae] sanitatem enim operari et conseruare promittit et exercere corpori; per quam . . . omnia meditatio et disciplina procedit et ipse animae operationes."

3. Cf. Pucci Donati, *Dieta*, 70, who finds no link between ethics and dietetics in medical texts of the early Middle Ages and states that self-discipline was to be found only within the monastery.

4. Walafrid, *De cultura hortorum* 20, line 334, ed. Berschin, 82. The stomach is the most prominent organ mentioned in the poem.

5. Quintus Serenus, *Liber medicinalis* 17, line 300, ed. Vollmer, 17.

6. *Epitome altera*, as found in St. Gall, SB 44, p. 206: "Sthomachum autem nostrum qui dominus est totius corporis et possidet alimenta et degerit." The text is no longer accepted as Vindicianus's (Chapter 3). See also a text preserved in Paris, BnF lat. 7027 (s.IX$^{med}$), *De natura generis humani* 23, ed. Buján, "Vindiciano," 54: "Stomachus autem noster, qui dominium totius corporis possidet, ad curis uoluntate alimenta digeruntur."

7. *Epistula de ratione ventris* 4.1, ed. Scherer, 63: "totius corporis prerogator" (on *praerogator* as a distributor see Souter, *Glossary*, 317).

8. Alcuin, *Disputatio Pippini* 30, ed. Orchard, 184.

9. Found as *stomachus, venter, ventriculus*. But *stomachus* could also refer to the esophagus and *venter* to the general intestinal area. On the difficulties with Latin and Greek terminology for these organs, see Powell, *Properties of Foodstuffs*, 22–26; Paolucci, *Profilo*, 123–25.

10. *Epistula de ratione ventris vel viscerum* (sometimes *Epistula de ratione organi*), preserved in: Vatican, BAV Pal. lat. 1088; Paris, BnF lat. 11219; Glasgow, UL Hunter 404; Montecassino, Archivio dell'Abbazia 97; London, BL Add. 8928; Karlsruhe, BLB 172; St. Gall, SB 761. Edited and discussed by Scherer, "Die *Epistula de ratione ventris vel viscerum*."

11. The text places the liver on the right side of the belly, the spleen on the left.

12. *Epistula de ratione ventris* 4.1, ed. Scherer, 64.

13. This third cooking seems to take place in the liver itself, but the heat comes from the gallbladder: *Epistula de ratione ventris* 4.3, ed. Scherer, 65. For Galen, digestion occurred in the stomach, liver, and tissues, with the spleen taking the dregs of blood for removal; Galen excluded a role for the gallbladder: Stewart, *Galen's Theory*, 76–109; Powell, *Properties of Foodstuffs*, 10–18; Siegel, *Galen's System*, 216–332; Scherer, "Die *Epistula*," 94–95.

14. This fourth cooking process and its results (whether black bile is produced in isolation or with a melancholic humor) are far from clear. *Epistula de ratione ventris* 4.3, ed. Scherer, 66: "Ex quibus coleribus operante calore nigra colera nasci permittit fecesque sordide sanguinis ex epate venientis partim melancolicum faciunt humorem, partim dimittit spleni." See also Scherer's brief discussion at pp. 94–95.

15. *Epistula de ratione ventris* 3, ed. Scherer, 62.

16. On Galen's theory of fevers, see Wittern, "Die Wechselfieber"; Demaitre, *Medieval Medicine*, 35–60. See also the pseudo-Galenic *Epistula de febribus* (transmitted in several Carolingian manuscripts), with the same causative schema of fevers and humors: Flammini, "L'*Epistula*," 245.

17. The ancient system of counting malarial fevers, such that tertian fever strikes every other day (with forty-eight hours in between paroxysms) allows the text to highlight the connection between concoction and fever.

18. *Epistula de ratione ventris* 5.1, ed. Scherer, 67–71. On fevers and plethora, see Pellegrin, "L'imaginaire de la fièvre."

19. *Epistula de ratione ventris* 6.3, ed. Scherer, 71.

20. *Epistula de ratione ventris* 6.4, ed. Scherer, 72 (reading *horripilans* for *obripilans*).

21. *Epistula Anthimi viri inlustris comitis et legatarii ad gloriosissimum Theudoricum regem Francorum de observatione ciborum*, ed. Rose, *Anecdota Graeca*, 2:41–102; ed. Liechtenhan, *De observatione ciborum*. Many elements of the title vary, with only two witnesses supplying "De observatione/m ciborum" and some giving Pliny as the author or Emperor Titus as the recipient. Translations are mine but draw on those by Weber, *Anthimus: De observatio[ne] ciborum*; Grant, *On the Observance*. Paolucci, *Profilo*, offers a close textual analysis.

22. Lorsch catalogue (ca. 860): Häse, *MBKL*, Ca 419. Murbach catalogue (ca. 875): Geith and Berschin, "Die Bibliothekskataloge," 67 no. 38. Walafrid: St. Gall, SB 878, pp. 352–65. Anthimus's text survives in eight full and five partial witnesses (including four full and two partial from the ninth century, and one copy of a ninth-century exemplar).

23. *LAB*, ff. 72r–75r, ed. Stoll, 392–406. St. Gall, SB 762 (*s*.IX$^{1/4}$), pp. 217–60; see *Codici* 137; *Katalog* 3.5848. Paris, BnF nouv. acq. lat. 229 (*s*.XII), f. 1v: toward the end of the preface is the insertion "o rex gloriose et invicte auguste Karole."

24. Rose, *Anecdota Graeca*, 2:44–52, first proposed this narrative based on the brief mention of a doctor Anthimus in a history of the fifth-century Byzantine Empire by Malchus of Philadelphia. Rose and others assume Anthimus became Theodoric's courtier based on his title *legatarius*. If this Anthimus was the author, the treatise dates to the Merovingian Theuderic I (r. 511–533); if not, it might be Theuderic II, III, or IV. Much hinges on the words *legatarii ad Theudoricum regem*, but given other epistolary titles (*Epistula Hippocratis ad Antiochum regem*, *Epistula Vindiciani ad Pentadium*), *legatarius* should not necessarily be read with *ad Theodoricum*.

25. See Anthimus, *DOC* 64, ed. Liechtenhan, 24: "quod nos Graeci dicimus alfita, Latine uero polenta, Gothi uero barbarice fenea." His slight derision toward the Goths militates

against his being Theodoric of Italy's legate. The name Anthimus was widespread among medical families of the Byzantine Empire: Paolucci, *Profilo*, 10.

26. Hen accepts Anthimus's identity but as a *legatarius* for the Byzantine Emperor Anastasius, not Theodoric of Italy: "Food and Drink," 102–3.

27. On *legatarius*, see Gillett, *Envoys*, 244, 265–66, who finds it in Frankish-Byzantine correspondence in the 540s–580s and, by the seventh century, interchangeable with *legatus* in Frankish sources. This might better support a date during Theuderic II's reign (r. 595–613). On Anthimus's unusual Latin vocabulary, see Messing, "Remarks on Anthimus"; Paolucci, *Profilo*, 83–91, 113–26.

28. Complete copies: *LAB*; St. Gall, SB 878 (Walafrid's *vademecum*); St. Gall, SB 762 (*s*.IX$^{1/4}$, entirely medical treatises); Paris, BnF lat. 6842B (*s*.IX$^{1}$, with Palladius on agriculture and Caesar on the Gallic wars). See Liechtenhan, *DOC*, xi–xx; Rose, *Anecdota Graeca*, 2:52. Fragmentary and revised copies: *De ratione omnium ciborum*, pp. 298–301 in St. Gall SB 44 (*s*.IX$^{2}$, entirely medical treatises); *De ciborum causis*, p. 395 in St. Gall, SB 751 (*s*.IX$^{med}$, entirely medical treatises).

29. Effros, *Creating Community*, 65, sees the letter as a gift showcasing the Ostrogoths' Roman *civilitas*.

30. Anthimus does not name his sources, but they almost certainly included Galen's *De alimentorum facultatibus* and versions of Dioscorides's *De materia medica* (perhaps even in the original Greek); whether he was also familiar with Oribasius, Pliny, Celsus, and Caelius Aurelianus is not clear. See Grant, *On the Observance*, esp. 84; cf. Paolucci, *Profilo*, 23–56.

31. Anthimus, *DOC* Preface, ed. Liechtenhan, 1. On digestion in Anthimus, see Deroux, "La digestion."

32. Anthimus, *DOC* Preface, ed. Liechtenhan, 3–4.

33. Anthimus, *DOC* Preface, ed. Liechtenhan, 3. Compare Agnellus, *Lectures* 9, ed. Westerink, 41.

34. Anthimus, *DOC* Preface, ed. Liechtenhan, 2–3 (singling out cautery as an offensive remedy).

35. Anthimus, *DOC* Preface, ed. Liechtenhan, 3.

36. Part of his appeal may have been his advice for cooking while on campaign: Anthimus, *DOC* Preface, ed. Liechtenhan, 2.

37. Only a few foods (e.g., lampreys) are categorically condemned; most are allowed on occasion or in a specific preparation. On the differences between Anthimus and popular late antique recipes (e.g., his condemnation of *liquamen/garum*, a Roman staple), see Anthimus, *DOC* 9, ed. Liechtenhan, 7; Grant, *On the Observance*, 89–90, 95–96, 105, 118; Deroux, "Franks and Bacon," 520–21.

38. For *humores boni*, see Anthimus, *DOC* Preface, 23, 33, ed. Liechtenhan, 2, 12, 16.

39. Deroux, "La digestion," 413–14, on too much liquid, which might cause food to float (*supernatare*) in the stomach.

40. The one exception is bacon, which Anthimus calls a Frankish delicacy and praises as a wondrous remedy for wounds and internal putridity: Deroux, "Franks and Bacon." Papal correspondence likewise suggests the eating of raw bacon: Boniface, Ep. 87, ed. Tangl, 199; Filotas, *Pagan Survivals*, 349.

41. Einhard, *Vita Karoli* 22, ed. Holder-Egger, 27.

42. On the *DOC*'s lack of Galenic theory: Grant, *On the Observance*, 40–44.

43. See Anthimus, *DOC* 14, 25, 27, 41, 47, ed. Liechtenhan, 8, 13, 14, 18, 19. On phlegmatic people and food: *DOC* 49, 60, 61, ed. Liechtenhan, 20, 23.

44. Deroux, "La digestion," 415–16. An exception is cabbage, which should only be eaten in winter because it produces melancholy in the summer: Anthimus, *DOC* 50, ed. Liechtenhan, 20.

45. Anthimus, *DOC* 23, ed. Liechtenhan, 12. On the term *corruptilla/corruptela* in Anthimus, see Paolucci, *Profilo*, 161–62.

46. Anthimus, *DOC* Preface, ed. Liechtenhan, 3.

47. See, for example, Anthimus, *DOC* 25 and 66, ed. Liechtenhan, 14, 25.

48. Anthimus, *DOC* Preface, ed. Liechtenhan, 1 (on *carbunculus* not as a skin lesion but as an *odor fumosus*, like a burning coal, see Deroux, "La digestion," 410–11; Paolucci, *Profilo*, 113–14; on *acidiuas*, see Grant, *On the Observance*, 85).

49. Mähl, *Quadriga virtutum*, 95–125.

50. Alcuin, *Ars grammatica*, col. 850D: "philosophicum illud valet elogium: *Ne quid nimis*. DIS. Notum est, omnia nimia nocere." *Omnia nimia nocere* is, to my knowledge, only found in Alcuin and Anthimus. For *ne quid nimis*, see also *Regula Benedicti* 64, ed. Venarde, 208; Alcuin, *Disputatio de rhetorica* 43, ed. Howell, 144; Paschasius, *Epitaphium Arsenii* 1.2 and 1.11, ed. Dümmler, 24 and 39; Astronomer, *Vita Hludowici* Prologue, ed. Tremp, 282.

51. On this interpretation of Genesis, see Hill, "Ooze of Gluttony."

52. Paulinus, *LE* 14 and 60, cols. 208C (borrowing from Pomerius's *De vita contemplativa*) and 269A.

53. See Alcuin's definition of fornication not as sex but as *omnis corporalis immunditia* (*DVV*, col. 633D). On marriage in the manuals, see Toubert, "La théorie du mariage"; Heene, *Legacy of Paradise*; cf. Stone, *Morality*, 285–89, 298–300.

54. For this reason, Duval says it is not a lay mirror: "Paulin d'Aquilée," 143–45. But this presupposes that marriage was seen as the most problematic aspect of the lay condition.

55. Paulinus, *LE* 36, cols. 234A–235A.

56. On the "Galenic" (reading Galen through Oribasius) monastic diets of Jerome, Paulinus of Nola, and Cassian, intended to counter the warm and wet foods that generated semen, see Rousselle, "Abstinence et continence."

57. Shaw, *Burden of the Flesh*, 80–24, 145.

58. *Admonitio ad filium* 13, ed. Lehmann, 52–54.

59. *Admonitio ad filium* 12–13, ed. Lehmann, 50–53.

60. Jonas, *DIL* 1.10, ed. Dubreucq, 1:208 (shifting from a rebuke of penitents to a general discussion of dietary habits, drawing on Pomerius).

61. Alcuin, *DVV* 28, col. 633C (associating gluttony with lust at col. 633D).

62. To my knowledge, Alcuin's source has not been identified: *DVV* 28, col. 633C.

63. Jonas, *DIL* 3.6, ed. Dubreucq, 2:232.

64. *Regula Benedicti* 39, ed. and trans. Venarde, 138–39 (with slight modification).

65. Smaragdus, *Expositio* 39.9, ed. Spannagel and Engelbert, 256 (borrowing from Isidore's *Etymologiae* 20.2.9). He contrasts the fullness of the belly with the emptiness of the soul: *Expositio* 4.36, ed. Spannagel and Engelbert, 118.

66. Smaragdus, *Expositio* 39.9, ed. Spannagel and Engelbert, 256.

67. In the sixth-century *Regula Magistri* 33, ed. Vogüé, 2:180: the brothers will be *crudi* if they wake before their members have finished cooking any digested food, and the ensuing indigestion will cause spiritual torpor.

68. Smaragdus, *Expositio* 4.12, ed. Spannagel and Engelbert, 96.

69. Hildemar, *Expositio regulae* 39, ed. Mittermüller, 438.

70. Hildemar, *Expositio regulae* 39, ed. Mittermüller, 438.

71. Hildemar, *Expositio regulae* 39, ed. Mittermüller, 439–42, discusses the need to abstain from meat and fowl, unless sick, because its sweetness is a spur of the flesh (citing Cassian).

72. Hildemar, *Expositio regulae* 39, ed. Mittermüller, 438.

73. *Epistola Yppocratis de quatuor humoribus*, in Paris, BnF lat. 11219, f. 18v: "Ut Yppocratis ait, quattuor humores sunt in corpore humano . . . qui si mensuram suam non excesserint perpetua sanitas est hominibus. Si vero minuuntur aut abundent plusquam oportet aut conspissantur aut extenuentur aut excedunt naturam suam aut acerbiores fuerint aut sedes suas reliquerint et incognitum occupaverint, varias exhibent hominibus valitudines."

74. Phelan, *Formation*, 137–41; Garipzanov, *Symbolic Language*, 88–89; Mähl, *Quadriga virtutum*, 83–156.

75. See *Epistola Yppocratis de observatione temporum*, in Paris, BnF lat. 11219, f. 17v: "Nulla res melior est quam purgaturius bonus et optimus: id est talia purgare expediunt . . . Nulla res melior est quam corporis abstinentia: id est talia comedent temporibus suis."

76. *Statuta Murbacensia* 12, ed. Semmler, in *Initia consuetudinis*, 445–46. The Synods of 816–817 discussed whether monks were permitted fowl.

77. Alcuin, Ep. 144, ed. Dümmler, 228–30, states that Christians should not fast on Lenten Sundays because that day honors the resurrection; this letter followed the *Epistula ad Antiochum* in Walafrid's *vademecum*: St. Gall, SB 878, pp. 335–39. Even monks forbidden meat and fowl were allowed it on eighty-six days a year (evidenced in Corbie's annual slaughter of some 600 pigs): McKitterick, *Frankish Kingdoms*, 116.

78. Heito, *Visio Wettini* 1, ed. Dümmler, 268. Wetti experienced his vision at Reichenau in 824, Heito's text was written shortly after, and Walafrid's verse version followed three years later: Dutton, *Politics of Dreaming*, 63–66.

79. Walafrid, *Visio Wettini*, lines 189–98, ed. and trans. Traill, 45–46, 191–92.

80. *Epistula ad Antiochum*, ed. Nelson, 213–14.

81. On sexual pollution, see Stone, *Morality*, 300–304.

82. Jonas, *DIL* 2.10, ed. Dubreucq, 1:400.

83. Firey, *Contrite Heart*, 94.

84. On Hrabanus's and Claudius of Turin's commentaries on Leviticus (the only ones from the early Middle Ages), see Firey, "Letter of the Law."

85. Firey, *Contrite Heart*, 64–83, with penitential dietary canons in Appendix A. Filotas, *Pagan Survivals*, 339–56, finds over 450 different food injunctions, with three-quarters of penitentials including at least one clause.

86. On horses in Irish penitentials: see Meens, "Pollution," 14, 18; Firey, *Contrite Heart*, 239. On Jewish laws, see Gn 9:4, Lv 11 and 17.

87. Biblical precedents in Lv 22:8 and Acts 15:20, 15:29, 21:25. On Louis the German's particular concern with how dietary laws related to meat caught in the hunt, see Goldberg's discussion of two treatises: "Hunt Belongs to Man," 33–41.

88. Meens, "Pollution"; Bonnassie, "Consommation," 1040–41, emphasizes the pagan/Christian boundary; Filotas, *Pagan Survivals*, 352–56, links the taboos with missionary activity.

89. Meens, "Pollution," 9–13; Firey, *Contrite* Heart, 74–76 (noting that dietary canons appear alongside postpartum issues and handling of the dead). On the frequency of carrion

stipulations, see Bonnassie, "Consommation," 1035–39. On the Irish origins of food taboos (especially the problem of coagulated blood), see Filotas, *Pagan Survivals*, 341–43.

90. For example, *Paenitentiale Pseudo-Bedae* 22.2, ed. Wasserschleben, *Die Bussordnungen*, 270; for others, see Filotas, *Pagan Survivals*, 349n62. On penitentials associated with Bede and Egbert, see Meens, *Penance*, 96–113; Haggenmüller, *Die Überlierferung.*

91. Anthimus, *DOC* 8–9, 23–24 and 41, ed. Liechtenhan, 6–7, 12–13 and 18. The exception is older peacocks, which should be killed five or six days before being eaten.

92. Anthimus, *DOC* 85, ed. Liechtenhan, 31.

93. The same for unknowingly drinking from a well that contains a dead animal.

94. Firey, *Contrite Heart*, 76.

95. *Capitulare de villis* 24, 34, 41, 48, ed. Boretius, Capit. 1, 85–87, at 86: "cum summo nitore."

96. Beer was mentioned, but wine was the archetypal alcoholic drink.

97. See Halitgar, *Paenitentiale Pseudo-Romanum*, Prologue, ed. Schmitz, *Die Bussbücher*, 292.

98. *Concilium Moguntinense* 46, ed. Werminghoff, Conc. 2.1, 272.

99. Einhard, *Vita Karoli* 24, ed. Holder-Egger, 28–29 (following Suetonius's *De vita Caesarum*). On ritual drunkenness, see Filotas, *Pagan Survivals*, 185–90.

100. *Capitulare missorum Aquigranense primum* (810) 7, ed. Boretius, Capit. 1, 153; Nelson, "Voice of Charlemagne," 79–80. On production of wine, see Campbell, "*Capitulare de villis.*"

101. Alcuin, *Disputatio de rhetorica* 39, ed. and trans. Howell, 136–39 (with slight modification, translating *mens* as soul).

102. Alcuin, Ep. 8, ed. Dümmler, 34.

103. *De virtute vini*, in St. Gall, SB 44, pp. 279–80. This excerpt derives from a fragmentary Latin translation of Dioscorides's *De materia medica*: Ferraces Rodríguez, "Tradición indirecta." Compare with the *Diaeta Theodori* (extant from *s.*XI): Sudhoff, "*Diaeta Theodori,*" 393–94.

104. See St. Gall, SB 44, p. 220: "ideo vinum album bibimus ad sanguinem firmandum," and at 269: "Si ex percusso caput dolet, vinum ab initio prohibendum est et omnes carnes et omnes cibus fortiores."

105. Jonas, *DIL* 1.10, ed. Dubreucq, 1:210 (drawing on Pomerius's *De vita contemplativa*).

106. Paulinus, *LE* 37, col. 236A.

107. Hildemar spent his early life at Corbie before moving to Civate. Medical manuscripts associated with Corbie's library (some questionably) include: Paris, BnF nouv. acq. lat. 1619 (*s.*VIII); St. Petersburg, National Library, lat. F.v.VI. 3 (*s.*VIII$^{ex}$/IX$^{in}$); Paris, BnF lat. 12958 (*s.*IX$^{in}$); Paris, BnF lat. 13403 (*s.*IX$^{in}$); Paris, BnF lat. 6842B (*s.*IX$^{1}$); Paris, BnF lat. 13955 (*s.*IX$^{3/4}$). On these, see *CLA* 5:688, 11:1611; *Katalog* 3.4416, 3.4850, 3.4924, 3.4948; Ganz, *Corbie*, 49, 79, 152–53; Baader, "Die Anfänge," 713, 715, 716; *Codici* 23, 36, 38, 39, 145.

108. An exception is Pilsworth, *Healthcare.*

109. See Choy, *Intercessory Prayer*, 175–77, 181–83; Romig, *Perfect Man*, 71–75.

110. On the move from material text to immaterial presence, see Polanichka, "Maternity," 12–18.

111. Dhuoda, *LM*, Epigrama and Prologus, ed. Riché, 72 and 80; trans. Neel, 2 and 5.

112. The *Epistula ad Maecenatem* circulated independently and within Marcellus's *De medicamentis*. See Opsomer and Halleux, "La lettre d'Hippocrate," 341–43; *BTML*, 96–100. Cf. Sconocchia, "La lettera di Diocle."

113. *Epistula ad Maecenatem* in Marcellus, *De medicamentis*, ed. Niedermann, 1:26, 32.

114. See Wiedemann, "Untersuchungen," 23–81; Boscherini, "La dottrina medica," 1–11; Baader, "Lehrbrief und Kurztraktat."

115. Date and authorship drawn from Paris, BnF lat. 6880, f. 1r (*s*.IX$^{2/4}$, Fulda): *Marcellus vir inluster ex magno officio Theodosii sen<ioris>*. On the manuscript, see *Codici* 25; *Katalog* 3.4418. On Marcellus (not necessarily from Bordeaux), see Cilliers, "Forgery"; Stannard, "Marcellus of Bordeaux"; *BTML*, 111.

116. Baader, "Die Anfänge," 691–97; Wiedemann, "Untersuchungen," 5–55; Scherer, "Die *Epistula de ratione ventris*," 8–31.

117. Brussels, BR 3701-15, ff. 7r–8r: prefaces of Oribasius's *Synopsis* and *Ad Eunapium*. Paris, BnF lat. 11219, ff. 12r–41v: entitled *Liber epistolarum*. On medical epistles, see Weidemann, "Untersuchungen," 50–69.

118. On medical letters in the ancient world, see Langslow, "The Epistula."

119. Jonas, *DIL* Preface, ed. Dubreucq, 1:122–24. Compare with Marcellus's preface: *De medicamentis*, ed. Niedermann, 1:2–4.

120. See the Introduction.

121. Wallis, "Experience of the Book," 107.

122. Beccaria, *I codici*, 455, lists nearly twenty (full or partial) witnesses, nine from *s*.VIII$^{ex}$–X$^{in}$. The Latin translation of the *De methodo medendi ad Glauconem* was an abridged version of the Greek and circulated with a spurious third book (the *Liber tertius*): see Fischer, "Die spätlateinische Übersetzung"; Fischer, "Der pseudogalenische *Liber tertius*"; Peterson, "Galen's *Therapeutics*"; *BTML*, 85. The Galenic commentaries extant in Milan, BA G.108 inf. (*s*.IX$^{2}$) indicate that Latin translations of Galen's *De sectis*, *Ars medica*, and *De pulsibus ad Tirones* also *may* have circulated.

123. Nothing indicates that Pentadius was a physician, though he was learned in Greek.

124. On the project of condensing useful medical knowledge, see Oribasius, *Synopsis*, Preface, ed. Mørland, *Oribasius Latinus*, 29–31.

125. *Medicina Plinii*, Prologue, ed. and trans. Hunt, 14–15.

126. On the prefaces of the *Medicina Plinii*, *Herbarius* of Pseudo-Apuleius, and Marcellus's *De medicamentis*, see Buffa Giolito, "*Topoi*"; essays in Santini, Scivoletto, and Zurli, *Prefazioni*, 3 vols.

127. *Epistula de ratione ventris* 5.1 and 7.1, ed. Scherer, 68 and 74.

128. Marcellus, *De medicamentis*, Preface, ed. Niedermann, 1:2.

129. *Epistula ad Antiochum*, ed. Nelson, 216. See also Stadler, "*Epistola Pseudohippocratis*," 25.

130. St. Gall, SB 217 (*s*.IX$^{in}$); Modena, Archivio Capitolare MS O. I.11 (*s*.VIII$^{ex}$/IX$^{in}$, northern Italy, possibly Nonantola); Vatican, BAV Pal. lat. 187 (*s*.VII/VIII, northern Italy). On the latter two, see Pilsworth, *Healthcare*, 79–96; Everett, *Alphabet of Galen*, 121–23; *Codici* 93; *Katalog* 2.2796 and 3.6474; *CLA*, 1:80a–81 and 3:368.

131. On Vatican, BAV Reg. lat. 846 (*s*.IX$^{1/4}$), often ascribed to a *leges* scriptorium based in Tours, see *Codici* 105; *Katalog* 3.6736–38; Faulkner, *Law and Authority*, 195–96, 200, 228–31, 246; cf. Ubl, "Gab es das Leges-Skriptorium," esp. 52–63. The codex consists of three units (with the medical texts at the end), but these are linked by the use of Tironian notes throughout.

132. On the medical items, see Bricout, "Note sur deux laïcs," 458–61. On the wills, see Riché, "Les bibliothèques"; McKitterick, *Written Word*, 244–50.

133. On Eberhard and Gisela, see La Rocca and Provero, "The Dead"; Kershaw, "Eberhard of Friuli" (with the caution that book ownership does not indicate literacy).

134. *Recueil des chartes*, ed. Prou and Vidier, 1:66. On Theutberga: Stafford, *Queens*, 75–76, 180.

135. *Recueil des chartes*, ed. Prou and Vidier, 1:65.

136. *Cartulaire de l'abbaye de Cysoing*, ed. de Coussemaker, 3–4.

137. Cf. the certainty of Bricout, "Note sur deux laïcs."

138. The *Liber bestiarum* (remedies from animals and birds, drawn from Sextus Placitus, *Liber medicinae ex animalibus*) is found in St. Gall, SB 217, pp. 288–92, 323–32. Only one Carolingian witness of the *Physiologus* includes the exact phrase *Liber bestiarum*; three survive in manuscripts with medical writings. Thanks to Anna Dorofeeva for sharing her research.

139. Bricout, "Note sur deux laïcs," 459, proposes a two-part pseudo-Hippocratic text. I incline to a collection of prognostics and computus materials, monthly dietetic calendars, and Egyptian Days. On connections between agriculture and prognostics, see Chardonnens, "Do Anglo-Saxons Dream."

140. Taking *Lopi* as *Loxi*, the "Loxus *medicus*" mentioned as a source in the first line of the *De physiognomonia*: Bricout, "Note sur deux laïcs," 460–61; Riché, "Les bibliothèques," 100. On a date ca. 400, see André, *Traité de physiognomonie*, 31–34. On the preface, see Stok, "Il prologo."

141. On late medieval medical physiognomy, see Ziegler, "Philosophers and Physicians."

142. We also have evidence of a (likely lay) *medicus* donating a book to Reichenau (823–838), which *may* have been a medical volume: see Lehmann, *MBDS*, 238; Zettler, "Exkurs I," 268.

143. St. Gall, SB 44 consists of two codicological units, likely bound together under Abbot Grimald of Saint-Gall, 841–872. The second, medical unit (pp. 185–368, *s*.IX$^2$), written by multiple hands in a small, dense Caroline minuscule, is one of several manuscripts written in northern Italy that later made its way into northern libraries (see Old High German glosses throughout and marginalia at pp. 195, 197, 337, 340, 348). On dating, see Bischoff, "Italienische Handschriften," 178, 190; *Katalog* 3.5530; *Codici* 129; on the binding, see Autenrieth "*Medicus*," 1–4.

144. See, for example, the line added to the end of the *Epitome altera* (p. 217) and the title that follows: "Omnium autem infirmitatis origo in stomacho incidi . . . Superius diximus de caput, pectus, vente atque vissica, nunc dicimus de cetera que obmisimus et de stomacho."

145. St. Gall SB 44, p. 246: "In Christi nomine Alberici comes g<r>acia dei et do<mi>ni i<m>peratori<s>." The reading is uncertain and the end of the line is obscured by the centerfold (though the following word may read "deligatus"). On the phrase *comes gratia Dei*, see Koziol, *Begging Pardon*, 27–33, with examples as early as the late eighth century.

146. One Albrich, Count of Breisgau and Alpgau, is attested in several Alemannic charters from the middle decades of the ninth century, as identified by Borgolte, *Die Grafen Alemanniens*, 52–54. An "Alberih comes" appears in the St. Gall confraternity book: Borgolte et al., eds., *Subsidia Sangallensia I*, 118; and an "Albirich comes" and "Alberichcus comes" in the Reichenau confraternity book: *Das Verbrüderungsbuch*, ed. Autenrieth et al., 216. The marginal notation, however, is likely an Italian hand.

147. Alcuin, Ep. 224, ed. Dümmler, 367–68.

148. Alcuin, Ep. 281, ed. Dümmler, 439.

149. Karlsruhe, BLB 172 (*s*.IX$^1$, southwest Germany) consists of four units, the first three of which (at least) were joined and at Reichenau by 822 (see Lehmann, *MBDS*, 249: "De temporibus et chronica et dialectica Aristotelis liber I et dicta Sibyllae in codice I"). The fourth

unit (ff. 57–77), with medical and moral works, shares similar decorative schemes (compare the titles at f. 14v and f. 74r), which may indicate that it was added early. On the manuscript, see *Codici* 57; *Katalog* 1.1678.

150. The recipes (covering wounds, broken bones, and the preparation of nuts) may hint at a lay audience.

151. The hand that wrote the *Liber ad Gregoriam* and the two hands that copied the medical texts are distinct, but the transition is seamless and the overall appearance is similar.

152. On the dating, see Cooper, "Concord and Martyrdom," 108–11. English translation: Cooper, *Fall of the Roman Household*, 239–83. It shares a basic resemblance with the Carolingian lay manuals but does not seem to have influenced these later works.

153. Cooper, *Fall of the Roman Household*, 88, raises the possibility of female ownership. It might also have been intended for secular clergy to use in offering pastoral care to noblewomen.

154. *Liber ad Gregoriam*, in Karlsruhe, BLB 172, f. 74r: "Explicit libellum Iohannis episcopi Constantinopolitani scribtum ad Gregoria de officiis matronalibus vel quid uxor deo omnipotenti debeat quid marito."

155. On wife as household manager, see Garver, *Women*, 170–88.

156. Mistry, "'There are three reasons why *sterilitas* affects women': Thinking about Fertility in Carolingian Monasteries" (delivered at Leeds IMC, 2017). See also Horden, "What's Wrong," 12–13.

157. On such masses, see de Jong, *In Samuel's Image*, 140.

158. See Devroey, "Monastic Economics"; Choy, *Intercessory Prayer*, 115–20.

159. Coon, *Dark Age Bodies*, 165–215; de Jong, "Internal Cloisters"; Collins, *Carolingian Debate*, 67–87.

160. Debate centers on whether the plan represents an architectural schema for renovations, a reforming ideal, or a contemplative device, but, for my purposes, the plan still evinces a concern with medicine in any of these scenarios. See Horn and Born, *Plan of St. Gall*, 3 vols.; Sanderson, "Plan of St. Gall"; Jacobsen, *Der Klosterplan*; Ochsenbein and Schmuki, *Studien zum St. Galler Klosterplan II*; Coon, *Dark Age Bodies*, 165–215.

161. See the digitalized version at: http://www.stgallplan.org/en/index_plan.html (accessed July 2021). On medical care: D'Aronco, "Benedictine Rule."

162. Horn and Born, *Plan of St. Gall*, 2:175–88 and 3:52–59, with the bloodletting building described as "fleotomatis hic gustandum vel potionariis." Numerous latrines indicate the taking of purgative medicines here. On fencing, see Zettler, "Spaces for Servants."

163. Horn and Born, *Plan of St. Gall*, 3:59, but here following the digitized plan: "coquina eorundem et sanguinem minuentium."

164. For laymen as *medici*, see Zettler, "Spaces for Servants," 11; for clergy, see Pilsworth, *Healthcare*, 201. On the segregation of visitors, pilgrims, and the poor to spaces not directly linked to the main church, see Collins, *Carolingian Debate*, 76–79. On the spiritual liminality of the sick and novices, see Coon, *Dark Age Bodies*, 165–71, 205–8.

165. Horn and Born, *Plan of St. Gall*, 3:53, believe this housed serfs and workmen. In their commentaries, neither Smaragdus nor Hildemar suggest that outsiders could be treated within the monastery.

166. On these charters, see Erhart, *Lebenswelten*, 115–18.

167. Assuming that Bricout's identification is correct and that the text owned by Eberhard resembled the earliest extant witness (*s.*XII).

168. *De physiognomonia* 12, ed. André, 60.

169. *De physiognomonia* 2, ed. André, 50–51.

170. *De physiognomonia* 12, ed. André, 60.

171. Recall that Rodolphus received the *Physionomia*, his sister Judith received Alcuin's *DVV.*

172. For the term *vitia*, see *De physiognomonia* 7, 27, 29, 104, ed. André, 55, 74, 75, 127.

173. *Duplex legationis edictum* 19, ed. Boretius, Capit. 1, 63.

174. *Synodi primae Aquisgranensis* 10, *Statuta Murbacensia* 12, *Regula sancti Benedicti abbatis Anianensis* 7, ed. Semmler, *Initia consuetudinis*, 445–46, 459–60, 518.

175. Adalhard, *Consuetudines Corbeienses* 33, ed. Semmler, *Initia consuetudinis*, 413.

176. Yearl also associates bloodletting with the alleviation of *acedia* (spiritual indifference): "Time of Bloodletting," 122–51.

177. If the laity, not just monastics, practiced phlebotomy, it becomes more difficult to interpret it as dampening semen production.

178. *Epistula ad Maecenatem*, ed. Niedermann, 1:26–28.

179. Isidore, *Etymologiae* 11.1.123: "Proprie autem sanguis animae possessio est."

180. See also *De temperamentis temporum anni*, Karlsruhe, BLB 172, f. 74v: bloodletting and purging cannot be undertaken without due precaution to temperature and season because otherwise the practitioners "breathe out the soul (*animam ex<h>alaverunt*)."

181. Paris, BnF lat. 4883 is the exception; St. Gall, SB 762 and Paris, BnF lat. 11218 have the same bloodletting treatise following the *Disputatio*; Brussels, BR 3701-15 gives the greatest weight to bloodletting (with one treatise preceding the *Disputatio* and then eleven treatises grouped at ff. 10v–14v).

182. Evaluating (and challenging) this: Horden and Hsu, *Body in Balance.*

183. Kuriyama, *Expressiveness of the Body*; Kuriyama, "Forgotten Fear."

184. *De physiognomonia* 116, ed. André, 132–33.

185. See *De physiognomonia* 12, ed. André, 61.

186. Paris, BnF lat. 6842B (s.IX$^{1}$, possibly Corbie) contains Palladius's *De agricultura*, Caesar's *De bello gallico*, and Anthimus's *DOC*, but an eighteenth-century list of contents (f. Ar) includes also Alcuin's *De fide sanctae Trinitatis*, *De Trinitate ad Fredegisum quaestiones*, and *De animae ratione* (three works that often traveled together in that order: Mattter, "A Carolingian Schoolbook?"). On the manuscript: *Katalog* 3.4416; *Codici* 23; Wickersheimer, *Manuscrits latins*, 67.

## Conclusion

1. On Hincmar, health, and ecclesial ministry, see Morrison, "*Unum ex multis*," 594–96, 616–32.

2. See the edition of Pardulus's letter in Contreni, "Masters and Medicine," 349–50.

3. On medieval *regimen sanitatis* literature, see Adamson, *Medieval Dietetics.*

4. Smaragdus, *Expositio* 4.36, ed. Spannagel, 118–9; trans. Barry, 205–6 (quoting, in part, Isidore's *Sententiae*).

5. But note that Einhard praises Charlemagne for his moderation in drink: *Vita Karoli* 22, 24, and 32, ed. Holder-Egger, 27–29, 36–37.

6. For responses to Colin Morris's *The Discovery of the Individual, 1050–1200*, see Rosenwein, "Y avait-il un *moi*"; Pohl, "Introduction: Ego Trouble?"; Choy, "The Brother."

7. Choy, *Intercessory Prayer*, 203.

8. Hildegard, *Cause et cure* 2.63–68, 2.99–121, 2.171–75, ed. Moulinier, 62–66, 86–90, 125–29.

9. On complexion theory and gender, see Cadden, *Meanings of Sex Difference*, 169–227.

10. On gynecological literature circulating in the Carolingian period, see Green, "Transmission," 130–94. An extant manuscript from Corbie showcases a particular interest in diseases affecting women: St. Petersburg, National Library, F.v.VI.3 (*s*.VIII$^{ex}$/IX$^{in}$); see *Codici* 145.

11. This is the perspective from medical codices, but, of course, this discourse vied with competing theological models of women's bodies as looser and leakier (states denoting sinfulness), as argued by Coon, *Dark Age Bodies*.

12. The parallel between husband-wife and soul-body is highlighted by Hincmar, *De divortio Lotharii*, Responsio 5, ed. Böhringer, 144 (drawing on Eph 5:23–33).

13. Riddle, "Theory and Practice," 171, categorizes Hildegard as early medieval because of the "practical" orientation of her medical writings (vs. the theory-laden texts of the post-1100s).

14. On her medical sources, see Moulinier, *Cause et Cure*, lxiii–ci; Glaze, "Medical Writer," 138–43.

15. Similarly, Pucci Donati, *Dieta*, 62–69, describes how Galen's dietetics, focused on individual temperament and life stages, displaced a Hippocratic dietetics focused on seasonal change.

16. Perkins, *Suffering Self*.

17. Rom 12:4–5 and 1 Cor 12:12. On Isidore's influence, see Moore, *Sacred Kingdom*, 153–60, 318–20. On the medieval application of Paul's metaphor, see Sălăvăstru, "Biblical Origins."

18. See de Jong, "*Ecclesia* and the Early Medieval Polity," 115–23. Not until several centuries later, in John of Salisbury's *Policraticus*, does one find an attempt to associate each particular body part (such as an arm, leg, or organ) with a precise political role.

19. Jonas, *De institutione regia* 1, ed. Dubreucq, 176. See also Pope Gregory IV, Ep. 17, ed. Dümmler, Epp. 5, 231.

20. Jonas, *De institutione regia* 8, ed. Dubreucq, 222–24; quoted by Guillot, "Une *ordinatio* méconnue," 469n72.

21. Hrabanus, *Commentaria in Paralipomena*, col. 279D. On this text, see de Jong "Empire as *ecclesia*." Another exegetical tradition (employed by Hrabanus and Claudius of Turin) likened the state and its secular officials (soldiers, counts, tribunes) to members of the emperor's own body: see Wemple, "Claudius."

22. Guillot, "Une *ordinatio* méconnue"; de Jong, *Penitential State*, 132–35.

23. See Hrabanus, *Expositio in epistulam ad Corinthios primam* 12, cols. 113C–115D. On the unity of the body of Christ, see Morrison, "*Unum ex multis*," 595–619; its opposition to the body of Satan, Moore, *Sacred Kingdom*, 301–4, 353–62.

24. Alcuin, Ep. 198, ed. Dümmler, 327.

25. See Chazelle, *Crucified God*, 209–38; "Exegesis"; "The Eucharist."

26. Paschasius, *De corpore et sanguine* 7, ed. Paulus, 39; trans. Vaillancourt, 79.

27. Paschasius, *De corpore et sanguine* 7, ed. Paulus, 40; Chazelle, "Figure, Character," 9–15.

28. See Phelan, "Horizontal and Vertical Theologies."

29. As detailed by Alcuin in *Primo paganus* (798), the most popular Carolingian baptismal commentary: Phelan, *Formation*, 121–35.

30. Historiography on the Carolingian state has long utilized medical metaphors: see Booker, *Past Convictions*, 1–10.

31. Astronomer, *Vita Hludowici* 3 and 43, ed. Tremp, 290 and 452. Isidore explains that *cancer* is so named because it moves like a crab: *Etymologiae* 4.8.14.

32. *Libellus sacrosyllabus episcoporum Italiae*, ed. Werminghoff, Conc. 2.1, 131.

33. Agobard, *Liber apologeticus I* 6, ed. van Acker, 312.

34. Regino of Prüm, *Chronicon* (841 and 888), ed. Kurze, 75 and 129. On Regino's metaphors, see Dutton, *Charlemagne's Mustache*, 153–58; Meens, "Rise and Fall."

35. Jonas, *DIL* 1.10, ed. Dubreucq, 1:204.

36. On the concern with self-diagnosis, see Booker, "Hypocrisy," 200–202; Firey, "Blushing," 176–80.

# BIBLIOGRAPHY

## Manuscripts


Bamberg, Staatsbibliothek
Msc. med. 1

Bern, Burgerbibliothek
Cod. 109
Cod. 363
Cod. F. 219 III

Brussels, Bibliothèque royale de Belgique
Ms. 3701–15

Berlin, Staatsbibliothek
Ms. Phillipps 1790

Chartres, Bibliothèque municipale
Ms. 62

Einsiedeln, Stiftsbibliothek
Cod. 304

Glasgow, University Library
Ms. Hunter 96 (formerly T. 4. 13)
Ms. Hunter 404 (formerly V. 3. 2)

Karlsruhe, Badische Landesbibliothek
Aug. perg. 120
Aug. perg. 172

Kassel, Universitätsbibliothek, Landesbibliothek und Murhardsche Bibliothek der Stadt Kassel
2° Ms. phys. et hist. nat. 10

Laon, Bibliothèque municipale
Ms. 426 bis.

London, British Library
Arundel Ms. 166
Add. Ms. 8928
Sloane Ms. 2839

Milan, Biblioteca Ambrosiana
Ms. G. 108 inf.
Ms. C. 74 sup.

Modena, Archivio capitolare
Cod. O. I. 11

Montecassino, Archivio dall'Abbazia
Cod. 69
Cod. 97

Paris, Bibliothèque nationale de France
Ms. lat. 4883
Ms. lat. 6842B
Ms. lat. 6862
Ms. lat. 6880
Ms. lat. 6882A
Ms. lat. 7027
Ms. lat. 9332
Ms. lat. 10233
Ms. lat. 11218
Ms. lat. 11219
Ms. lat. 11379
Ms. lat. 12958
Ms. lat. 13403
Ms. lat. 13955
Ms. nouv. acq. lat. 203
Ms. nouv. acq. lat. 1619

St. Gall, Stiftsbibliothek
Cod. sang. 44
Cod. sang. 217
Cod. sang. 265
Cod. sang. 751
Cod. sang. 752
Cod. sang. 759
Cod. sang. 761
Cod. sang. 762
Cod. sang. 877
Cod. sang. 878

St. Petersburg, National Library of Russia
Ms. lat. F. v. VI. 3
Ms. lat. O. v. I. 5

Uppsala, Universitetsbiblioteket
Ms. C. 664

Vatican, Biblioteca Apostolica Vaticana
Pal. lat. 187
Pal. lat. 276
Pal. lat. 485
Pal. lat. 1088
Reg. lat. 846
Urb. lat. 293

Zurich, Zentralbibliothek
Ms. C. 78

## Printed Primary Sources

(Anonymous medical texts without a standardized title listed by editor)

Adalhard of Corbie. *Consuetudines Corbeienses*. Ed. J. Semmler, in *Initia consuetudinis Benedictinae: Consuetudines saeculi octavi et noni*. CCM 1:365–422. Siegburg: F. Schmitt, 1963.

*Admonitio generalis*. Ed. H. Mordek, K. Zechiel-Eckes, and M. Glatthaar, in *Die Admonitio generalis Karls des Großen*. MGH Fontes iuris Germanici antiqui in usum scholarum, separatim editi 16. Hanover: Hahn, 2012.

*Admonitio ad filium spiritualem [Pseudo-Basilii]*. Ed. Paul Lehmann, in *Die Admonitio S. Basilii ad filium spiritualem*. Sitzungsberichte der Bayerischen Akademie der Wissenschaften. Munich: C. H. Beck, 1955.

Agnellus of Ravenna. *Lectures on Galen's De sectis*. Ed. and trans. L. G. Westerink et al. Buffalo: SUNY, 1981.

Agobard of Lyon. *Epistolae*. Ed. E. Dümmler. MGH Epp. 5:150–239. Berlin: Weidmann, 1899.

———. *Opera omnia*. Ed. L. van Acker. CCCM 52. Turnhout: Brepols, 1981.

Alcuin. *Ad pueros Sancti Martini*. Ed. Michael S. Driscoll, in "*Ad pueros Sancti Martini*: A Critical Edition, English Translation, and Study of the Manuscript Transmission." *Traditio* 53 (1998): 37–61.

———. *Ars grammatica*. PL 101, cols. 854–902.

———. *Carmina*. Ed. E. Dümmler. MGH Poetae 1:160–351. Berlin: Weidmann, 1881. Select trans. Peter Godman, in *Poetry of the Carolingian Renaissance*. London: Duckworth, 1985.

———. *De ratione animae*. Ed. James J. Curry, in "Alcuin, *De ratione animae*: A Text with Introduction, Critical Apparatus, and Translation." Ph.D. Diss., Cornell, 1966.

———. *De virtutibus et vitiis*. PL 101, cols. 613–638.

———. *Disputatio de rhetorica et de virtutibus sapientissimi regis Karli et Albini magistri*. Ed. and trans. W. Howell, in *The Rhetoric of Alcuin and Charlemagne*. Princeton: Princeton University Press, 1941.

———. *Disputatio Pippini cum Albino*. Ed. and trans. Andy Orchard, in "Alcuin's Educational Dispute: The Riddle of Teaching and the Teaching of Riddles." In *Childhood and Adolescence in Anglo-Saxon Literary Culture*, ed. S. Irvine and W. Rudolf, 162–201. Toronto: University of Toronto Press, 2018.

———. *Disputatio puerorum*. Ed. Andrew Rabin and Liam Felsen, in *The Disputatio puerorum: A Ninth-Century Monastic Instructional Text*. Toronto: Pontifical Institute of Mediaeval Studies, 2017.

———. *Epistolae*. Ed. E. Dümmler. MGH Epp. 4. Berlin: Weidmann, 1895.

———. *Vita Willibrordi*. Ed. W. Levison. MGH SS rer. Merov. 7: 81–141. Hanover: Hahn, 1920. Trans. C. H. Talbot. In *Soldiers of Christ: Saints and Saints' Lives from Late Antiquity and the Early Middle Ages*, ed. T. Head and T. Noble. University Park: Pennsylvania State University Press, 1995.

*The Alphabet of Galen. Pharmacy from Antiquity to the Middle Ages: A Critical Edition of the Latin Text with English Translation and Commentary*. Ed. and trans. Nicholas Everett. Toronto: University of Toronto Press, 2012.

Amalarius of Metz. *Liber officialis*. Ed. and trans. Eric Knibbs, in *On the Liturgy*, 2 vols. Cambridge, MA: Harvard University Press, 2014.

*Annales Bertiniani*. Ed. F. Grat, J. Vielliard, and S. Clémencet, in *Annales de Saint-Bertin*. Paris: Klincksieck, 1964.

*Annales Fuldenses*. Ed. F. Kurze and G. Pertz. MGH SS rer. Germ. 7. Hanover: Hahn, 1891.

*Annales regni Francorum*. Ed. G. Pertz and F. Kurze. MGH SS rer. Germ. 6. Hanover: Hahn, 1895.

Anthimus. *De observatione ciborum ad Theodoricum regem Francorum epistula*. Ed. E. Liechtenhan. CML 8.1. Berlin: Akademie-Verlag, 1963. Trans. Mark Grant, in *Anthimus: On the Observance of Foods*. Blackawton: Prospect Books, 1996.

———. *De observatio[ne] ciborum: Text, Commentary, and Glossary, with a Study of the Latinity*. Ed. and trans. Shirley H. Weber. Leiden: Brill, 1924.

Pseudo-Apuleius. *Herbarius*. Ed. E. Howald and H. Sigerist, in *Antonii Musae De herba vettonica liber; Pseudoapulei Herbarius; Anonymi De taxone liber; Sexti Placiti Liber medicinae ex animalibus etc*. CML 4. Leipzig: Teubner, 1927.

Ardo. *Vita Benedicti abbatis Anianensis et Indensis*. Ed. G. Waitz. MGH SS 15.1:198–220. Hanover: Hahn, 1887. Trans. Allen Cabaniss, in *Benedict of Aniane, the Emperor's Monk: Ardo's* Life. Kalamazoo: Cistercian Publications, 2008.

Astronomer. *Vita Hludowici imperatoris*. Ed. E. Tremp. MGH SS rer. Germ. 64. Hanover: Hahn, 1995.

Augustine of Hippo. *Confessionum libri XIII*. Ed. L. Verheijen. CCSL 27. Turnhout: Brepols, 1981.

———. *De anima et eius origine libri quattuor*. Ed. C. Urba and J. Zycha. CSEL 60. Vienna: Tempsky, 1913.

———. *De bono coniugali*. Ed. J. Zycha. CSEL 41. Vienna: Tempsky, 1900.

———. *De civitate Dei*. Ed. B. Dombart and A. Kalb. CCSL 47–48. Turnhout: Brepols, 1955.

———. *De doctrina christiana*. Ed. G. Green. CSEL 80. Vienna: Tempsky, 1963.

———. *Enarrationes in psalmos, CI–CL*. Ed. E. Dekkers and J. Fraipont. CCSL 40. Turnhout: Brepols, 1956.

———. *Enchiridion ad Laurentium, de fide et spe et caritate*. Ed. E. Evans. CCSL 46. Turnhout: Brepols, 1969.

——. *Epistulae, pars II* and *III*. Ed. Al. Goldbacher. CSEL 34/2 and 44. Vienna: Tempsky, 1898–1904.

——. *Expositio epistolae ad Galatas*. Ed. J. Divjak. CSEL 84. Vienna: Hoelder-Pichler-Tempsky, 1971.

——. *In Johannis Evangelium*. Ed. R. Williams. CCSL 36. Turnhout: Brepols, 1954.

Basil of Caesarea. *Regulae fusius tractatae*. PG 31, cols. 889–1052.

Bede. *De natura rerum*. Ed. C. W. Jones, in *Opera didascalica, pars I*. CCSL 123A. Turnhout: Brepols, 1975. Trans. Calvin Kendall and Faith Wallis. *Bede: On the Nature of Things and On Times*. Liverpool: Liverpool University Press, 2010.

——. *De schematibus et tropis*. Ed. C. Kendall, in *Opera didascalica, pars I*. CCSL 123A. Turnhout: Brepols, 1975.

——. *De temporum ratione*. Ed. C. W. Jones, in *Opera didascalica, pars 2*. CCSL 123B. Turnhout: Brepols, 1977. Trans. Faith Wallis. *Bede: The Reckoning of Time*. Liverpool: Liverpool University Press, 1999.

——. *Expositio Actuum Apostolorum*. Ed. M. L. W. Laistner. CCSL 121. Turnhout: Brepols, 1983.

——. *Expositio Apocalypseos*. Ed. R. Gryson. CCSL 121A. Turnhout: Brepols, 2001. Trans. Faith Wallis. *Bede: Commentary on Revelation*. Liverpool: Liverpool University Press, 2013.

——. *In Marcum evangelium expositio*. Ed. D. Hurst. CCSL 120. Turnhout: Brepols, 1960.

Pseudo-Bede. *De minutione sanguinis sive de phlebotomia*. Ed. J. A. Giles, in *The Miscellaneous Works of Venerable Bede*, 6:349–52. London: Whittaker, 1843.

Boniface. *Epistolae*. Ed. M. Tangl. MGH Epp. sel. 1. Berlin: Weidmann, 1916.

*Die Bussbücher und das kanonische Bussverfahren*, vol. 2. Ed. H. J. Schmitz. Düsseldorf: L. Schwann, 1898.

*Die Bussordnungen der abendländlischen Kirche*. Ed. F. W. H. Wasserschleben. Halle: Graeger, 1851.

Caelius Aurelianus. *De morbis acutis, De morbus chronicis*. Ed. and trans. I. E. Drabkin, in *On Acute Diseases and On Chronic Diseases*. Chicago: University of Chicago Press, 1950.

Candidus Wizo. "Num Christus corporeis oculis Deum videre potuerit (Ep. 39)." Ed. E. Dümmler. MGH Epp. 4:557–61. Berlin: Weidmann, 1895.

*Die Canones Theodori Cantuariensis und ihre Überlieferungsformen*. Ed. P. W. Finsterwalder. Weimar: H. Böhlaus, 1929.

*Capitula episcoporum*. Ed. P. Brommer, R. Pokorny, M. Stratmann, and V. Lukas. MGH, 4 vols. Hanover: Hahn, 1984–2005.

*Capitularia regum Francorum*, vol. 1. Ed. A. Boretius MGH Capit. 1. Hanover: Hahn, 1883.

*Capitularia regum Francorum*, vol. 2. Ed. A. Boretius and V. Krause. MGH Capit. 2. Hanover: Hahn, 1897.

*Cartulaire de l'abbaye de Cysoing et ses dépendances*. Ed. Ignace de Coussemaker. Lille: Saint-Augustin, 1883.

Cassiodorus. *De anima*. Ed. J. W. Halporn. CCSL 96. Turnhout: Brepols, 1958.

——. *Institutiones divinarum et saecularium litterarum*. Ed. R. A. B. Mynors. Oxford: Clarendon Press, 1937.

——. *Variae*. Ed. A. J. Fridh. CCSL 96. Turnhout: Brepols, 1973.

*Chronica monasterii Casinensis*. Ed. H. Hoffmann. MGH SS 34. Hanover: Hahn, 1980.

*Chronicon Hildesheimense*. Ed. G. Pertz. MGH SS 7:847–73. Hanover: Hahn, 1846.

*Concilia aevi Karolini [742–842]*. Ed. A. Werminghoff. MGH Conc. 2.1 and 2.2. Hanover: Hahn, 1906–1908.

*Concilia aevi Karolini, 843–859.* Ed. W. Hartmann, in *Die Konzilien der karolingischen Teilreiche, 843–859.* MGH Conc. 3. Hanover: Hahn, 1984.

*De physiognomonia.* Ed. J. André, in *Traité de physiognomonie: Anonyme latin texte établi, traduit et commenté.* Paris: Les Belles Lettres, 1981.

Dhuoda. *Liber manualis.* Ed. Pierre Riché, in *Manuel pour mon fils*, 2nd ed. SC 225bis. Paris: Éditions du Cerf, 1997. Trans. Carol Neel, in *Handbook for William: A Carolingian Woman's Counsel for her Son.* Washington, DC: Catholic University of America Press, 1991.

Eigil of Fulda. *Vita Sturmi.* Ed. P. Engelbert, in *Die Vita Sturmi des Eigil von Fulda: Literarkritisch-historische Untersuchung und Edition.* Marburg: N. G. Elwert, 1968.

Einhard. *Charlemagne's Courtier: The Complete Einhard.* Trans. Paul E. Dutton. Peterborough: Broadview, 1998.

———. *Epistolae.* Ed. K. Hampe. MGH, Epp. 5:105–45. Berlin: Weidmann, 1899.

———. *Translatio et miracula Sanctorum Marcellini et Petri.* Ed. G. Waitz. MGH SS 15.1: 238–64. Hanover: Hahn, 1888.

———. *Vita Karoli Magni.* Ed. O. Holder-Egger. MGH SS rer. Germ. 25. Hanover: Hahn, 1911.

Ermenrich of Ellwangen. *Lettre à Grimald.* Ed. Monique Goullet. Paris: CNRS Éditions, 2008.

*Formulae Merowingici et Karolini aevi.* Ed. K. Zeumer. MGH Formulae. Hanover: Hahn, 1886.

*Gesta abbatum Fontanellensium.* Ed. F. Lohier and J. Laporte, in *Gesta sanctorum patrum Fontanellensis coenobii.* Rouen: Lestringant, 1936.

Gottschalk of Orbais. *Oeuvres théologiques et grammaticales de Godescalc d'Orbais.* Ed. C. Lambot. Louvain: Spicilegium sacrum Lovaniense, 1945.

Gregory of Tours. *De virtutibus Sancti Martini episcopi.* Ed. B. Krusch. MGH SS rer. Merov. 1.2:134–211. Hanover: Hahn, 1885.

———. *Historiae.* Ed. B. Krusch and W. Levison. MGH SS rer. Merov. 1.1. Hanover: Hahn, 1951.

———. *Liber in gloria martyrum.* Ed. B. Krusch. MGH SS rer. Merov. 1.2:34–111. Hanover: Hahn, 1969. Trans. R. Van Dam. *The Glory of the Martyrs.* Liverpool: Liverpool University Press, 1988.

Gregory the Great. *Dialogi.* Ed. A. de Vogüé, in *Grégoire le Grand: Dialogues.* SC 251, 260, 265. Paris: Éditions du Cerf, 1978–80.

———. *Moralia in Iob.* Ed. M. Adriaen. CCSL 143, 143A, 143B. Turnhout: Brepols, 1979–1985.

———. *Regula pastoralis.* Ed. F. Rommel, in *Règle pastorale.* SC 381–82. Paris: Éditions du Cerf, 1992.

Groenke, Frank-Dieter. "Die frühmittelalterlichen lateinischen Monatskalendarien: Text, Übersetzung, Kommentar." Diss., Freie Universität Berlin, 1986.

Hartmann, Wilfried. "Unbekannte Kanones aus dem Westfrankenreich des 10. Jahrhunderts." *Deutsches Archiv für Erforschung des Mittelalters* 43 (1987): 28–45.

Heiric of Auxerre. *Miracula Sancti Germani.* PL 124, cols. 1207–1272.

Heito. *Visio Wettini.* Ed. E. Dümmler. MGH Poetae 2:267–75. Berlin: Weidmann, 1884.

Hibernicus Exul. *Carmina de artibus liberalibus.* Ed. E. Dümmler. MGH Poetae 1:408–10. Berlin: Weidmann, 1881.

Hildegard of Bingen. *Cause et cure.* Ed. Laurence Moulinier and Rainer Berndt, in *Beate Hildegardis Cause et cure.* Berlin: Akademie Verlag, 2003.

Hildemar of Civate. *Expositio regulae Sancti Benedicti.* Ed. R. Mittermüller, in *Vita et regula SS. P. Benedicti.* Regensburg: Pustet, 1880.

Hincmar of Reims. *De cavendis vitiis et virtutibus exercendis*. Ed. D. Nachtmann. MGH Quellen zur Geistesgeschichte des Mittelalters 16. Munich: MGH, 1998.
——. *De diversa et multiplici animae ratione ad Carolum calvum regem*. PL 125, cols. 929–952.
——. *De divortio Lotharii regis et Theutbergae reginae*. Ed. L. Böhringer. MGH, Conc. 4.1. Hanover: Hahn, 1992.
——. *De praedestinatione*. PL 125, cols. 65–474.
Hirschfeld, Ernst. "Deontologische Texte des frühen Mittelalters." *AGM* 20 (1928): 353–71.
Hrabanus Maurus. *Commentaria in Ecclesiasticum*. PL 109, cols. 763–1126.
——. *Commentaria in libros duos Paralipomenon*. PL 109, cols. 279–540.
——. *De magicis artibus*. PL 110, cols. 1095–1110.
——. *De rerum naturis [De universo]*. PL 111, cols. 9–614.
——. *Enarrationum in epistolas beati Pauli libri triginta*. PL 111, cols. 1273–616.
——. *Epistolae*. Ed. E. Dümmler. MGH Epp. 5:379–516. Berlin: Weidmann, 1899.
——. *Expositio in epistolam ad Corinthios primam*. PL 112, cols. 9–160.
——. *In honorem sanctae crucis*. Ed. M. Perrin. CCCM 100, 100A. Turnhout: Brepols, 1997.
——. *Tractatus de anima*. PL 110, cols. 1109–1120.
Isidore of Seville. *De natura rerum*. Ed. J. Fontaine, in *Traité de la nature*. Bordeaux: Féret, 1960.
——. *Etymologiarum sive originum libri XX*. Ed. W. M. Lindsay. Oxford: Clarendon Press, 1911. Trans. Stephen A. Barney et al. *The Etymologies of Isidore of Seville*. Cambridge: Cambridge University Press, 2006.
——. *Isidori Hispalensis Versus*. Ed. J. M. Sánchez Martín. Turnhout: Brepols, 2000.
——. *Liber differentiarum II*. Ed. M. A. Andrés Sanz. CCSL 111A. Turnhout: Brepols, 2006.
——. *Sententiae*. Ed. P. Cazier. CCSL 111. Turnhout: Brepols, 1998.
Jacobus. *Versus ad Carolum*. Ed. E. Dümmler. MGH Poetae 1:97–98. Berlin: Weidmann, 1881.
Jerome. *Adversus Jovinianum libri duo*. PL 23, cols. 211–338.
——. *Commentarii in epistulas Pauli apostoli ad Titum et ad Philemonem*. Ed. F. Bucchi. CCSL 77C. Turnhout: Brepols, 2003.
——. *Epistulae*. Ed. I. Hilberg and M. Kamptner. CSEL 54–56. Vienna: Tempsky, 1910–1918.
——. *Tractatuum in psalmos series altera*. Ed. G. Morin, in *S. Hieronymi presbyteri opera, pars II*. CCSL 78. Turnhout: Brepols, 1958.
Jonas of Orléans. *De institutione laicali*. Ed. O. Dubreucq, in *Instruction des laïcs*. SC 549, 550. Paris: Éditions du Cerf, 2012–2013.
——. *De institutione regia*. Ed. A. Dubreucq, in *Le métier de roi*. SC 407. Paris: Éditions du Cerf, 1995.
——. *Vita secunda et translatio Sancti Huberti*. *Acta Sanctorum*, Nov. 1. Brussels: Société des Bollandistes, 1887, cols. 806–18.
Jörimann, Julius. *Frühmittelalterliche Rezeptarien*. Zurich: O. Füssli, 1925.
Julian Pomerius. *De vita contemplativa*. PL 59, cols. 415–520.
Köpp, Peter. *Vademecum eines frühmittelalterlichen Arztes: Die gefaltete lateinische Handschrift medizinischen Inhalts im Codex 217 und der Fragmentensammlung 1396 der Stiftsbibliothek in St. Gallen*. Aarau: Sauerländer, 1980.
Laux, Rudolf. "*Ars medicinae*: Ein frühmittelalterliches Kompendium der Medizin." *Kyklos* 3 (1930): 417–34.
*Legislatio Aquisgranensis*. Ed. J. Semmler, in *Initia consuetudinis Benedictinae: Consuetudines saeculi octavi et noni*. CCM 1:423–582. Siegburg: F. Schmitt, 1963.

*Lex Alamannorum*. Ed. K. Lehmann and K. Eckhardt. MGH LL nat. Germ. 5.1. Hanover: Hahn, 1966.

*Lex Baiwariorum*. Ed. E. von Schwind. MGH LL nat. Germ. 5.2. Hanover: Hahn, 1926.

*Liber accipitrum*. Ed. An Smets, in *Le* Liber accipitrum *de Grimaldus: Un traité d'autourserie du haut Moyen Âge*. Nogent-le-Roi: Laget, 1999.

*Liber Aurelii*. Ed. Charles Daremberg, in "Aurelius: *De acutis passionibus*." *Janus* 2 (1847): 468–96, 705–31.

*Liber sacramentorum Romanae aeclesiae ordinis anni circuli (Cod. Vat. Reg. lat. 316/Paris Bibl. Nat. 7193, 41/56) (Sacramentarium Gelasianum)*, 2nd ed. Ed. L. C. Mohlberg, L. Eisenhöfer, and P. Siffrin. Rome: Herder, 1968.

López Figueroa, Laura. "Estudio y edición crítica de la compilación médica latina denominada *Tereoperica*." Ph.D. Diss., Santiago de Compostela, 2011.

*Das "Lorscher Arzneibuch": Ein medizinisches Kompendium des 8. Jahrhunderts (Codex Bambergensis medicinalis 1): Text, Übersetzung und Fachglossar*. Ed. Ulrich Stoll. Stuttgart: F. Steiner, 1992.

Lupus of Ferrières. *Epistolae*. Ed. E. Dümmler. MGH Epp. 6:1–126. Berlin: Weidmann, 1925. Trans. G. W. Regenos. *The Letters of Lupus of Ferrières*. The Hague: Martinus Nijhoff, 1966.

Marcellus of Bordeaux. *De medicamentis liber*, 2 vols. Ed. M. Niedermann and E. Liechtenhan. CML 5. Berlin: Akademie-Verlag, 1968.

*Medicina Plinii*. Ed. A. Önnerfors, in *Plinii Secundi Iunioris qui feruntur de medicina libri tres*. CML 3. Berlin: Akademie-Verlag, 1964. Trans. Yvette Hunt. *The* Medicina Plinii*: Latin Text, Translation, and Commentary*. New York: Routledge, 2020.

*Miracula Sancti Quintini*. Ed. O. Holder-Egger. MGH SS 15.1:265–70. Hanover: Hahn, 1887.

Nelson, Axel. "Zur pseudohippokratischen *Epistula ad Antiochum Regem*." In *Symbolae Philologicae O. A. Danielsson octogenario dicatae*, 203–17. Uppsala: Lundequistska, 1932.

Nithard. *Historiarum libri IV*. Ed. P. Lauer. *Histoire des fils de Louis le Pieux*. Paris: H. Champion, 1926.

Normann, Herbert. "*Disputatio Platonis et Aristotelis:* Ein apokrypher Dialog aus dem frühen Mittelalter." *SAGM* 23 (1930): 68–86.

Oribasius. *Euporista ad Eunapium*. Ed. A. Molinier, in *Oeuvres d'Oribase*, 6:403–626.

———. *Oeuvres d'Oribase*, 6 vols. Ed. U. C. Bussemaker and C. Daremberg. Paris: Imprimerie nationale, 1851–1876.

———. *Synopsis ad Eustathium*. Ed. U. C. Bussemaker, C. Daremberg, and A. Molinier, in *Oeuvres d'Oribase*, 5:799–927 and 6:1–402.

———. *Synopsis ad Eustathium*. Ed. H. Mørland, in *Oribasius Latinus*. Oslo: Brøgger, 1940.

*Pactus legis Salicae*. Ed. K. Eckhardt. MGH LL nat. Germ. 4.1:1–236. Hanover: Hahn, 1962.

Paschasius Radbertus. *De corpore et sanguine Domini*. Ed. B. Paulus. CCCM 16. Turnhout: Brepols, 1969. Trans. M. G. Vaillancourt. *On the Body and the Blood of the Lord with the Letter to Fredugard*. Turnhout: Brepols, 2020.

———. *Epitaphium Arsenii*. Ed. E. Dümmler. *Abhandlungen der Königlichen Akademie der Wissenschaften zu Berlin, Philologische und historische Klasse* 2 (1900): 1–98.

Paulinus of Aquilea. *Liber exhortationis*. PL 99, cols. 197–282.

———. *Liber exhortationis* (chapters 1–9). Ed. A. de Nicola, in "Sancti Paulini Patriarchae Aquileiensis *Liber exhortationis*: Editio critica." *Atti e Memorie della Società Istriana di Archeologia e Storia Patria* 101 (2001): 187–213.

*Physica Plinii*. Ed. A. Önnerfors, in *Physica Plinii Bambergensis (Cod. Bamb. Med. 2, fol. 93v–232r)*. Hildesheim: G. Olms, 1975.

Pliny the Elder. *Historia naturalis*. Ed. and trans. H. Rackham, W. H. S. Jones, and D. E. Eicholz, in *Natural History*, 10 vols. Loeb Classical Library. Cambridge, MA: Harvard University Press, 1938–1963.

*Polyptyque de l'abbé Irminon*, 2 vols. Ed. B. Guérard. Paris: Imprimerie royale, 1836–1844.

*Precum libelli quattuor aevi Karolini*. Ed. A. Wilmart. Rome: Ephemerides Liturgicae, 1940.

Quintus Serenus. *Liber medicinalis*. Ed. F. Vollmer. CML 2.3. Leipzig: Teubner, 1916.

Ratramnus of Corbie. *Liber de anima ad Odonem Bellovacensem*. Ed. D. C. Lambot. Namur: Éditions Godenne, 1952.

———. *De anima*. Ed. A. Wilmart, in "L'opuscule inédit de Ratramne sur la nature de l'âme." *Revue Bénédictine* 43 (1931): 207–23.

———. "De cynocephalis (Ep. 12)." Ed. E. Dümmler. MGH Epp. 6:155–57. Berlin: Weidmann, 1925.

*Recueil des chartes de l'abbaye de Saint-Benoît-sur-Loire*, 2 vols. Ed. M. Prou and A. Vidier. Paris: Picard, 1900–1907.

Regino of Prüm. *Chronicon*. Ed. F. Kurze. MGH SS rer. Germ. 50. Hanover: Hahn, 1890.

*Regula Benedicti*. Ed. and trans. Bruce L. Venarde, in *The Rule of Saint Benedict*. Cambridge, MA: Harvard University Press, 2011.

*Regula Magistri*. Ed. A. de Vogüé, in *La règle de maître*. SC 105–7. Paris: Éditions du Cerf, 1964–1965.

Rose, Valentin. *Anecdota graeca et graecolatina: Mitteilungen aus Handschriften zur Geschichte der griechischen Wissenschaft*, 2 vols. Berlin: Dümmler, 1864–1870.

———. *Theodori Prisciani Euporiston libri III*. Leipzig: Teubner, 1894.

Rudolf of Fulda, *Miracula sanctorum in ecclesias Fuldenses translatorum*. Ed. G. Waitz. MGH SS 15.1:328–41. Hanover: Hahn, 1887.

———. *Vita Leobae abbatissae Biscofesheimensis*. Ed. G. Waitz. MGH SS 15.1:121–31. Hanover: Hahn, 1887.

*Le sacramentaire grégorien: Ses principales formes d'après les plus anciens manuscrits*, 3 vols. Ed. Jean Deschusses. Fribourg: Éditions universitaires, 1971–1982.

Sallust. *Bellum Catilinae*. Trans. J. T. Ramsey and J. C. Rolfe, in *The War with Catiline. The War with Jugurtha*. Loeb Classical Library 116. Cambridge, MA: Harvard University Press, 2013.

Scherer, Veit. "Die *Epistula de ratione ventris vel viscerum*: Ein Beitrag zur Geschichte des Galenismus im frühen Mittelalter." Diss., Freie Universität Berlin, 1976.

Schubring, Konrad. "*Epistula Paraxagorae*." *SAGM* 46 (1962): 295–310.

Sedulius Scottus. *Carmina*. Ed. L. Traube. MGH Poetae 3:166–240. Berlin: Weidmann, 1896. Trans. E. G. Doyle. *Sedulius Scottus* On Christian Rulers *and* The Poems. Binghamton: Center for Medieval and Early Renaissance Studies, 1983.

Sigerist, Henry. "Die *Lecciones Heliodori*." *AGM* 13 (1921): 145–56.

———. "Die *Prognostica Democriti* im Cod. Hunterian T. 4, 13, S. IX/X." *AGM* 13 (1921): 157–59.

———. "Fragment einer unbekannten lateinischen Übersetzung des hippokratischen Prognostikon." *SAGM* 23 (1930): 87–90.

———. *Studien und Texte zur frühmittelalterlichen Rezeptliteratur*. Leipzig: J. A. Barth, 1923.

Smaragdus of Saint-Mihiel. *Expositio in regulam Sancti Benedicti*. Ed. A. Spannagel and P. Engelbert. CCM 8. Siegburg: F. Schmitt, 1974. Trans. David Barry. *Smaragdus of Saint-Mihiel: Commentary on the Rule of Saint Benedict*. Kalamazoo: Cistercian Publications, 2007.

Sophronius of Jerusalem. *Miracula Cyri et Iohannis*. Ed. A. Mai, in *Spicilegium Romanum*, 3:97–669. Rome: Typis collegii urbani, 1840.

Stadler, Hermann. "Epistola Pseudohippocratis." *Archiv für lateinische Lexikographie und Grammatik* 12 (1902): 21–25.

Sudhoff, Karl. "*Diaeta Theodori*." *AGM* 8 (1915): 377–403.

———. "Die pseudohippokratische Krankheitsprognostik nach dem Auftreten von Hautausschlägen, *Secreta Hippocratis* oder *Capsula eburnea* benannt." *AGM* 9 (1915): 79–116.

*Translatio Sancti Germani Parisiensis*. Ed. C. de Smedt. *Analecta Bollandiana* 2 (1883): 69–98.

Ulmarus of Saint-Vaast. *Miraculorum S. Vedasti liber II*. Ed. O. Holder-Egger. MGH SS 15.1:399–402. Hanover: Hahn, 1887.

*Vita Adae et Evae*. Ed. W. Lechner-Schmidt (Latin version). Trans. B. Custis, G. Anderson, and R. Layton, at http://www2.iath.virginia.edu/anderson/vita/english/vita.lat.html#per2. Electronic edition prepared by Gary Anderson and Michael Stone, at http://www2.iath.virginia.edu/anderson/iath.report.html (copyright 1995)

Venantius Fortunatus. *Vita Sanctae Radegundis*. Ed. B. Krusch. MGH SS rer. Merov. 2:364–95. Hanover: Hahn, 1888.

*Das Verbrüderungsbuch der Abtei Reichenau*. Ed. Johanne Autenrieth, Dieter Geuenich and Karl Schmid. MGH Libri memoriales, Nova series 1. Hanover: Hahn, 1979.

Vindicianus. *Epistula ad Pentadium*. Ed. V. Rose, in *Theodori Prisciani*, 484–92.

———. *Epitome altera*. Ed. V. Rose, in *Theodori Prisciani*, 467–83

———. *Gynaecia*. Ed. V. Rose, in *Theodori Prisciani*, 426–66.

———. *Gynaecia*. Ed. L. Cilliers, in "Vindicianus's *Gynaecia*: Text and Translation of the Codex Monacensis." *Journal of Medieval Latin* 15 (2005): 153–236.

*Visio Baronti monachi Longoretensis*. Ed. W. Levison. MGH SS rer. Merov. 5:368–94. Hanover: Hahn, 1910.

Walafrid Strabo. *De cultura hortorum*. Ed. W. Berschin, in *De cultura hortorum (Hortulus): Das Gedicht vom Gartenbau*. Heidelberg: Mattes, 2007.

———. *Visio Wettini*. Ed. and trans. D. A. Traill, in *Walafrid Strabo's* Visio Wettini: *Text, Translation, and Commentary*. Bern: Herbert Lang, 1974.

———. *Vita sancti Galli confessoris*. Ed. B. Krusch. MGH SS rer. Merov. 4:280–337. Hanover: Hahn, 1902.

Wallis, Faith, trans. *Medieval Medicine: A Reader*. Toronto: University of Toronto Press, 2010.

Wlaschky, M. "*Sapientia artis medicinae*. Ein frühmittelalterliches Kompendium der Medizin." *Kyklos* 1 (1928): 103–113.

Wolfhard of Herrieden. *Miracula S. Walburgis Monheimensia*. Ed. O. Holder-Egger. MGH SS 15.1:535–55. Hanover: Hahn, 1887.

## Secondary Literature

Adams, J. N. *The Regional Diversification of Latin, 200 B.C.-A.D. 600*. Cambridge: Cambridge University Press, 2007.

Adamson, Melitta Weiss. *Medieval Dietetics: Food and Drink in Regimen Sanitatis Literature from 800 to 1400*. Frankfurt am Main: Peter Lang, 1995.

Agamben, Giorgio. *State of Exception*. Trans. K. Attell. Chicago: University of Chicago Press, 2005.

Airlie, Stuart. "'I, Agobard, Unworthy Bishop.'" In Corradini, *Ego Trouble*, 175–83.

———. "The Palace of Memory: The Carolingian Court as Political Centre." In *Courts and Regions in Medieval Europe*, ed. S. Jones, R. Marks, and A. Minnis, 1–20. Rochester: York Medieval Press, 2000.

———. "Private Bodies and the Body Politic in the Divorce Case of Lothar II." *Past and Present* 161 (1998): 3–38.

Alberi, Mary. "'The Better Paths of Wisdom': Alcuin's Monastic 'True Philosophy' and the Worldly Court." *Speculum* 76 (2001): 896–910.

———. "The 'Mystery of the Incarnation' and Wisdom's House (Prov. 9:1) in Alcuin's *Disputatio de vera philosophia*." *Journal of Theological Studies* 48 (1997): 505–16.

———. "'The Sword Which You Hold in Your Hand': Alcuin's Exegesis of the Two Swords and the Lay *Miles Christi*." In Chazelle and Edwards, *Study of the Bible*, 117–31.

Alibert, Dominique. "La transmission des textes patristiques à l'époque carolingienne." *Revue des sciences philosophiques et théologiques* 91 (2007): 7–21.

Amos, Thomas. "Augustine and the Education of the Early Medieval Preacher." In *Reading and Wisdom: The* De doctrina christiana *of Augustine in the Middle Ages*, ed. E. English, 23–40. Notre Dame: University of Notre Dame Press, 1995.

Amundsen, Darrel W. *Medicine, Society, and Faith in the Ancient and Medieval Worlds*. Baltimore: Johns Hopkins University Press, 1996.

———. "Visigothic Medical Legislation." *Bulletin of the History of Medicine* 45 (1971): 553–69.

Andrés Sanz, María A. "Isidoro de Sevilla como fuente de una falsa *Epistula* del evangelista Lucas." In Ferraces Rodríguez, *Isidorus medicus*, 39–64.

Angenendt, Arnold. "Corpus incorruptum: Eine Leitidee der mittelalterlichen Reliquienverehrung." *Saeculum* 42 (1991): 320–48.

Anton, Hans H. *Fürstenspiegel und Herrscherethos in der Karolingerzeit*. Bonn: L. Röhrscheid, 1968.

Appleby, David. "Beautiful on the Cross, Beautiful in His Torments: The Place of the Body in the Thought of Paschasius Radbertus." *Traditio* 60 (2005): 1–46.

———. "Hagiography and Ideology in the Ninth Century: The Narrative Descriptions of the Translation of Relics." Ph.D. Diss., University of Virginia, 1989.

Arbesmann, Rudolph. "The Concept of 'Christus medicus' in St. Augustine." *Traditio* 10 (1954): 1–28.

Arnaud-Lindet, Marie-Pierre. *Orose: Histoires (Contre les Païens)*, vol. 1. Paris: Les Belles Lettres, 1990.

Ashley, Scott. "The Power of Symbols: Interpreting Portents in the Carolingian Empire." *Medieval History* 4 (1994): 34–50.

———. "What Did Louis the Pious See in the Night Sky? A New Interpretation of the Astronomer's Account of Halley's Comet, 837." *EME* 21 (2013): 27–49.

Autenrieth, Johanne. "*Medicus—vir iustus et bonus*. Zu einer lateinischen Version des hippokratischen Prognostikon im Codex Sangallensis 44." In *Florilegium Sangallense: Festschrift für Johannes Duft zum 65. Geburtstag*, ed. O. Clavadetscher, H. Maurer, and S. Sonderegger, 1–13. St. Gall: Verlag Ostschweiz, 1980.

Baader, Gerhard. "Die Anfänge der medizinischen Ausbildung im Abendland bis 1100." In *La scuola nell'occidente latino dell'alto medioevo*, 669–718. Spoleto: Centro italiano di studi sull'alto Medioevo, 1972.

———. "Early Medieval Latin Adaptations of Byzantine Medicine in Western Europe." *Dumbarton Oaks Papers* 38 (1984): 251–59.

———. "Lehrbrief und Kurztraktat in der medizinischen Wissensvermittlung des Früh- und Hoch-Mittelalters." In *Wissensorganisierende und wissensvermittelnde Literatur im Mittelalter*, ed. N. Wolf, 246–54. Wiesbaden: L. Reichert, 1987.

Bachrach, Bernard. *Early Medieval Jewish Policy in Western Europe*. Minneapolis: University of Minnesota Press, 1977.

Baldwin, Barry. "The Career of Oribasius." *Acta Classica* 18 (1975): 85–97.

Banham, Debby. "Investigating the Anglo-Saxon *materia medica:* Latin, Old English, and Archaeobotany." In *The Archaeology of Medicine*, ed. R. Arnott, 95–99. Oxford: Archaeopress, 2002.

Barrow, Julia. "Ideas and Applications of Reform." In Noble and Smith, *Cambridge History of Christianity*, 345–62.

Bartlett, Robert. *The Natural and the Supernatural in the Middle Ages*. Cambridge: Cambridge University Press, 2008.

Beagon, Mary. "Science and Medicine in the Roman Encyclopedists: Patronage for Praxis." In Keyser, *Oxford Handbook*, 655–76.

Beccaria, Augusto. *I codici di medicina del periodo presalernitano (secoli IX, X e XI)*. Rome: Edizioni di storia e letteratura, 1956.

———. "Sulle tracce di un antico canone latino di Ippocrate e di Galeno." I, II, and III. *Italia medioevale e umanistica* 2 (1959): 1–56; 4 (1961) 1–73; 14 (1971) 1–23.

Becker, Julia, Tino Licht, and Stefan Weinfurter, eds. *Karolingische Klöster: Wissenstransfer und kulturelle Innovation*. Berlin: De Gruyter, 2015.

Bejczy, István P. *The Cardinal Virtues in the Middle Ages: A Study in Moral Thought from the Fourth to the Fourteenth Century*. Leiden: Brill, 2011.

Berschin, Walter. *Greek Letters and the Latin Middle Ages: From Jerome to Nicholas of Cusa*. Trans. J. Frakes. Washington, DC: Catholic University of America Press, 1988.

———. "Lateinische Kultur im Benediktinerkloster Lorsch (764–1231)." *Studien und Mitteilungen zur Geschichte des Benediktinerordens und seiner Zweige* 131 (2020): 1–32.

Biller, Peter, and Joseph Ziegler, eds. *Religion and Medicine in the Middle Ages*. Rochester: York Medieval Press, 2001.

Bischoff, Bernhard. *Die Abtei Lorsch im Spiegel ihrer Handschriften*, 2nd ed. Lorsch: Laurissa, 1989.

———. "Italienische Handschriften des neunten bis elften Jahrhunderts in frühmittelalterlichen Bibliotheken außerhalb Italiens." In *Il Libro e il testo*, ed. C. Questa and R. Raffaelli, 169–94. Urbino: Università degli studi di Urbino, 1984.

———. *Katalog der festländlischen Handschriften des neunten Jahrhunderts (mit Ausnahme der wisigotischen)*, 3 vols. Wiesbaden: Harrasowitz, 1998–2014.

———. *Manuscripts and Libraries in the Age of Charlemagne*. Trans. and ed. M. Gorman. Cambridge: Cambridge University Press, 1994.

———. *Mittelalterliche Studien: Ausgewählte Aufsätze zur Schriftkunde und Literaturgeschichte*, 3 vols. Stuttgart: Hiersemann, 1966–1981.

Blanchard, Yves-Marie. "Le Christ médecin et la relecture augustinienne du prologue johannique." In Boudon-Millot, *Les Pères de l'Église*, 477–95.

Bloomfield, Morton W. *The Seven Deadly Sins: An Introduction to the History of a Religious Concept, with Special Reference to Medieval English Literature.* East Lansing: Michigan State College Press, 1952.

Blumenkranz, Bernhard. *Juifs et chrétiens dans le monde occidental, 430–1096.* Paris: Mouton, 1960.

Bochet, Isabelle. "Maladie de l'âme et thérapeutique scripturaire selon Augustin." In Boudon-Millot, *Les Pères de l'Église*, 379–400.

Bonnassie, Pierre. "Consommation d'aliments immondes et cannibalisme de survie dans l'Occident du haut Moyen Âge." *Annales ESC* 44 (1989): 1035–56.

Booker, Courtney M. "By the Body Betrayed: Blushing in the Penitential State." In *Carolingian Experiments*, ed. M. Gillis. Turnhout: Brepols, forthcoming.

———. "Hypocrisy, Performativity, and the Carolingian Pursuit of Truth." *EME* 26 (2018): 174–202.

———. "A New Prologue of Walafrid Strabo." *Viator* 36 (2005): 83–105.

———. *Past Convictions: The Penance of Louis the Pious and the Decline of the Carolingians.* Philadelphia: University of Pennsylvania Press, 2009.

Borgolte, Michael. *Die Grafen Alemanniens in merowingischer und karolingischer Zeit: Eine Prosopographie.* Sigmaringen: J. Thorbecke, 1986.

Borgolte, Michael, Dieter Geuenich, and Karl Schmid, eds. *Subsidia Sangallensia I: Materialien und Untersuchungen zu den Verbrüderungsbüchern und zu den älteren Urkunden des Stiftarchivs St. Gallen.* St. Gall: Staatsarchiv und Stiftsarchiv St. Gallen, 1986.

Born, Lester. "The *Specula principis* of the Carolingian Renaissance." *Revue belge de philologie et d'histoire* 12 (1933): 583–612.

Borst, Arno. *Das Buch der Naturgeschichte: Plinius und seine Leser im Zeitalter des Pergaments.* Heidelberg: C. Winter, 1994.

———. *Die karolingische Kalenderreform.* Hanover: Hahn, 1998.

———. *Der Streit um den karolingischen Kalender.* Hanover: Hahn, 2004.

———. *The Ordering of Time: From the Ancient Computus to the Modern Computer.* Trans. A. Winnard. Cambridge: Polity, 1993.

Boscherini, Silvano. "La dottrina medica comunicata *per epistulam*: Struttura e storia di un genere." In Pigeaud, *Les textes médicaux*, 1–11.

———. *Parole e cose: Raccolta di scritti minori*, ed. I. Mazzini, A. Ciabatti, and G. Volante. Florence: Firenze University Press, 2016.

Boucaud, Pierre. "*Factus est homo in animam viventem*: Anthropologie chrétienne et psychologie dans l'exégèse de Claude de Turin." In *The Multiple Meanings of Scripture: The Role of Exegesis in Early-Christian and Medieval Culture*, ed. I. van't Spijker, 125–51. Leiden: Brill, 2009.

Boudon-Millot, V., and B. Pouderon, eds. *Les Pères de l'Église face à la science médicale de leur temps.* Paris: Beauchesne, 2005.

Bouhot, Jean-Paul. *Ratramne de Corbie: Histoire littéraire et controverses doctrinales.* Paris: Études augustiniennes, 1976.

Bourbon, Florence. "Necessity and Timeliness in Hippocratic Gynaecological Treatises." In *Asklepios: Studies on Ancient Medicine*, ed. L. Cilliers, 19–28. Bloemfontein: Classical Association of South Africa, 2008.

Bourgain, Pascale. "The Works of Gregory of Tours: Manuscripts, Language, and Style." In Murray, *A Companion*, 141–88.

Bradley, Rita M. "Backgrounds of the Title *Speculum* in Mediaeval Literature." *Speculum* 29 (1954): 100–115.

Brakke, David. *Demons and the Making of the Monk: Spiritual Combat in Early Christianity.* Cambridge, MA: Harvard University Press, 2006.

Bricout, Sébastien. "Note sur deux laïcs carolingiens et la médecine au IXe siècle." *Latomus* 65 (2006): 458–61.

Broszinski, Hartmut. *Kasseler Handschriftenschätze.* Kassel: Johannes Stauda Verlag, 1985.

Brown, Giles. "Introduction: The Carolingian Renaissance." In *Carolingian Culture: Emulation and Innovation*, ed. R. McKitterick, 1–51. Cambridge: Cambridge University Press, 1994.

Brown, Peter. *The Body and Society: Men, Women, and Sexual Renunciation in Early Christianity*, 2nd ed. New York: Columbia University Press, 2008.

———. "The End of the Ancient Other World: Death and the Afterlife Between Late Antiquity and the Early Middle Ages." *Tanner Lectures on Human Values.* New Haven: Yale University, 1996.

———. *The Ransom of the Soul: Afterlife and Wealth in Early Western Christianity.* Cambridge, MA: Harvard University Press, 2015.

———. *The Rise of Western Christendom: Triumph and Diversity, A.D. 200–1000*, 2nd ed. Malden: Blackwell, 2003.

Brown, Warren, Marios Costambeys, Matthew Innes, and Adam Kosto, eds. *Documentary Culture and the Laity in the Early Middle Ages.* Cambridge: Cambridge University Press, 2013.

Brubaker, Leslie, and Julia M. H. Smith, eds. *Gender in the Early Medieval World: East and West, 300–900.* Cambridge: Cambridge University Press, 2004.

Bücker, Andreas. "Christianizing the Arts: From Augustine's *De ordine* to Carolingian Thought." In *Signs of Change: Transformations of Christian Traditions and Their Representation in the Arts, 1000–2000*, ed. N. H. Petersen, C. Clüver, and N. Bell, 173–89. Amsterdam: Rodopi, 2004.

Buffa Giolito, M. F. "*Topoi* della tradizione letteraria in tre prefazioni di testi medici latini." In Pigeaud, *Les textes médicaux*, 13–31.

Bullough, Donald A. *Alcuin: Achievement and Reputation.* Leiden: Brill, 2004.

———. "Alcuin and Lay Virtue." In *Predicazione e società nel medioevo: Riflessione etica, valori e modelli di comportamento*, ed. L. Gaffuri and R. Quinto, 71–91. Padua: Centro Studi Antoniani, 2002.

———. "'*Aula renovata*': The Carolingian Court Before the Aachen Palace." *Proceedings of the British Academy* 71 (1985): 267–301.

Burgess, R. "The Date, Purpose, and Historical Context of the Original Greek and the Latin Translation of the So-Called *Excerpta latina barbari.*" *Traditio* 68 (2013): 1–56.

Burnett, Charles. "The Legend of Constantine the African." *Micrologus* 21 (2013): 277–94.

Burnett, Charles, and Danielle Jacquart, eds. *Constantine the African and ʿAlī Ibn al-ʿAbbās al-Magūsī: The Pantegni and Related Texts.* Leiden: Brill, 1994.

Burns, J. Patout, Jr., ed. and trans. *Romans: Interpreted by Early Christian Commentators.* Grand Rapids: Eerdmans, 2012.

Burridge, Claire. "Incense in Medicine: An Early Medieval Perspective." *EME* 28 (2020): 219–55.

Byers, Sarah. "Augustine and the Philosophers." In *A Companion to Augustine*, ed. M. Vessey, 175–87. Malden: Wiley-Blackwell, 2012.

Bynum, Caroline W. *The Resurrection of the Body in Western Christianity, 200–1336*. New York: Columbia University Press, 1995.

———. "Why All the Fuss About the Body? A Medievalist's Perspective." *Critical Inquiry* 22 (1995): 1–33.

Caciola, Nancy M. *Afterlives: The Return of the Dead in the Middle Ages*. Ithaca: Cornell University Press, 2016.

———. *Discerning Spirits: Divine and Demonic Possession in the Middle Ages*. Ithaca: Cornell University Press, 2003.

Cadden, Joan. *Meanings of Sex Difference in the Middle Ages: Medicine, Science, and Culture*. Cambridge: Cambridge University Press, 1993.

Cameron, Averil. *Dialoguing in Late Antiquity*. Cambridge, MA: Harvard University Press, 2014.

Cameron, M. L. *Anglo-Saxon Medicine*. Cambridge: Cambridge University Press, 1993.

———. "Bald's *Leechbook* and Cultural Interactions in Anglo-Saxon England." *Anglo-Saxon England* 19 (1990): 5–12.

Campbell, Darryl. "The *Capitulare de villis*, the *Brevium exempla*, and the Carolingian Court at Aachen." *EME* 18 (2010): 243–64.

Cappuyns, Maïeul. *Jean Scot Érigène: Sa vie, son œuvre, sa pensée*. Brussels: Culture and Civilisation, 1964.

Carozzi, Claude. "Les carolingiens dans l'au-delà." In *Haut Moyen-Âge: Culture, éducation et société*, ed. M. Sot, 367–76. Nanterre: Publidix, 1990.

———. *Le voyage de l'âme dans l'au-delà d'après la littérature latine (V$^{e}$-XIII$^{e}$ siècle)*. Rome: École française de Rome, 1994.

Cavadini, John C. "From Letter to Spirit: The Multiple Senses of Scripture." In *The Oxford Handbook of Early Christian Biblical Interpretation*, ed. P. Blowers and P. Martens, 126–48. Oxford: Oxford University Press, 2019.

———. *The Last Christology of the West: Adoptionism in Spain and Gaul, 785–820*. Philadelphia: University of Pennsylvania Press, 1993.

———. "Reconsidering Augustine on Marriage and Concupiscence." *Augustinian Studies* 48 (2017): 183–99.

Chandler, Cullen J. "Barcelona BC 569 and a Carolingian Programme on the Virtues." *EME* 18 (2010): 265–91.

Chardonnens, László S. *Anglo-Saxon Prognostics, 900–1100: Study and Texts*. Leiden: Brill, 2007.

———. "Do Anglo-Saxons Dream of Exotic Sheep?" In *Representing Beasts in Early Medieval England and Scandinavia*, ed. M. Bintley and T. Williams, 131–50. Woodbridge: Boydell, 2015.

Chazelle, Celia. *The Crucified God in the Carolingian Era: Theology and Art of Christ's Passion*. Cambridge: Cambridge University Press, 2001.

———. "The Eucharist in Early Medieval Europe." In *A Companion to the Eucharist in the Middle Ages*, ed. I. Levy, G. Macy, and K. van Ausdall, 205–49. Leiden: Brill, 2012.

———. "Exegesis in the Ninth-Century Eucharist Controversy." In Chazelle and Edwards, *Study of the Bible*, 167–87.

———. "Figure, Character, and the Glorified Body in the Carolingian Eucharistic Controversy." *Traditio* 47 (1992): 1–36.

———. "Images, Scripture, the Church, and the *Libri Carolini*." *Proceedings of the PMR Conference* 16/17 (1993): 53–76.

———. "Matter, Spirit, and Image in the *Libri Carolini*." *Recherches Augustiniennes* 21 (1986): 163–84.

Chazelle, C., and B. van Name Edwards, eds. *The Study of the Bible in the Carolingian Era*. Turnhout: Brepols, 2003.

Chélini, Jean. *L'aube du Moyen Âge: Naissance de la chrétienté occidentale: La vie religieuse des laïcs dans l'Europe carolingienne (750–900)*. Paris: Picard, 1991.

Cherewatuk, Karen. "*Speculum matris*: Duoda's Manual." *Florilegium* 10 (1988–1991): 49–63.

Choy, Renie S. "'The Brother Who May Wish to Pray by Himself': Sense of Self in Carolingian Prayers of Private Devotion." In *Prayer and Thought in Monastic Tradition*, ed. S. Bhattacharji, R. Williams, and D. Mattos, 101–20. New York: Bloomsbury, 2014.

———. *Intercessory Prayer and the Monastic Ideal in the Time of the Carolingian Reform*. Oxford: Oxford University Press, 2016.

Ciccarese, Maria P. "La *Visio Baronti* nella tradizione letteraria delle visioni dell'Aldilà." *Romanobarbarica* 6 (1981/82): 25–52.

Cilliers, Louise. "The Contribution of the 4th Century North African Physician, Helvius Vindicianus." In *Medicine and Healing in the Ancient Mediterranean*, ed. D. Michaelides, 122–28. Oxford: Oxbow Books, 2014.

———. "Forgery, Fiction and Pseudonym in the Collection of Medical Letters Prefacing Marcellus's *De medicamentis*." *Acta Academica* 38 (2006): 91–110.

———. "Medical Writing in the Late Roman West." In Keyser, *Oxford Handbook*, 1013–33.

Claszen, David and J. M. J. G. Kats. "*Chronicon Moissiacense Maius:* A Carolingian World Chronicle from Creation Until the First Years of Louis the Pious," 2 vols. M.Phil. Thesis, Leiden University, 2012.

Claussen, M. A. "Fathers of Power and Mothers of Authority: Dhuoda and the *Liber manualis*." *French Historical Studies* 19 (1996): 785–809.

———. "God and Man in Dhuoda's *Liber manualis*." *Studies in Church History* 27 (1990): 43–52.

Cohen-Hanegbi, Naama. *Caring for the Living Soul: Emotions, Medicine and Penance in the Late Medieval Mediterranean*. Leiden: Brill, 2017.

Colish, Marcia. *The Stoic Tradition from Antiquity to the Early Middle Ages*, 2 vols. Leiden: Brill, 1985.

Collins, Minta. *Medieval Herbals: The Illustrative Traditions*. Toronto: University of Toronto Press, 2000.

Collins, Samuel. *The Carolingian Debate over Sacred Space*. New York: Palgrave Macmillan, 2012.

Conti, Aidan. "Scribes as Authors, Transmission as Composition: Towards a Science of Copying." In *Modes of Authorship in the Middle Ages*, ed S. Ranković, 267–88. Toronto: Pontifical Institute of Medieval Studies, 2012.

Contreni, John J. "'Building Mansions in Heaven': The *Visio Baronti*, Archangel Raphael, and a Carolingian King." *Speculum* 78 (2003): 673–706.

———. "The Carolingian Renaissance: Education and Literary Culture." In *The New Cambridge Medieval History*, vol. 2, ed. R. McKitterick, 709–57. Cambridge: Cambridge University Press, 1995.

———. *The Cathedral School of Laon from 850 to 930: Its Manuscripts and Masters.* Munich: Arbeo-Gesellschaft, 1978.
———. "John Scottus, Martin Hiberniensis, the Liberal Arts, and Teaching." In *Carolingian Learning, Masters and Manuscripts*, VI:1–22. Aldershot: Variorum, 1992.
———. "Masters and Medicine in Northern France during the Reign of Charles the Bald." In *Charles the Bald: Court and Kingdom*, ed. J. Nelson and M. Gibson, 333–50. Oxford: B. A. R., 1981.
———. "What Was Emperor Augustus Doing at a Carolingian Banquet (Anth. Lat.[2] 719[f])?" *Rheinisches Museum für Philologie* 146 (2003): 372–94.
Coon, Lynda L. *Dark Age Bodies: Gender and Monastic Practice in the Early Medieval West.* Philadelphia: University of Pennsylvania Press, 2011.
———. "Gendering Dark Age Jesus." *Gender & History* 28 (2016): 8–33.
———. "Somatic Styles of the Early Middle Ages." *Gender & History* 20 (2008): 463–86.
———. "'What Is the Word If Not Semen?' Priestly Bodies in Carolingian Exegesis." In Brubaker and Smith, *Gender*, 278–300.
Cooper, Kate. "Concord and Martyrdom: Gender, Community, and the Uses of Christian Perfection in Late Antiquity." Ph.D. Diss., Princeton University, 1993.
———. *The Fall of the Roman Household.* Cambridge: Cambridge University Press, 2007.
Cordoliani, A. "Une encyclopédie carolingienne de comput: Les *Sententiae in laude computi.*" *Bibliothèque de l'École des chartes* 104 (1943): 237–43.
Corradini, Richard. "The Rhetoric of Crisis: *Computus* and *Liber annalis* in Early Ninth-Century Fulda." In Corradini, *Construction of Communities*, 269–321.
Corradini, Richard, et al., eds. *Ego Trouble: Authors and Their Identities in the Early Middle Ages.* Vienna: Verlag der österreichischen Akademie der Wissenschaften, 2010.
Corradini, Richard, Max Diesenberger, and Helmut Reimitz, eds. *The Construction of Communities in the Early Middle Ages: Texts, Resources and Artefacts.* Leiden: Brill, 2003.
Costambeys, Marios, Matthew Innes, and Simon MacLean. *The Carolingian World.* Cambridge: Cambridge University Press, 2011.
Courcelle, Pierre. *Late Latin Writers and Their Greek Sources.* Trans. H. Wedeck. Cambridge, MA: Harvard University Press, 1969.
Cramer, Peter. *Baptism and Change in the Early Middle Ages, c.200–c.1150.* Cambridge: Cambridge University Press, 2003.
Crislip, Andrew T. *Thorns in the Flesh: Illness and Sanctity in Late Ancient Christianity.* Philadelphia: University of Pennsylvania Press, 2013.
Cristiani, Marta. "L'espace de l'âme: La controverse sur la corporéité des esprits, le *De statu animae* de Claudien Mamert et le *Periphyseon.*" In *Eriugena: Studien zu seinen Quellen*, ed. W. Beierwaltes, 149–63. Heidelberg: C. Winter, 1980.
Cross, J. E. "Cosmas and Damian in the *Old English Martyrology.*" *Notes and Queries* 30 (1983): 15–18.
Curry, Janie. "The Illustrated *Visio Baronti*: A Carolingian Manuscript from Reims." *Athanor* 11 (1992): 6–11.
Dal Santo, Matthew. *Debating the Saints' Cult in the Age of Gregory the Great.* Oxford: Oxford University Press, 2012.
Darby, Peter. "The Codex Amiatinus *Maiestas Domini* and the Gospel Prefaces of Jerome." *Speculum* 92 (2017): 343–71.

D'Aronco, Maria. "The Benedictine Rule and the Care of the Sick: The Plan of St Gall and Anglo-Saxon England." In *The Medieval Hospital and Medical Practice*, ed. B. Bowers, 235–251. Aldershot: Ashgate, 2007.

Davis, Jennifer R. *Charlemagne's Practice of Empire*. Cambridge: Cambridge University Press, 2015.

DeGregorio, Scott, ed. *The Cambridge Companion to Bede*. Cambridge: Cambridge University Press, 2010.

Deichgräber, Karl. *Medicus gratiosus: Untersuchungen zu einem griechischen Arzbild*. Mainz: Akademie der Wissenschaften und der Literatur, 1970.

de Jong, Mayke. "Carolingian Monasticism: The Power of Prayer." In *The New Cambridge Medieval History*, vol. 2, ed. R. McKitterick, 622–53. Cambridge: Cambridge University Press, 1995.

———. "*Ecclesia* and the Early Medieval Polity." In *Staat im frühen Mittelalter*, ed. S. Airlie, W. Pohl, and H. Reimitz, 113–32. Vienna: Verlag der österreichischen Akademie der Wissenschaften, 2006.

———. "The Emperor Lothar and his *Bibliotheca Historiarum*." In *Media Latinitas*, ed. R. Nip et al., 229–35. Turnhout: Brepols, 1996.

———. "The Empire as *ecclesia*: Hrabanus Maurus and Biblical Historia for Rulers." In *The Uses of the Past in the Early Middle Ages*, ed. Y. Hen and M. Innes, 191–226. Cambridge: Cambridge University Press, 2000.

———. "Growing Up in a Carolingian Monastery: Magister Hildemar and his Oblates." *Journal of Medieval History* 9 (1983): 99–128.

———. *In Samuel's Image: Child Oblation in the Early Medieval West*. Leiden: Brill, 1996.

———. "Internal Cloisters: The Case of Ekkehard's *Casus sancti Galli*." In *Grenze und Differenz im frühen Mittelalter*, ed. W. Pohl and H. Reimitz, 209–21. Vienna: Verlag der österreichischen Akademie der Wissenschaften, 2000.

———. *The Penitential State: Authority and Atonement in the Age of Louis the Pious, 814–840*. Cambridge: Cambridge University Press, 2009.

Delaruelle, Étienne. "Jonas d'Orléans et le moralisme carolingien." *Bulletin de littérature ecclésiastique* 55 (1954): 129–43.

Delhaye, Philippe. *Une controverse sur l'âme universelle au IXe siècle*. Namur: Centre d'études médiévales, 1950.

Demaitre, Luke. *Medieval Medicine: The Art of Healing, from Head to Toe*. Santa Barbara: Praeger, 2013.

Dendle, Peter. "Plants in the Early Medieval Cosmos: Herbs, Divine Potency, and the *Scala natura*." In *Health and Healing from the Medieval Garden*, ed. P. Dendle and A. Touwaide, 47–59. Woodbridge: Boydell, 2008.

de Nie, Giselle, Karl Morrison, and Marco Mostert, eds. *Seeing the Invisible in Late Antiquity and the Early Middle Ages*. Turnhout: Brepols, 2005.

Depreux, Philippe. "Ambitions et limites des réformes culturelles à l'époque carolingienne." *Revue historique* 304 (2002): 721–53.

———. "Le comte Matfrid d'Orléans (av. 815–836)." *Bibliothèque de l'École des chartes* 152 (1994): 331–74.

———. *Prosopographie de l'entourage de Louis le Pieux (781–840)*. Sigmaringen: Thorbecke, 1997.

Deroux, Carl. "La digestion dans la *Diététique* d'Anthimus: Langage, mythe et réalités." In *Le latin médical: La constitution d'un langage scientifique*, ed. G. Sabbah, 407–16. Saint-Étienne: Université de Saint-Étienne, 1991.

———. "The Franks and Bacon according to Doctor Anthimus (*De obs. cib.* 14)." In *Studies in Latin Literature and Roman History XIV*, ed. C. Deroux, 518–28. Brussels: Latomus, 2008.

Deug-Su, I. "Il *Liber exhortationis* di Paolino d'Aquileia nella cultura carolingia." In Leonardi, *Un ponte*, 285–342.

———. "La *saecularis potestas* nei primi *specula* carolingi." In Leonardi, *Un ponte*, 343–424.

Devisse, Jean. *Hincmar, archevêque de Reims, 845–882*, 3 vols. Geneva: Droz, 1975–1976.

de Vogüé, A. "Entre Basile et Benoît: L'*Admonitio ad filium spiritualem* du Pseudo-Basile." *Regulae Benedicti Studia* 10/11 (1981/82): 19–34.

Devroey, Jean-Pierre. "Monastic Economics in the Carolingian Age." In *The Cambridge History of Medieval Monasticism in the Latin West*, ed. A. Beach and I. Cochelin, 466–84. Cambridge: Cambridge University Press, 2020.

Diebold, William. "The Artistic Patronage of Charles the Bald." Ph.D. Diss., Johns Hopkins University, 1990.

Diem, Albrecht. "The Carolingians and the *Regula Benedicti*." In *Religious Franks: Religion and Power in the Frankish Kingdoms*, ed. R. Meens et al., 243–61. Manchester: Manchester University Press, 2016.

———. *Das monastische Experiment: Die Rolle der Keuschheit bei der Entstehung des westlichen Klosterwesens*. Münster: LIT, 2005.

———. "On Opening and Closing the Body: Techniques of Discipline in Early Monasticism." In *Körper er-fassen: Körperfahrungen, Körpervorstellungen, Körperkonzepte*, ed. K. Schnegg and E. Grabner-Nie, 89–112. Munich: Studien Verlag, 2010.

Dierkens, Alain. "Superstitions, christianisme et paganisme à la fin de l'époque mérovingienne: À propos de l'*Indiculus superstitionum et paganiarum*." In *Magie, sorcellerie, parapsychologie*, ed. H. Hasquin, 9–26. Brussels: Éditions de l'Université de Bruxelles, 1984.

Diesenberger, Maximilian. "Hair, Sacrality and Symbolic Capital in the Frankish Kingdoms." In Corradini, *Construction of Communities*, 173–212.

Di Marco, Michele. *La polemica sull'anima tra "Fausto di Riez" e Claudiano Mamerto*. Rome: Institutum Patristicum Augustinianum, 1995.

Doody, Aude. "Authority and Authorship in the *Medicina Plinii*." In *Authorial Voices in Greco-Roman Technical Writing*, ed. A. Doody and L. Taub, 93–105. Trier: WVT, 2009.

Drews, Wolfram. *Die Karolinger und die Abbasiden von Bagdad: Legitimationsstrategien frühmittelalterlicher Herrscherdynastien im transkulturellen Vergleich*. Berlin: Akademie-Verlag, 2009.

Dronke, Peter. *Women Writers of the Middle Ages: A Critical Study of Texts from Perpetua (†203) to Marguerite Porete (†1310)*. Cambridge: Cambridge University Press, 1984.

Dubreucq, Alain. "Autour du *De virtutibus et vitiis* d'Alcuin." *Annales de Bretagne et des pays de l'Ouest* 111 (2004): 269–88.

———. "La littérature des *specula*: Délimitation du genre, contenu, destinataires et réception." In *Guerriers et moines: Conversion et sainteté aristocratique dans l'occident médiéval (IXe-XIIe siècle)*, ed. M. Lauwers, 17–39. Antibes: APDCA, 2002.

Duden, Barbara. *The Woman Beneath the Skin: A Doctor's Patients in Eightheenth-Century Germany*. Trans. T. Dunlap. Cambridge, MA: Harvard University Press, 1991.

Dutton, Paul E. "Carolingian Invisibles and Eriugena's Lost *Vision of God*." In de Nie, *Seeing the Invisible*, 463–78.

———. *Charlemagne's Mustache and Other Cultural Clusters of a Dark Age*. New York: Palgrave Macmillan, 2004.

———. "Observations on Early Medieval Weather in General, Bloody Rain in Particular." In *The Long Morning of Medieval Europe: New Directions in Early Medieval Studies*, ed. J. Davis and M. McCormick, 167–80. Burlington: Ashgate, 2008.

———. *The Politics of Dreaming in the Carolingian Empire*. Lincoln: University of Nebraska Press, 1994.

Dutton, Paul, and Herbert Kessler. *The Poetry and Paintings of the First Bible of Charles the Bald*. Ann Arbor: University of Michigan Press, 1997.

Duval, Yves-Marie. "Paulin d'Aquilée et le duc Éric: Des clercs et moines aux laïcs et des laïcs aux clercs et moines." In *Aquileia e le Venezie nell'alto medioevo*, 115–47. Udine: Arti Grafiche Friulane, 1988.

Eastwood, Bruce S. *Ordering the Heavens: Roman Astronomy and Cosmology in the Carolingian Renaissance*. Leiden: Brill, 2007.

Edelstein, Ludwig. *Ancient Medicine: Selected Papers of Ludwig Edelstein*, ed. O. Temkin and L. Temkin. Baltimore: Johns Hopkins University Press, 1967.

Edelstein, Wolfgang. *Eruditio und sapientia. Weltbild und Erziehung in der Karolingerzeit: Untersuchungen zu Alcuins Briefen*. Freiburg: Rombach, 1965.

Effros, Bonnie. *Caring for Body and Soul: Burial and the Afterlife in the Merovingian World*. University Park: Pennsylvania State University Press, 2002.

———. *Creating Community with Food and Drink in Merovingian Gaul*. New York: Palgrave Macmillan, 2002.

Erhart, Peter, ed. *Lebenswelten des frühen Mittelalters*. St. Gallen: Kunstverlag Fink, 2019.

Elsakkers, Marianne. "The Early Medieval Latin and Vernacular Vocabulary of Abortion and Embryology." In *Science Translated: Latin and Vernacular Translations of Scientific Treatises in Medieval Europe*, ed. M. Goyens, P. de Leemans, and A. Smets, 377–413. Leuven: Leuven University Press, 2008.

Elukin, Jonathan. *Living Together, Living Apart: Rethinking Jewish-Christian Relations in the Middle Ages*. Princeton: Princeton University Press, 2007.

Englisch, Brigitte. "Realitätsorientierte Wissenschaft oder praxisfernes Traditionswissen? Inhalte und Probleme mittelalterlicher Wissenschaftsvorstellungen am Beispiel von *De temporum ratione* des Beda Venerabilis." In *Dilettanten und Wissenschaft: Zur Geschichte und Aktualität eines wechselvollen Verhältnisses*, ed. E. Strauss, 11–34. Amsterdam: Rodopi, 1996.

Esders, Stefan. "'Faithful Believers': Oaths of Allegiance in Post-Roman Societies as Evidence for Eastern and Western 'Visions of Community.'" In *Visions of Community in the Post-Roman World: The West, Byzantium and the Islamic World, 300–1100*, ed. W. Pohl, C. Gantner, and R. Payne, 357–74. Burlington: Ashgate, 2012.

———. "Rechtliche Grundlagen frühmittelalterlicher Staatlichkeit: Der allgemeine Treueid." In *Der frühmittelalterliche Staat–Europäische Perspectiven*, ed. W. Pohl and V. Weiser, 423–34. Vienna: Verlag der österreichischen Akademie der Wissenschaften, 2009.

———. *Sacramentum fidelitatis: Treueid, Militärwesen und Formierung mittelalterlicher Staatlichkeit*. Habilitationsschrift, Bochum, 2003.

Everett, Nicholas. "Paulinus, the Carolingians and *famosissima* Aquileia." In *Paolino d'Aquileia e il contributo italiano all'Europa carolingia*, ed. P. Chiesa, 115–54. Udine: Forum, 2003.

Faulkner, Thomas. *Law and Authority in the Early Middle Ages: The Frankish leges in the Carolingian Period*. Cambridge: Cambridge University Press, 2016.

Fees, Irmgard. "War Walahfrid Strabo der Lehrer und Erzieher Karls des Kahlen?" In *Studien zur Geschichte des Mittelalters*, ed. M. Thumser, A. Wenz-Haubfleisch, and P. Wiegand, 42–61. Stuttgart: Theiss, 2000.

Ferngren, Gary. *Medicine & Health Care in Early Christianity*. Baltimore: Johns Hopkins University Press, 2009.

Ferngren, Gary, and Darrel Amundsen. "Virtue and Health/Medicine in Pre-Christian Antiquity" and "Virtue and Medicine from Early Christianity Through the Sixteenth Century." In *Virtue and Medicine*, ed. E. Shelp, 3–61. Boston: D. Reidel, 1985.

Ferraces Rodríguez, Arsenio. "Isidoro de Sevilla y los textos de medecina." In Ferraces Rodríguez, *Isidorus medicus*, 11–37.

———, ed. *Isidorus Medicus: Isidoro de Sevilla y los textos de medicina*. La Coruña: Universidade da Coruña, 2005.

———. "Problemas de edición y límites en la enmienda de recetarios de tradición difusa: El *De herbis femininis* y las *Curae herbarum*." In *Fito-zooterapia antigua y altomedieval: textos y doctrinas*, ed. A. Ferraces Rodríguez, 61–78. La Coruña: Universidade da Coruña, 2009.

———. "Tradición indirecta del *De materia medica* de Dioscórides y del *De plantis* atribuido a Tésalo de Tralles: La reutilización de dos fragmentos en traducción latina." In *Body, Disease and Treatment in a Changing World: Latin Texts and Contexts in Ancient and Medieval Medicine*, ed. D. Langslow and B. Maire, 201–12. Lausanne: Éditions BHMS, 2010.

———. "Un recetario médico inexplorado: Los *Teraupetica* (con una tentative de restitución y traducción del prefacio)." *Revue des Études Tardo-Antiques* 8 (2018): 25–65.

Filotas, Bernadette. *Pagan Survivals, Superstitions and Popular Cultures in Early Medieval Pastoral Literature*. Toronto: Pontifical Institute of Mediaeval Studies, 2005.

Finot, André. "Les médecins de rois Mérovingiens et Carlovingiens." *Histoire des sciences médicales* 4 (1970): 41–48.

Firey, Abigail. "Blushing Before the Judge and the Physician: Moral Arbitration in the Carolingian Empire." In *A New History of Penance*, ed. A. Firey, 173–200. Leiden: Brill, 2008.

———. *A Contrite Heart: Prosecution and Redemption in the Carolingian Empire*. Leiden: Brill, 2009.

———. "The Letter of the Law: Carolingian Exegetes and the Old Testament." In *With Reverence for the Word: Medieval Scriptural Exegesis in Judaism, Christianity, and Islam*, ed. J. McAuliffe, B. Walfish, and J. Goering, 204–224. Oxford: Oxford University Press, 2003.

Fischer, Klaus-Dietrich. "Beiträge zu den pseudosoranischen *Quaestiones medicinales*." In *Text and Tradition: Studies in Ancient Medicine and its Transmission*, ed. K.-D. Fischer, D. Nickel, and P. Potter, 1–54. Leiden, Brill, 1998.

———. "De coelo uita–de terra mors. Zwei Zeugnisse zur physischen Anthropologie aus dem frühen Mittelalter." In *Worte, Bilder, Töne: Studien zur Antike und Antikerezeption*, ed. R. Faber and B. Seidensticker, 213–29. Würzburg: Königshausen & Neumann, 1996.

———. "De epistulis XVIII et XVIIII codicis Bruxellensis 3701." In Ferraces Rodríguez, *Isidorus Medicus*, 263–69.

———. "Dr Monk's Medical Digest." *SHM* 13 (2000): 239–51.

———. "*Ex occidente lux*: Greek Medical Works as Represented in Pre-Salernitan Latin Translations." In *Officina Hippocratica: Beiträge zu Ehren von Anargyros Anastassiou und Dieter Irmer*, ed. L. Perilli et al., 29–56. Berlin: De Gruyter, 2011.

———. "Gesund durchs Jahr mit Dr. Hippokrates—Monat für Monat!" In *The Frontiers of Ancient Science: Essays in Honor of Heinrich von Staden*, ed. B. Holmes and K.-D. Fischer, 111–38. Berlin: De Gruyter, 2015.

———. "The *Isagoge* of Pseudo-Soranus: An Analysis of the Contents of a Medieval Introduction to the Art of Medicine." *Medizinhistorisches Journal* 35 (2000): 3–30.

———. "Die lateinischen Fassungen des dem Diokles von Karystos zugeschriebenen diätetischen Briefes." In *Conserver la santé ou la rétablir: Le rôle de l'environnement dans la médecine antique et médiévale*, ed. N. Palmieri, 335–58. Saint-Étienne: Université de Saint-Étienne, 2012.

———. "Das *Lorscher Arzneibuch* im Widerstreit der Meinungen." *Medizinhistorisches Journal* 45 (2010): 165–88.

———. "Neue oder vernachlässigte Quellen der *Etymologien* Isidors von Sevilla (Buch 4 und 11)." In Ferraces Rodríguez, *Isidorus Medicus*, 129–74.

———. "Der pseudogalenische *Liber tertius*." In *Galenismo e medicina tardoantica: Fonti greche, latine e arabe*, ed. I. Garofalo and A. Roselli, 101–32. Naples: Istituto Universitario Orientale, 2003.

———. "Die spätlateinische Übersetzung von Galen, *Ad Glauconem* (Kühn 11.1–146)." *Galenos* 6 (2012): 103–16.

———. "Two Latin Pre-Salernitan Medical Manuals, the *Liber passionalis* and the *Tereoperica* (Ps. Petroncellus)." In *Medical Books in the Byzantine World*, ed. B. Zipser, 35–56. Bologna: Eikasmós, 2013.

Fisher, Matthew. *Scribal Authorship and the Writing of History in Medieval England*. Columbus: Ohio State University Press, 2012.

Flammini, Giuseppe. "L'*Epistula* pseudogalenica *de febribus*." In Santini, *Prefazioni*, 3:237–57.

Flint, Valerie. "The Early Medieval *Medicus*, the Saint—and the Enchanter." *SHM* 2 (1989): 127–45.

———. *The Rise of Magic in Early Medieval Europe*. Princeton: Princeton University Press, 1991.

Folliet, G. "La fortune du dit de Virgile 'Aurum colligere de stercore' dans la littérature chrétienne." *Sacris Erudiri* 41 (2002): 31–53.

Fort, Gavin. "Penitents and Their Proxies: Penance for Others in Early Medieval Europe." *Church History* 86 (2017): 1–32.

Foucault, Michel. *The History of Sexuality: The Care of the Self*. Trans. R. Hurley. New York: Pantheon Books, 1986.

———. "What Is an Author?" In *Language, Counter-Memory, Practice*. Trans. D. Bouchard and S. Simon, 113–38. Ithaca: Cornell University Press, 1977.

Fouracre, Paul. "The Origins of the Carolingian Attempt to Regulate the Cult of Saints." In *The Cult of Saints in Late Antiquity and the Middle Ages*, ed. J. Howard-Johnston and P. Hayward, 143–65. Oxford: Oxford University Press, 1999.

Franklin, C. V. "The Date of Composition of Bede's *De schematibus et tropis* and *De arte metrica*." *Revue Bénédictine* 110 (2000): 199–203.

Freeman, Ann. "Carolingian Orthodoxy and the Fate of the *Libri Carolini*." *Viator* 16 (1985): 65–108.

French, Roger. "Astrology in Medical Practice." In García-Ballester, *Practical Medicine*, 30–59.

———. *Medicine Before Science: The Rational and Learned Doctor from the Middle Ages to the Enlightenment*. Cambridge: Cambridge University Press, 2003.

Fricke, Beate, and Theresa Holler. "Rosenrot: Die Bildwelt von Flora, Fauna und *fons vitae* im Godesscalc-Evangelistar als Heilsruam." In *Die Handschriften der Hofschule Kaiser Karls des Großen*, ed. M. Embach, C. Moulin, and H. Wolter-von dem Knesebeck, 97–127. Trier: Verlag für Geschichte und Kultur, 2019.

Galvão-Sobrinho, C. R. "Hippocratic Ideals, Medical Ethics, and the Practice of Medicine in the Early Middle Ages: The Legacy of the Hippocratic Oath." *JHMAS* 51 (1996): 438–55.

Gantner, Clemens, Rosamond McKitterick, and Sven Meeder, eds. *The Resources of the Past in Early Medieval Europe*. Cambridge: Cambridge University Press, 2015.

Ganz, David. *Corbie in the Carolingian Renaissance*. Sigmaringen: Thorbecke, 1990.

———. "The Debate on Predestination." In *Charles the Bald: Court and Kingdom*, ed. J. Nelson and M. Gibson, 353–73. Oxford: B. A. R., 1981.

García-Ballester, Luis, et al., eds. *Practical Medicine from Salerno to the Black Death*. Cambridge: Cambridge University Press, 1994.

Garipzanov, Ildar H. *The Symbolic Language of Authority in the Carolingian World (c. 751–877)*. Leiden: Brill, 2008.

Garrison, Mary. "The Social World of Alcuin: Nicknames at York and at the Carolingian Court." In *Alcuin of York: Scholar at the Carolingian Court*, ed. L. Howen and A. MacDonald, 59–79. Groningen: Forsten, 1998.

Garver, Valerie L. "Childbearing and Infancy in the Carolingian World." *Journal of the History of Sexuality* 21 (2012): 208–44.

———. *Women and Aristocratic Culture in the Carolingian World*. Ithaca: Cornell University Press, 2009.

Gastgeber, Christian. "The Aristotle of Pippin III: Greek Books Sent to the Frankish Court (ca. 758 A.D.)." *Medieval Worlds* 8 (2018): 42–65.

Geary, Patrick J. *Furta sacra: Thefts of Relics in the Central Middle Ages*, rev. ed. Princeton: Princeton University Press, 2011.

———. *Living with the Dead in the Middle Ages*. Ithaca: Cornell University Press, 1994.

Geith, Karl-Ernst, and Walter Berschin. "Die Bibliothekskataloge des Klosters Murbach aus dem IX. Jahrhundert." *Zeitschrift für Kirchengeschichte* 83 (1972): 61–87.

Gillett, Andrew. *Envoys and Political Communication in the Late Antique West, 411–533*. Cambridge: Cambridge University Press, 2003.

Gillis, Matthew B. *Heresy and Dissent in the Carolingian Empire: The Case of Gottschalk of Orbais*. Oxford: Oxford University Press, 2017.

Glaze, Florence Eliza. "Master-Student Medical Dialogues: The Evidence of London, British Library, Sloane 2839." In *Form and Content of Instruction in Anglo-Saxon England in the Light of Contemporary Manuscript Evidence*, ed. P. Lendinara, L. Lazzari, and M. D'Aronco, 467–94. Turnhout: Brepols, 2007.

———. "Medical Writer: 'Behold the Living Creature.'" In *Voice of the Living Light: Hildegard of Bingen and Her World*, ed. B. Newman, 125–48. Berkeley: University of California Press, 1998.

———. "The Perforated Wall: The Ownership and Circulation of Medical Books in Medieval Europe, ca. 800–1200." Ph.D. Diss., Duke University, 1999.

———. "Salerno's Lombard Prince: Johannes 'Abbas de Curte' as Medical Practitioner." *Early Science and Medicine* 23 (2018): 177–216.

Glaze, F. Eliza, and Brian Nance, eds. *Between Text and Patient: The Medical Enterprise in Medieval & Early Modern Europe*. Florence: SISMEL, 2011.

Godden, M. R. "Anglo-Saxons on the Mind." In *Learning and Literature in Anglo-Saxon England*, ed. M. Lapidge and H. Gneuss, 271–98. Cambridge: Cambridge University Press, 1985.

Goldberg, Eric. "'The Hunt Belongs to Man': Some Neglected Treatises Related to Hunting and Falconry from the Court of Louis the German." In *Discovery and Distinction in the Early Middle Ages*, ed. C. Chandler and S. Stofferahn, 31–57. Kalamazoo: Medieval Institute, 2013.

———. *In the Manner of the Franks: Hunting, Kingship, and Masculinity in Early Medieval Europe*. Philadelphia: University of Pennsylvania Press, 2020.

Green, Monica H. *Making Women's Medicine Masculine: The Rise of Male Authority in Pre-Modern Gynaecology*. Oxford: Oxford University Press, 2008.

———. "Medical Books." In *The European Book in the Twelfth Century*, ed. E. Kwakkel and R. Thomson, 277–92. Cambridge: Cambridge University Press, 2018.

———. "Rethinking the Manuscript Basis of Salvatore De Renzi's *Collectio Salernitana*: The Corpus of Medical Writings in the 'Long' Twelfth Century." In *La "Collectio Salernitana" di Salvatore De Renzi*, ed. D. Jacquart and A. Bagliani, 15–60. Florence: SISMEL, 2008.

———. "The Transmission of Ancient Theories of Female Physiology and Disease Through the Early Middle Ages." Ph.D. Diss., Princeton University, 1985.

Griffin, Carl, and David Paulsen. "Augustine and the Corporeality of God." *Harvard Theological Review* 95 (2002): 97–118.

Guillot, Olivier. "Une *ordinatio* méconnue: Le capitulaire de 823–825." In *Charlemagne's Heir: New Perspectives on the Reign of Louis the Pious (814–840)*, ed. P. Godman and R. Collins, 455–86. Oxford: Clarendon Press, 1990.

Gutas, Dimitri. *Greek Thought, Arabic Culture: The Graeco-Arabic Translation Movement in Baghdad and Early 'Abbāsid Society (2nd–4th/8th–10th Centuries)*. London: Routledge, 1998.

Hack, Achim Thomas. *Alter, Krankheit, Tod und Herrschaft im frühen Mittelalter: Das Beispiel der Karolinger*. Stuttgart: Hiersemann, 2009.

Haggenmüller, Reinhold. *Die Überlieferung der Beda und Egbert zugeschriebenen Bussbücher*. Frankfurt am Main: Peter Lang, 1991.

Halkias, Georgios. "From Reflections to Membranes: Transcripts on the Body in Religious Discourse." In *Religious Boundaries for Sex, Gender, and Corporeality*, ed. A. Cuffel, A. Echevarria, and G. Halkias, 1–10. New York: Routledge, 2019.

Hanson, Ann, and Monica Green. "Soranus of Ephesus: *Methodicorum princeps*." In *Aufstieg und Niedergang der römischen Welt*, ed. W. Haase and H. Temporini, 968–1075. Berlin: De Gruyter, 1994.

Harrold, Jillian. "Saintly Doctors: The Early Iconography of SS. Cosmas and Damian in Italy." Ph.D. Diss., University of Warwick, 2007.

Hartmann, Wilfried. *Die Synoden der Karolingerzeit im Frankenreich und in Italien*. Paderborn: F. Schöningh, 1989.

Harvey, Susan Ashbrook. "The Sense of a Stylite: Perspectives on Simeon the Elder." *Vigiliae Christianae* 42 (1988): 376–94.

Häse, Angelika. *Mittelalterliche Bücherverzeichnisse aus Kloster Lorsch: Einleitung, Edition, und Kommentar*. Wiesbaden: Harrassowitz, 2002.

Haverkamp, Symke. "Making Something from Nothing: Content and Context of Fredegisus of Tours' *De substantia nihili et tenebrarum*." M.A. Thesis, Universiteit Utrecht, 2006.

Head, Thomas. *Hagiography and the Cult of Saints: The Diocese of Orléans, 800–1200*. Cambridge: Cambridge University Press, 1990.

Heene, Katrien. *The Legacy of Paradise: Marriage, Motherhood and Woman in Carolingian Edifying Literature*. Frankfurt am Main: Peter Lang, 1997.

Heinzelmann, Martin. *Translationsberichte und andere Quellen des Reliquienkultes*. Turnhout: Brepols, 1979.

Hen, Yitzhak. "The *Annals of Metz* and the Merovingian Past." In *The Uses of the Past in the Early Middle Ages*, ed. Y. Hen and M. Innes, 175–90. Cambridge: Cambridge University Press, 2000.

———. "The Early Medieval West." In *The Cambridge History of Magic and Witchcraft in the West: From Antiquity to the Present*, ed. D. Collins, 183–206. Cambridge: Cambridge University Press, 2015.

———. "Food and Drink in Merovingian Gaul." In *Tätigkeitsfelder und Erfahrungshorizonte des ländlichen Menschen in der frühmittelalterlichen Grundherrschaft (bis ca. 1000)*, ed. B. Kasten, 99–110. Stuttgart: Steiner, 2006.

———. "The Structure and Aims of the *Visio Baronti*." *Journal of Theological Studies* 47 (1996): 477–97.

Hennings, Ralph. "*Disputatio de origine animae* (CPL 623,37—or the Victory of Creatianism in the Fifth Century." *Studia Patristica* 29 (1997): 260–68.

Herren, Michael. "Pelasgian Fountains: Learning Greek in the Early Middle Ages." In *Learning Latin and Greek from Antiquity to the Present*, ed. E. Archibald, W. Brockliss, and J. Gnoza, 65–82. Cambridge: Cambridge University Press, 2015.

Herrin, Judith. *Ravenna: Capital of Empire, Crucible of Europe*. Princeton: Princeton University Press, 2020.

Heydemann, Gerda. "The People of God and the Law: Biblical Models in Carolingian Legislation." *Speculum* 95 (2020): 89–131.

———. "Relics and Texts: Hagiography and Authority in Ninth-Century Francia." In *An Age of Saints? Power, Conflict, and Dissent in Early Medieval Christianity*, ed. P. Sarris, M. Dal Santo, and P. Booth, 187–204. Leiden: Brill, 2011.

Heyse, Elisabeth. *Hrabanus Maurus' Enzyklopädie* De rerum naturis*: Untersuchungen zu den Quellen und zur Methode der Kompilation*. Munich: Arbeo-Gesellschaft, 1969.

Hildebrandt, M. M. *The External School in Carolingian Society*. Leiden: Brill, 1992.

Hill, Susan E. "'The Ooze of Gluttony': Attitudes Toward Food, Eating, and Excess in the Middle Ages." In *The Seven Deadly Sins: From Communities to Individuals*, ed. R. Newhauser, 57–70. Leiden: Brill, 2007.

Hillgarth, J. N. *Christianity and Paganism, 350–750*. Philadelphia: University of Pennsylvania Press, 1986.

Hillner, Julia. *Prison, Punishment and Penance in Late Antiquity*. Cambridge: Cambridge University Press, 2015.

Holmes, Brooke. "Disturbing Connections: Sympathetic Affections, Mental Disorder, and the Elusive Soul in Galen." In *Mental Disorders in the Classical World*, ed. W. V. Harris, 147–76. Leiden: Brill, 2013.

———. *The Symptom and the Subject: The Emergence of the Physical Body in Ancient Greece*. Princeton: Princeton University Press, 2010.

Horden, Peregrine. "Medieval Medicine." In *The Oxford Handbook of the History of Medicine*, ed. M. Jackson, 40–59. Oxford: Oxford University Press, 2011.

———. "Sickness and Healing." In Noble and Smith, *Cambridge History of Christianity*, 416–32.

———. "What's Wrong with Early Medieval Medicine?" *SHM* 24 (2011): 5–25.

Horden, Peregrine, and Elisabeth Hsu, eds. *The Body in Balance: Humoral Medicines in Practice*. New York: Berghahn Books, 2013.

Horn, Walter, and Ernest Born. *The Plan of St. Gall: A Study of the Architecture and Economy of and Life in a Paradigmatic Carolingian Monastery*, 3 vols. Berkeley: University of California Press, 1979.

Hubert, J., J. Porcher, and W. Volbach. *L'Empire carolingien*. Paris: Gallimard, 1968.

Ineichen-Eder, Christine. "The Authenticity of the *Dicta Candidi, Dicta Albini*, and Some Related Texts." In *Insular Latin Studies: Papers on Latin Texts and Manuscripts of the British Isles, 550–1066*, ed. M. Herren, 179–93. Toronto: Pontifical Institute of Mediaeval Studies, 1981.

Innes, Matthew. "Keeping It in the Family: Women and Aristocratic Memory, 700–1200." In *Medieval Memories: Men, Women and the Past, 700–1300*, ed. E. van Houts, 17–35. Harlow: Longman, 2001.

———. "'A Place of Discipline': Carolingian Courts and Aristocratic Youth." In *Court Culture in the Early Middle Ages: The Proceedings of the First Alcuin Conference*, ed. C. Cubitt, 59–76. Turnhout: Brepols, 2003.

———. "Kings, Monks and Patrons: Political Identities and the Abbey of Lorsch." In *La royauté et les élites dans l'Europe carolingienne*, ed. R. Le Jan, 301–24. Villeneuve d'Ascq: Centre d'histoire de l'Europe du Nord-Ouest, 1998.

Jacobsen, Werner. *Der Klosterplan von St. Gallen und die karolingische Architektur: Entwicklung und Wandel von Form und Bedeutung im fränkischen Kirchenbau zwischen 751 und 840*. Berlin: Deutscher Verlag für Kunstwissenschaft, 1992.

Jaffe, Clella I. "Dhuoda's *Handbook for William* and the Mother's Manual Tradition." In *Listening to Their Voices: The Rhetorical Activities of Historical Women*, ed. M. Wertheimer, 177–98. Columbia: University of South Carolina Press, 1997.

James, Edward. "A Sense of Wonder: Gregory of Tours, Medicine and Science." In *The Culture of Christendom*, ed. M. Meyer, 45–60. London: Hambledon Press, 1993.

Jolly, Karen L. *Popular Religion in Late Saxon England: Elf Charms in Context*. Chapel Hill: University of North Carolina Press, 1996.

Jones, Allen E. *Social Mobility in Late Antique Gaul: Strategies and Opportunities for the Non-Elite*. Cambridge: Cambridge University Press, 2009.

Jones, Christopher A. "Candidus Wizo, Arn of Salzburg and the Treatise *De sole et luna*." *EME* 27 (2019): 546–66.

Jones, Peter Murray. "Image, Word, and Medicine in the Middle Ages." In *Visualizing Medieval Medicine and Natural History, 1200–1550*, ed. J. Givens, K. Reeds, and A. Touwaide, 1–24. Aldershot: Ashgate, 2006.

———. *Medieval Medical Miniatures*. Austin: University of Texas Press, 1985.

Jouanna, Jacques. *Greek Medicine from Hippocrates to Galen: Selected Papers*, ed. P. van der Eijk, trans. N. Allies. Leiden: Brill, 2012.

———. "La théorie des quatre humeurs et des quatre tempéraments dans la tradition latine (Vindicien, Pseudo-Soranos) et une source grecque retrouvée." *Revue des Études Grecques* 118 (2005): 138–67.

Juste, David, and Hilbert Chiu, "The *De tonitruis* Attributed to Bede: An Early Medieval Treatise on Divination by Thunder Translated from Irish." *Traditio* 68 (2013): 97–124.

Kaczynski, Bernice. *Greek in the Carolingian Age: The St. Gall Manuscripts*. Cambridge, MA: Medieval Academy of America, 1988.

Kaye, Joel. *A History of Balance, 1250–1375: The Emergence of a New Model of Equilibrium and Its Impact on Medieval Thought*. Cambridge: Cambridge University Press, 2014.

Keefe, Susan A. *Water and the Word: Baptism and the Education of the Clergy in the Carolingian Empire*. Notre Dame: University of Notre Dame Press, 2002.

Keil, Gundolf. "Einleitung." In Keil and Schnitzer, *Das Lorscher Arzneibuch*, 7–28.

———. "Klostermedizin im frühen Mittelalter dokumentiert am *Lorscher Arzneibuch* von etwa 790." In *Geistliche Aspekte mittelalterlicher Naturlehre*, ed. B. Vollmann, 11–25. Wiesbaden: Reichert, 1993.

———. "Möglichkeiten und Grenzen frühmittelalterlicher Medizin." In Keil and Schnitzer, *Das Lorscher Arzneibuch*, 219–52.

Keil, Gundolf, and Paul Schnitzer, eds. *Das Lorscher Arzneibuch und die frühmittelalterliche Medizin: Verhandlungen des medizinhistorischen Symposiums im September 1989 in Lorsch*. Lorsch: Laurissa, 1991.

Kershaw, Paul. "Eberhard of Friuli, a Carolingian Lay Intellectual." In Wormald, *Lay Intellectuals*, 77–105.

Kesling, Emily. *Medical Texts in Anglo-Saxon Literary Culture*. Woodbridge: Boydell & Brewer, 2020.

Keyser, Paul, with John Scarborough, eds. *The Oxford Handbook of Science and Medicine in the Classical World*. Oxford: Oxford University Press, 2018.

Kibre, Pearl. *Hippocrates Latinus: Repertorium of Hippocratic Writings in the Latin Middle Ages*. New York: Fordham University Press, 1985.

Kieckhefer, Richard. "The Specific Rationality of Medieval Magic." *American Historical Review* 99 (1994): 813–36.

King, Helen. "Female Fluids in the Hippocratic Corpus: How Solid Was the Humoral Body?" In Horden, *Body in Balance*, 25–49.

Kitchen, J. K. "Gregory of Tours, Hagiography, and the Cult of the Saints in the Sixth Century." In Murray, *Companion*, 375–426.

Kitzinger, Beatrice E. *The Cross, the Gospels, and the Work of Art in the Carolingian Age*. Cambridge: Cambridge University Press, 2019.

Klibansky, Raymond, Erwin Panofsky, and Fritz Saxl. *Saturn and Melancholy: Studies in the History of Natural Philosophy, Religion, and Art*. London: Nelson, 1964.

Klingshirn, William E. "Divination and the Disciplines of Knowledge According to Augustine." In Pollman, *Augustine*, 113–40.

Knipp, David. "The Chapel of Physicians at Santa Maria Antiqua." *Dumbarton Oaks Papers* 56 (2002): 1–23.

Kosto, Adam J. *Hostages in the Middle Ages*. Oxford: Oxford University Press, 2012.

Kottje, Raymund. *Die Bussbücher Halitgars von Cambrai und des Hrabanus Maurus: Ihre Überlieferung und ihre Quellen*. Berlin: De Gruyter, 1980.

Koziol, Geoffrey. *Begging Pardon and Favor: Ritual and Political Order in Early Medieval France*. Ithaca: Cornell University Press, 1992.

———. "Leadership: Why We Have Mirrors for Princes but None for Presidents." In *Why the Middle Ages Matter: Medieval Light on Modern Injustice*, ed. C. Chazelle et al., 183–98. New York: Routledge, 2012.

———. "Truth and Its Consequences: Why Carolingianists Don't Speak of Myth." In *Myth in Early Northwest Europe*, ed. S. Glosecki, 71–104. Turnhout: Brepols, 2007.

Kramer, Rutger. *Rethinking Authority in the Carolingian Empire: Ideals and Expectations during the Reign of Louis the Pious (813–828)*. Amsterdam: Amsterdam University Press, 2019.

Kreiner, Jamie. "Autopsies and Philosophies of a Merovingian Life: Death, Responsibility, Salvation." *Journal of Early Christian Studies* 22 (2014): 113–52.

———. *Legions of Pigs in the Early Medieval West*. New Haven: Yale University Press, 2020.

Kroll, Jerome and Bernard Bachrach. "Sin and the Etiology of Disease in Pre-Crusade Europe." *JHMAS* 41 (1986): 395–414.

Kühnel, Bianca. "Carolingian Diagrams, Images of the Invisible." In de Nie, *Seeing the Invisible*, 359–89.

———. *The End of Time in the Order of Things: Science and Eschatology in Early Medieval Art*. Regensburg: Schnell & Steiner, 2003.

Kuriyama, Shigehisa. *The Expressiveness of the Body and the Divergence of Greek and Chinese Medicine*. New York: Zone Books, 1999.

———. "The Forgotten Fear of Excrement." *Journal of Medieval and Early Modern Studies* 38 (2008): 413–42.

Kwakkel, Erik, and Francis Newton. *Medicine at Monte Cassino: Constantine the African and the Oldest Manuscript of his Pantegni*. Turnhout: Brepols, 2019.

Laistner, M. L. W. "Some Early Medieval Commentaries on the Old Testament." *Harvard Theological Review* 46 (1953): 27–46.

Lake, Justin. *Richer of Saint-Rémi: The Methods and Mentality of a Tenth-Century Historian*. Washington, DC: Catholic University of America Press, 2013.

Langslow, D. R. "The *Epistula* in Ancient Scientific and Technical Literature, with Special Reference to Medicine." In *Ancient Letters: Classical and Late Antique Epistolography*, ed. R. Morello and A. Morrison, 211–34. Oxford: Oxford University Press, 2007.

———. *The Latin Alexander Trallianus: The Text and Transmission of a Late Latin Medical Book*. London: Society for the Promotion of Roman Studies, 2006.

Langum, Virginia. *Medicine and the Seven Deadly Sins in Late Medieval Literature and Culture*. New York: Palgrave Macmillan, 2016.

Lapidge, Michael. *Hilduin of Saint-Denis: The* Passio S. Dionysii *in Prose and Verse*. Leiden: Brill, 2017.

———. "The School of Theodore and Hadrian." *Anglo-Saxon England* 15 (1986): 45–72.

La Rocca, C., and L. Provero. "The Dead and Their Gifts: The Will of Eberhard, Count of Friuli, and his Wife, Gisela, Daughter of Louis the Pious (863–864)." In *Rituals of Power from Late Antiquity to the Early Middle Ages*, ed. F. Theuws and J. Nelson, 225–80. Leiden: Brill, 2000.

Lebech, Mette, James McEvoy, with John Flood. "*De dignitate conditionis humanae*: Translation, Commentary, and Reception History of the *Dicta Albini* (Ps.-Alcuin) and the *Dicta Candidi*." *Viator* 40 (2009): 1–34.

Le Bourdellès, H. *L'Aratus Latinus: Étude sur la culture et la langue latines dans le nord de la France au VIIIe siècle*. Lille: Université de Lille III, 1985.

Lee, Christina. "Disease." In *Oxford Handbook of Anglo-Saxon Archaeology*, ed. H. Hamerow, D. Hinton, and S. Crawford, 704–23. Oxford: Oxford University Press, 2011.

Lehmann, Paul. *Mittelalterliche Bibliothekskataloge Deutschlands und der Schweiz*, vol. 1: *Die Bistümer Konstanz und Chur*. Munich: C. H. Beck, 1918.

Le Jan, Régine. *Femmes, pouvoir et société dans le haut Moyen Âge*. Paris: Picard, 2001.

———. "The Multiple Identities of Dhuoda." In Corradini, *Ego Trouble*, 211–19.

Leonardi, C., F. Stella, and P. Stoppacci, eds. *Un ponte fra le culture: Studi medievistici di e per I Deug-Su*. Florence: SISMEL, 2009.

Levy, Ian. "Commentaries on the Pauline Epistles in the Carolingian Era." In *A Companion to St. Paul in the Middle Ages*, ed. S. Cartwright, 145–74. Leiden: Brill, 2013.

Lifshitz, Felice. *The Name of the Saint: The Martyrology of Jerome and Access to the Sacred in Francia, 627–827*. Notre Dame: University of Notre Dame Press, 2006.

———. *Religious Women in Early Carolingian Francia: A Study of Manuscript Transmission and Monastic Culture*. New York: Fordham University Press, 2014.

Liuzza, R. M. *Anglo-Saxon Prognostics: An Edition and Translation of Texts from London, British Library, MS Cotton Tiberius A.iii*. Cambridge: D. S. Brewer, 2011.

Lockett, Leslie. *Anglo-Saxon Psychologies in the Vernacular and Latin Traditions*. Toronto: University of Toronto Press, 2011.

Lohrmann, Dietrich. "Alcuins Korrespondenz mit Karl dem Großen über Kalender und Astronomie." In *Science in Western and Eastern Civilization in Carolingian Times*, ed. D. Lohrmann and P. Butzer, 79–114. Basel: Birkhäuser, 1993.

López Figueroa, Laura. "From Cassius Felix to *Tereoperica*: New Considerations on Indirect Tradition." In *'Greek' and 'Roman' in Latin Medical Texts*, ed. B. Maire, 383–401. Leiden: Brill, 2014.

*Das Lorscher Arzneibuch. Klostermedizin in der Karolingerzeit: Ausgewählte Texte und Beiträge*. Lorsch: Laurissa, 1990.

Lowe, E. A. *The Beneventan Script: A History of the South Italian Minuscule*, rev. ed. V. Brown. Rome: Edizioni di storia e letteratura, 1980.

———. *Codices latini antiquiores: A Palaeographical Guide to Latin Manuscripts Prior to the Ninth Century*, 11 vols. Oxford: Clarendon Press, 1934–1966.

———. *Scriptura Beneventana: Facsimiles of South Italian and Dalmatian Manuscripts from the Sixth to the Fourteenth Century*. Oxford: Clarendon Press, 1929.

Lozovsky, Natalia. "Perceptions of the Past in Ninth-Century Commentaries on Martianus Capella." In Teeuwen, *Carolingian Scholarship*, 123–45.

Luhtala, Anneli. "On Early Medieval Divisions of Knowledge." In Teeuwen, *Carolingian Scholarship*, 75–98.

Luscombe, David. *Medieval Thought*. Oxford: Oxford University Press, 1997.

MacKinney, Loren C. "'Dynamidia' in Medieval Medical Literature." *Isis* 24 (1936): 400–414.

———. *Early Medieval Medicine, With Special Reference to France and Chartres*. Baltimore: Johns Hopkins University Press, 1937.

———. "Medical Ethics and Etiquette in the Early Middle Ages: The Persistence of Hippocratic Ideals." *Bulletin of the History of Medicine* 26 (1952): 1–31.

———. "Tenth-Century Medicine as Seen in the *Historia* of Richer of Rheims." *Bulletin of the Institute of the History of Medicine* 2 (1934): 347–75.

———. "An Unpublished Treatise on Medicine and Magic from the Age of Charlemagne." *Speculum* 18 (1943): 494–96.

Mähl, Sibylle. *Quadriga virtutum: Die Kardinaltugenden in der Geistesgeschichte der Karolingerzeit*. Vienna: Böhlau, 1969.

Marenbon, John. *Early Medieval Philosophy (480–1150): An Introduction*. London: Routledge & K. Paul, 1983.

———. *From the Circle of Alcuin to the School of Auxerre: Logic, Theology, and Philosophy in the Early Middle Ages*. Cambridge: Cambridge University Press 1981.

———. "Platonism—A Doxographic Approach: The Early Middle Ages." In *The Platonic Tradition in the Middle Ages: A Doxographic Approach*, ed. S. Gersh and M. Hoenen, 67–89. Berlin: De Gruyter, 2002.

Margalhan-Ferrat, Corinne. "Le concept de 'ministerium' entre littérature spéculaire et législation carolingienne." In *Specula principum: Riflesso della realtà giuridica*, ed. A. de Benedictis with A. Pisapia, 121–57. Frankfurt am Main: Klostermann, 1999.

Markus, Robert. "From Caesarius to Boniface: Christianity and Paganism in Gaul." In *Le septième siècle: Changements et continuités*, ed. J. Fontaine and J. Hilgarth, 154–72. London: Warburg Institute, 1992.

Maskarinec, Maya. *City of Saints: Rebuilding Rome in the Early Middle Ages*. Philadelphia: University of Pennsylvania Press, 2018.

Mathisen, Ralph W. *Ecclesiastical Factionalism and Religious Controversy in Fifth-Century Gaul*. Washington, DC: Catholic University of America Press, 1989.

Mathon, Gérard. "L'anthropologie chrétienne en Occident de Saint Augustin à Jean Scot Érigène," 3 vols. Ph.D. Diss., Lille 1964.

———. "Les attitudes de quelques théologiens carolingiens en face des indéterminations augustiniennes en matière d'anthropologie." *Mélanges de science religieuse* 22 (1965): 35–44.

Matter, E. Ann. "Alcuin's Question-and-Answer Texts." *Rivista di storia della filsofia* 45 (1990): 645–56.

———. "A Carolingian Schoolbook? The Manuscript Tradition of Alcuin's *De fide* and Related Treatises." In *The Whole Book: Cultural Perspectives on the Medieval Miscellany*, ed. S. Nichols and S. Wenzel, 145–52. Ann Arbor: University of Michigan Press, 1996.

———. "The Soul of the Dog-Man: Ratramnus of Corbie Between Theology and Philosophy." *Rivista di storia della filosofia* 61 (2006): 43–53.

Mattern, Susan. *Galen and the Rhetoric of Healing*. Baltimore: Johns Hopkins University Press, 2008.

Mauss, Marcel. "Techniques of the Body." *Economy and Society* 2 (1973): 70–88.

Mavroudi, Maria. "Translations from Greek into Latin and Arabic During the Middle Ages: Searching for the Classical Tradition." *Speculum* 90 (2015): 28–59.

Mayeski, Marie Anne. *Dhuoda: Ninth Century Mother and Theologian*. Scranton: University of Scranton Press, 1995.

Mazzini, Innocenzo. "Cristianesimo e scienza pagana: Tracce di un conflitto nelle traduzioni latine di Ippocrate eseguite nei secoli V e VI." In *Saggi di storia del pensiero scientifico dedicati a Valerio Tonini*, ed. V. Cappelletti et al., 69–77. Rome: Jouvence, 1983.

———. "*De natura humana*: Estratti di un'antica traduzione latina parzialmente inedita del *Peri physios anthropou* di Polibo." *Romanobarbarica* 7 (1983): 255–71.

Mazzini, I., and N. Palmieri, "L'école médicale de Ravenne: Programmes et méthodes d'enseignement, langue, hommes." In *Les écoles médicales à Rome*, ed. P. Mudry and J. Pigeaud, 285–310. Geneva: Droz, 1991.

McCluskey, Stephen. *Astronomies and Cultures in Early Medieval Europe*. Cambridge: Cambridge University Press, 1998.

———. "Natural Knowledge in the Early Middle Ages." In *The Cambridge History of Science, vol. 2*, ed. D. Lindberg and M. Shank, 286–301. Cambridge: Cambridge University Press, 2013.

McCormick, Michael. *Origins of the European Economy: Communications and Commerce, A.D. 300–900.* Cambridge: Cambridge University Press, 2001.
McEnerney, John. "Precatio terrae and Precatio omnium herbarum." *Rheinisches Museum für Philologie* 126 (1983): 175–87.
McKitterick, Rosamond. *The Carolingians and the Written Word.* Cambridge: Cambridge University Press, 1989.
———. *Charlemagne: The Formation of a European Identity.* Cambridge: Cambridge University Press, 2008.
———. "Charles the Bald (823–877) and His Library: The Patronage of Learning," *English Historical Review* 95 (1980): 28–47.
———. *The Frankish Kingdoms Under the Carolingians, 751–987.* London: Longman, 1983.
———. *History and Memory in the Carolingian Word.* Cambridge: Cambridge University Press, 2004.
McLaughlin, Megan. *Consorting with Saints: Prayer for the Dead in Early Medieval France.* Ithaca: Cornell University Press, 1994.
McNeill, John. "Medicine for Sin as Prescribed in the Penitentials." *Church History* 1 (1932): 14–26.
McVaugh, Michael R. *Medicine Before the Plague: Practitioners and their Patients in the Crown of Aragon, 1285–1345.* Cambridge: Cambridge University Press, 1993.
———. *The Rational Surgery of the Middle Ages.* Florence: SISMEL, 2006.
Meaney, Audrey L. "The Practice of Medicine in England about the Year 1000." *SHM* 13 (2000): 221–37.
Meens, Rob. "The Historiography of Early Medieval Penance." In *A New History of Penance*, ed. A. Firey, 73–95. Leiden: Brill, 2008.
———. "Magic and the Early Medieval World View." In *The Community, the Family, and the Saint: Patterns of Power in Early Medieval Europe*, ed. J. Hill and M. Swan, 285–95. Turnhout: Brepols, 1998.
———. *Penance in Medieval Europe, 600–1200.* Cambridge: Cambridge University Press, 2014.
———. "Politics, Mirrors of Princes and the Bible: Sins, Kings and the Well-Being of the Realm." *EME* 7 (1998): 345–57.
———. "Pollution in the Early Middle Ages: The Case of the Food Regulations in Penitentials." *EME* 4 (1995): 3–19.
———. "The Rise and Fall of the Carolingians: Regino of Prüm and his Conception of the Carolingian Empire." In *Faire lien: Aristocratie, réseaux et échanges compétitifs*, ed. L. Jégou et al., 315–24. Paris: Publications de la Sorbonne, 2015.
Messing, Gordon. "Remarks on Anthimus, *De observatione ciborum.*" *Classical Philology* 37 (1942): 150–58.
Metzler, Irina. *Disability in Medieval Europe: Thinking about Physical Impairment during the High Middle Ages, c. 1100–1400.* New York: Routledge, 2006.
Migliorini, Paola. "Alcune denominazioni della malattia nella letteratura latina." In *Studi di lessicologia medica antica*, ed. S. Boscherini, 93–132. Bologna: Pàtron, 1993.
Milde, Wolfgang. *Der Bibliothekskatalog des Klosters Murbach aus dem 9. Jahrhundert.* Heidelberg: C. Winter, 1968.
Miller, Harold. "*Dynamis* and *Physis* in *On Ancient Medicine.*" *Transactions and Proceedings of the American Philological Association* 83 (1952): 184–97.

Molland, Einar. "*Ut sapiens medicus*: Medical Vocabulary in St. Benedict's *Regula Monachorum*." *Studia Monastica* 6 (1964): 273–98.
Montero Cartelle, Enrique. "La medicina y las Artes liberales según Isidoro de Sevilla." In Ferraces-Rodríguez, *Isidorus medicus*, 227–242.
Moore, Michael E. *A Sacred Kingdom: Bishops and the Rise of Frankish Kingship, 300–850*. Washington, DC: Catholic University of America Press, 2011.
Moreira, Isabel. *Heaven's Purge: Purgatory in Late Antiquity*. Oxford: Oxford University Press, 2010.
Mørland, Henning. *Die lateinischen Oribasiusübersetzungen*. Oslo: Brøgger, 1932.
Morris, Colin. *The Discovery of the Individual, 1050–1200*. New York: Harper & Row, 1972.
Morrison, Karl. "'Know Thyself': Music in the Carolingian Renaissance." In *Committenti e produzione artistico-letteraria nell'alto medioevo occidentale*, 369–479. Spoleto: Presso la sede del Centro, 1992.
———. "*Unum ex multis*: Hincmar of Rheims' Medical and Aesthetic Rationales for Unification." In *Nascita dell'Europa ed Europa carolingia: Un'equazione da verificare*, 2:583–712. Spoleto: Presso la sede del Centro, 1981.
Murray, Alexander, ed. *A Companion to Gregory of Tours*. Leiden: Brill, 2016.
Nauta, Lodi. "The Preexistence of the Soul in Medieval Thought." *Recherches de théologie ancienne et médiévale* 63 (1996): 93–135.
Nees, Lawrence. *Frankish Manuscripts: The Seventh to the Tenth Century*. A Survey of Manuscripts Illuminated in France 1. Turnhout: Brepols, forthcoming.
———.*The Gundohinus Gospels*. Cambridge, MA: Medieval Academy of America, 1987.
———. "The Illustrated Manuscript of the *Visio Baronti* [*Revelatio Baronti*] in St. Petersburg (Russian National Library, cod. lat. Oct.v.I.5)." In *Court Culture in the Early Middle Ages*, ed C. Cubitt, 91–128. Turnhout: Brepols, 2003.
———. *A Tainted Mantle: Hercules and the Classical Tradition at the Carolingian Court*. Philadelphia: University of Pennsylvania Press, 1991.
Nelson, Janet L. *Charles the Bald*. London: Longman, 1992.
———. *Courts, Elites, and Gendered Power in the Early Middle Ages: Charlemagne and Others*. Aldershot: Ashgate Variorum, 2007.
———. "Dhuoda." In Wormald, *Lay Intellectuals*, 106–20.
———. "England and the Continent in the Ninth Century: IV, Bodies and Minds." *Transactions of the Royal Historical Society* 15 (2005): 1–27.
———. "Gendering Courts in the Early Medieval West." In Brubaker and Smith, *Gender*, 185–97.
———. "Kingship and Empire." In *The Cambridge History of Medieval Political Thought, c. 350–c. 1450*, ed. J. Burns, 211–51. Cambridge: Cambridge University Press, 1998.
———. "Monks, Secular Men and Masculinity, c. 900." In *Masculinity in Medieval Europe*, ed. D. Hadley, 121–42. London: Longman, 1999.
———. "La mort de Charles le Chauve." *Médiévales* 31 (1996): 53–66.
———. "On the Limits of the Carolingian Renaissance." In *Renaissance and Renewal in Christian History*, ed. D. Baker, 51–69. Oxford: Blackwell, 1977.
———. "Organic Intellectuals in the Dark Ages?" *History Workshop Journal* 66 (2008): 1–17.
———. "The Voice of Charlemagne." In Nelson, *Courts*, XIII: 76–88.
Newfield, Timothy. "The Contours of Disease and Hunger in Carolingian and Early Ottonian Europe (c. 750–c. 950 CE)." Ph.D. Diss., McGill University, 2010.

Newhauser, Richard. "Preaching the 'Contrary Virtues.'" *Mediaeval Studies* 70 (2008): 135–62.

———. *The Treatise on Vices and Virtues in Latin and the Vernacular.* Turnhout: Brepols, 1993.

Newton, Francis. "Arabic Medicine and Other Arabic Cultural Influences in Southern Italy in the Time of Constantine Africanus (saec. XI)." In Glaze and Nance, *Between Text*, 25–56.

Niederer, Monica. *Der St. Galler Botanicus: Ein frühmittelalterliches Herbar: Kritische Edition, Übersetzung und Kommentar.* Bern: Peter Lang, 2005.

Nightingale, Andrea. *Once Out of Nature: Augustine on Time and the Body.* Chicago: University of Chicago Press, 2011.

Noble, Thomas F. X. "Carolingian Religion." *Church History* 84 (2015): 287–307.

———. *Images, Iconoclasm, and the Carolingians.* Philadelphia: University of Pennsylvania Press, 2009.

———. "Lupus of Ferrières in His Carolingian Context." In *After Rome's Fall: Narrators and Sources of Early Medieval History*, ed. A. Murray, 232–50. Toronto: University of Toronto Press, 1998.

———. "The Monastic Ideal as a Model for Empire: The Case of Louis the Pious." *Revue Bénédictine* 86 (1976): 235–50.

———. "Secular Sanctity: Forging an Ethos for the Carolingian Nobility." In Wormald, *Lay Intellectuals*, 8–36.

Noble, Thomas, and Julia Smith, eds. *The Cambridge History of Christianity*, vol. 3: *Early Medieval Christianities, c.600–c.1100.* Cambridge: Cambridge University Press, 2008.

Nordhagen, P. J. *The Frescoes of John VII (A.D. 705-707) in S. Maria Antiqua in Rome.* Rome: L'Erma, 1968.

Nugent, Patrick. "Bodily Effluvia and Liturgical Interruption in Medieval Miracle Stories." *History of Religions* 41 (2001): 49–70.

Nutton, Vivian. *Ancient Medicine.* New York: Routledge, 2004.

———. "*Archiatri* and the Medical Profession in Antiquity." *Papers of the British School at Rome* 45 (1977): 191–226.

———. "The Fortunes of Galen." In *The Cambridge Companion to Galen*, ed. R. Hankinson, 355–90. Cambridge: Cambridge University Press, 2008.

———. "From Galen to Alexander, Aspects of Medicine and Medical Practice in Late Antiquity." *Dumbarton Oaks Papers* 38 (1984): 1–14.

Obrist, Barbara. "Le diagramme isidorien des saisons: Son contenu physique et les représentations figuratives." *Mélanges de l'École française de Rome: Moyen Âge* 108 (1996): 95–164.

Ochsenbein, Peter, and Karl Schmuki, eds. *Studien zum St. Galler Klosterplan II.* St. Gall: Historischer Verein des Kantons St. Gallen, 2002.

Oliver, Lisi. *The Body Legal in Barbarian Law.* Toronto: University of Toronto Press, 2011.

Oliver, Lisi, and Maria Mahoney. "Episcopal Anatomies of the Early Middle Ages." In *Rhetorics of Bodily Disease and Health in Medieval and Early Modern England*, ed. J. Vaught, 25–42. Burlington: Ashgate, 2010.

Olsen, Glenn W. "One Heart and One Soul (Acts 4:32 and 34) in Dhuoda's *Manual*." *Church History* 61 (1992): 23–33.

Opsomer, Carmélia, and Robert Halleux. "La lettre d'Hippocrate à Mécène et la lettre d'Hippocrate à Antiochus." In *I testi di medicina latini antichi: Problemi filologici e storici*, ed. I. Mazzini and F. Fusco, 339–64. Rome: Bretschneider, 1985.

———. "Marcellus ou le mythe empirique." In *Les écoles médicales à Rome*, ed. P. Mundry and J. Pigeaud, 159–78. Geneva: Droz, 1991.

O'Sullivan, Sinéad. *Early Medieval Glosses on Prudentius'* Psychomachia: *The Weitz Tradition.* Leiden: Brill, 2004.

Otten, Willemien. "The Texture of Tradition: The Role of the Church Fathers in Carolingian Theology." In *The Reception of the Church Fathers in the West: From the Carolingians to the Maurists*, ed. I. Backus, 1:3–51. Leiden: Brill, 1997.

Palazzo, Eric. "Art, Liturgy, and the Five Senses in the Early Middle Ages." *Viator* 41 (2010): 25–56.

Palmer, James T. "Calculating Time and the End of Time in the Carolingian World, c. 740–820." *English Historical Review* 126 (2011): 1307–31.

———. "Climates of Crisis: Apocalypse, Nature, and Rhetoric in the Early Medieval World," *Viator* 48 (2017): 1–20.

———. "Defining Paganism in the Carolingian World." *EME* 15 (2007): 402–25.

Palmieri, Nicoletta. "Nouvelles remarques sur les commentaires à Galien de l'école médicale de Ravenne." In *Docente natura: Mélanges de médecine ancienne et médiévale offerts à Guy Sabbah*, ed. A. Debru and N. Palmieri, 209–46. Saint-Étienne: Université de Saint-Étienne, 2001.

Paolucci, Paola. *Profilo di una dietetica tardoantica: Saggio sull'Epistula Anthimi de observatione ciborum ad Theodoricum regem Francorum.* Naples: Edizioni scientifiche italiane, 2002.

Park, Katharine. *Secrets of Women: Gender, Generation, and the Origins of Human Dissection.* New York: Zone Books, 2006.

Patterson, David. "*Adversus paganos*: Disaster, Dragons, and Episcopal Authority in Gregory of Tours." *Comitatus* 44 (2013): 1–28.

Patzold, Steffen. *Episcopus: Wissen über Bischöfe im Frankenreich des späten 8. bis frühen 10. Jahrhunderts.* Ostfildern: Thorbecke, 2008.

Paxton, Frederick S. "*Bonus liber*: A Late Carolingian Clerical Manual from Lorsch (Biblioteca Vaticana MS Pal. lat. 485)." In *The Two Laws: Studies in Medieval Legal History Dedicated to Stephan Kuttner*, ed. L. Mayali and S. Tibbetts, 1–30. Washington, DC: Catholic University of America Press, 1990.

———. *Christianizing Death: The Creation of a Ritual Process in Early Medieval Europe.* Ithaca: Cornell University Press, 1990.

———. "Curing Bodies—Curing Souls: Hrabanus Maurus, Medical Education, and the Clergy in Ninth-Century Francia." *JHMAS* 50 (1995): 230–52.

———. "*Signa Mortifera*: Death and Prognostication in Early Medieval Monastic Medicine." *Bulletin of the History of Medicine* 67 (1993): 631–50.

Pease, Arthur. "Medical Allusions in the Works of St. Jerome." *Harvard Studies in Classical Philology* 25 (1914): 73–86.

Pellegrin, Pierre. "L'imaginaire de la fièvre dans la médecine antique." *History and Philosophy of the Life Sciences* 10 (1988): 109–20.

Perkins, Judith. *The Suffering Self: Pain and Narrative Representation in the Early Christian Era.* New York: Routledge, 1995.

Peters, Edward. *The Shadow King: Rex inutilis in Medieval Law and Literature, 751–1327.* New Haven: Yale University Press, 1970.

Peterson, Donald W. "Galen's *Therapeutics to Glaucon* and Its Early Commentaries." Ph.D. Diss., Johns Hopkins University, 1974.

Petit, Caroline. "Galen, Pharmacology and the Boundaries of Medicine: A Reassessment." In *Collecting Recipes: Byzantine & Jewish Pharmacology in Dialogue*, ed. L. Lehmhaus and M. Martelli, 51–79. Berlin: De Gruyter, 2017.

Pezé, Warren. "Autorité royale et controverses théologiques sous Charles le Chauve (840–877)." *Hypothèses* 1 (2011): 209–24.

———. "Débat doctrinal et genre littéraire à l'époque carolingienne: Les opuscules théologiques de Gottschalk d'Orbais." *Revue de l'histoire des religions* 235 (2017): 25–72.

———. "Doctrinal Debate and Social Control in the Carolingian Age: The Predestination Controversy (840s–60s)." *EME* 25 (2017): 85–101.

———. *Le virus de l'erreur: La controverse carolingienne sur la double prédestination.* Turnhout: Brepols, 2017.

Phelan, Owen M. *The Formation of Christian Europe: The Carolingians, Baptism, and the Imperium Christianum.* Oxford: Oxford University Press, 2014.

———. "Horizontal and Vertical Theologies: 'Sacraments' in the Works of Paschasius Radbertus and Ratramnus of Corbie." *Harvard Theological Review* 103 (2010): 271–89.

———. "New Insights, Old Texts: Clerical Formation and the Carolingian Renewal in Hrabanus Maurus." *Traditio* 71 (2016): 63–89.

Pigeaud, Alfrieda, and Jackie Pigeaud, eds. *Les textes médicaux latins comme littérature.* Nantes: Université de Nantes, 2000.

Pilsworth, Clare. "Could You Just Sign This for Me, John? Doctors, Charters and Occupational Identity in Early Medieval Northern and Central Italy." *EME* 17 (2009): 363–88.

———. *Healthcare in Early Medieval Northern Italy: More to Life than Leeches.* Turnhout: Brepols, 2014.

———. "Medicine and Hagiography in Italy, c. 800–c. 1000." *SHM* 13 (2000): 253–64.

Platte, Adelheid. "Der Weg des Arzneibuchs von Lorsch nach Bamberg." In *Das Lorscher Arzneibuch*, 23–27.

Pohl, Walter. "Introduction: Ego Trouble?" In Corradini, *Ego Trouble*, 9–22.

Polanichka, Dana M. "Maternity and Spiritual Progression in Dhuoda's *Liber manualis* (840s C.E.)." *Mediaevalia* 41 (2020): 7–41.

———. "'Quasi per speculum': Vision, Viligance and the Natural World in Dhuoda's *Liber manualis*." *Journal of Medieval History* 46 (2020): 1–22.

Polanichka, Dana, and Alex Cilley. "The Very Personal History of Nithard: Family and Honour in the Carolingian World." *EME* 22 (2014): 171–200.

Pollman, Karla, and Mark Vessey, eds. *Augustine and the Disciplines from Cassiciacum to Confessions.* Oxford: Oxford University Press, 2005.

Pomata, Gianna. *Contracting a Cure: Patients, Healers, and the Law in Early Modern Bologna.* Baltimore: Johns Hopkins University Press, 1998.

Ponesse, Matthew. "Smaragdus of St Mihiel and the Carolingian Monastic Reform." *Revue Bénédictine* 116 (2006): 367–92.

Pormann, Peter, and Emilie Savage-Smith. *Medieval Islamic Medicine.* Washington, DC: Georgetown University Press, 2007.

Poschmann, Bernhard. *Penance and the Anointing of the Sick.* Trans. F. Courtney. New York: Herder and Herder, 1964.

Pouchelle, Marie-Christine. *The Body and Surgery in the Middle Ages*. Trans. R. Morris. Cambridge: Polity Press, 1990.

Powell, Owen. *Galen: On the Properties of Foodstuffs (De alimentorum facultatibus)*. Cambridge: Cambridge University Press, 2003.

Probst, Otto. "Isidors Schrift *De medicina*." *AGM* 8 (1914): 22–38.

Pucci Donati, Francesca. *Dieta, salute, calendari: Dal regime stagionale antico ai regimina mensium medievali*. Spoleto: Centro italiano di studi sull'alto Medioevo, 2007.

Raaijmakers, Janneke. *Making of the Monastic Community of Fulda, c. 744–c. 900*. Cambridge: Cambridge University Press, 2012.

Ramírez-Weaver, Eric. *A Saving Science: Capturing the Heavens in Carolingian Manuscripts*. University Park: Pennsylvania State University Press, 2017.

Rankin, Alisha. *Panaceia's Daughters: Noblewomen as Healers in Early Modern Germany*. Chicago: University of Chicago Press, 2013.

Rapp, Claudia. "Holy Texts, Holy Men, and Holy Scribes: Aspects of Scriptural Holiness in Late Antiquity." In *The Early Christian Book*, ed. W. Klingshirn and L. Safran, 194–222. Washington, DC: Catholic University of America Press, 2007.

Reid, Shelley. "'The First Dispensation of Christ Is Medicinal': Augustine and Roman Medical Culture." Ph.D. Diss., University of British Columbia, 2008.

Reimitz, Helmut. "Conversion and Control: The Establishment of Liturgical Frontiers in Carolingian Pannonia." In *The Transformation of Frontiers from Late Antiquity to the Carolingians*, ed. W. Pohl, I. Wood, and H. Reimitz, 189–207. Leiden: Brill, 2001.

———. *History, Frankish Identity and the Framing of Western Ethnicity, 550–850*. Cambridge: Cambridge University Press, 2015.

———. "Transformations of Late Antiquity: The Writing and Re-writing of Church History at the Monastery of Lorsch, c. 800." In Gantner, *Resources of the Past*, 262–82.

Rembold, Ingrid. *Conquest and Christianization: Saxony and the Carolingian World, 772–888*. Cambridge: Cambridge University Press, 2018.

Riché, Pierre. "Les bibliothèques de trois aristocrates laïcs carolingiens." *Le Moyen Âge* 69 (1963): 87–104.

———. "La magie à l'époque carolingienne." *Comptes-rendus de l'Académie des inscriptions et belles-lettres* 1 (1973): 127–38.

Riddle, John M. "Pseudo-Dioscorides' *Ex herbis femininis* and Early Medieval Medical Botany." *Journal of the History of Biology* 14 (1981): 43–81.

———. "Theory and Practice in Medieval Medicine." *Viator* 5 (1974): 157–84.

Rider, Catherine. *Magic and Impotence in the Middle Ages*. Oxford: Oxford University Press, 2006.

Robinson, I. S. "Church and Papacy." In *The Cambridge History of Medieval Political Thought, c.350–c. 1450*, ed. J. Burns, 252–305. Cambridge: Cambridge University Press, 1988.

Rochais, H.-M. "Le *Liber de virtutibus et vitiis* d'Alcuin: Note pour l'étude des sources." *Revue Mabillon* 41 (1951): 77–86.

Romig, Andrew J. *Be a Perfect Man: Christian Masculinity and the Carolingian Aristocracy*. Philadelphia: University of Pennsylvania Press, 2017.

Rose, Els. "*Emendatio* and *effectus* in Frankish Prayer Traditions." In *Religious Franks: Religion and Power in the Frankish Kingdoms*, ed. R. Meens et al., 128–47. Manchester: Manchester University Press, 2016.

Rosenwein, Barbara H. *Generations of Feeling: A History of Emotions, 600–1700*. Cambridge: Cambridge University Press, 2016.

———. "Rereading *Askese und Laster*: The Case of Alcuin." In *Urkunden-Schriften-Lebensordnungen: Neue Beiträge zur Mediävistik*, ed. A. Schwarcz and K. Kaska, 77–90. Vienna: Böhlau, 2015.

———. "Y avait-il un 'moi' au haut Moyen Âge?" *Revue Historique* 307 (2005): 31–52.

Rouche, Michel. "Miroirs des princes ou miroir du clergé?" In *Committenti e produzione artistico-letteraria nell'alto medioevo occidentale*, 1:341–64. Spoleto: Presso la sede del Centro, 1992.

Roumy, Franck "L'origine et la diffusion de l'adage canonique *Necessitas non habet legem* (VIIIe–XIIIe s.)." In *Medieval Church Law and the Origins of the Western Legal Tradition*, ed. W. Müller and M. Sommar, 301–19. Washington, DC: Catholic University of America Press, 2006.

Rouse, R. H. "Quintus Serenus." In *Texts and Transmission: A Survey of the Latin Classics*, ed. L.D. Reynolds, 381–85. Oxford: Clarendon Press, 1983.

Rousselle, Aline. "Abstinence et continence dans les monastères de Gaule méridionale à la fin de l'Antiquité et au début du Moyen Âge: Étude d'un régime alimentaire et de sa fonction." In *Hommage à André Dupont*, 239–54. Montpellier: Fédération historique du Languedoc méditerranéen et du Roussillon, 1974.

———. *Croire et guérir: La foi en Gaule dans l'antiquité tardive*. Paris: Fayard, 1990.

Rubenson, Samuel. "Anthony and Pythagoras: A Reappraisal of the Appropriation of Classical Biography in Athanasius' *Vita Antonii*." In *Beyond Reception: Mutual Influences between Antique Religion, Judaism, and Early Christianity*, ed. D. Brakke et al., 191–208. Frankfurt am Main: Peter Lang, 2006.

Sabbah, Guy, Pierre-Paul Corsetti, and Klaus-Dietrich Fischer. *Bibliographie des textes médicaux latins: Antiquité et haut Moyen Âge*. Saint-Étienne: Université de Saint-Étienne, 1987.

Sălăvăstru, Andrei C. "The Biblical Origins of the 'Body Politic': Saint Paul's Corporal Analogies in Western European Political Thought from the Twelfth to the Early Seventeenth Centuries." *Biblicum Jassyense* 6 (2015): 19–32.

Saliba, George. *Islamic Science and the Making of the European Renaissance*. Cambridge, MA: MIT Press, 2007.

Sanderson, Warren. "The Plan of St. Gall Reconsidered." *Speculum* 60, no. 3. (1985): 615–32.

Santini, C., N. Scivoletto, and L. Zurli, eds. *Prefazioni, prologhi, proemi di opere tecnico-scientifiche latine*, 3 vols. Rome: Herder, 1990–1998.

Savigni, Raffaele. "Esegesi medievale ed antropologia biblica: L'interpretazione di Genesi 1–3 nei commentari carolingi ed i suoi fondamenti patristici." *Annali di storia dell'esegesi* 10 (1993): 571–614.

———. "L'immagine del santo fondatore nelle *Vitae* di Benedetto di Aniane e di Adalardo di Corbie (secolo IX)." In *Sant'Anselmo di Nonantola e i santi fondatori nella tradizione monastica tra Oriente e Occidente*, ed. R. Fangarezzi, P. Golinelli, and A. Orselli, 109–80. Rome: Viella, 2006.

———. "Les laïcs dans l'ecclésiologie carolingienne: Normes statutaires et idéal de 'conversion.'" In *Guerriers et moines: Conversion et sainteté aristocratiques dans l'occident médiéval (IXe-XIIe siècle)*, ed. M. Lauwers, 41–92. Antibes: APDCA, 2002.

Scheck, Helene. *Reform and Resistance: Formations of Female Subjectivity in Early Medieval Ecclesiastical Culture*. Albany: SUNY Press, 2008.

Schmidt, A. Jordan. *Wisdom, Cosmos, and Cultus in the Book of Sirach*. Berlin: De Gruyter, 2019.

Schmidt, Paul G. "Karolingische Autographen." In *Gli autografi medievali: Problemi paleografici e filologici*, ed. P. Chiesa and L. Pinelli, 137–48. Spoleto: Centro italiano di studi sull'alto Medioevo, 1994.

Schmitt, Charles, and Dilwyn Knox. *Pseudo-Aristoteles Latinus: A Guide to Latin Works Falsely Attributed to Aristotle Before 1500*. London: Warburg Institute, 1985.

Scholz, Sebastian. "Bemerkungen zur Bildungsentwicklung im frühen Mittelalter: Zusammenfassung." In Becker, *Karolingische Klöster*, 275–90.

Schöner, Erich. *Das Viererschema in der antiken Humoralpathologie*. Wiesbaden: Steiner, 1964.

Schröder, Isolde. "Zur Überlieferung von *De institutione laicali* des Jonas von Orléans." *Deutsches Archiv für Erforschung des Mittelalters* 44 (1988): 83–97.

Sconocchia, Sergio. "La lettera di Diocle ad Antigono e le sue traduzioni latine." In Santini, *Prefazioni*, 2:113–32.

Sedlmeier, Franz. *Die laienparänetischen Schriften der Karolingerzeit: Untersuchungen zu ausgewählten Texten des Paulinus von Aquileia, Alkuins, Jonas' von Orleans, Dhuodas und Hinkmars von Reims*. Neuried: Ars Una, 2000.

Segoloni, Maria Paola. "Il *prologus* della *Medicina Plinii*." In Santini, *Prefazioni*, 1:361–66.

Serralda, Vincent. *La philosophie de la personne chez Alcuin*. Paris: Nouvelles éditions latines, 1978.

Shanzer, Danuta. "Augustine's Disciplines: *Silent diutius musae Varronis*?" In Pollman, *Augustine*, 69–112.

Shaw, Teresa M. *The Burden of the Flesh: Fasting and Sexuality in Early Christianity*. Minneapolis: Fortress, 1998.

Shimahara, Sumi. *Haymon d'Auxerre: Exégète carolingien*. Turnhout: Brepols, 2013.

Siegel, Rudolph. *Galen's System of Physiology and Medicine*. New York: Karger, 1968.

Sigerist, Henry E. "The Latin Medical Literature of the Early Middle Ages." *JHMAS* 13 (1958): 127–46.

———. "The *Sphere of Life and Death* in Early Mediaeval Manuscripts." *Bulletin of the History of Medicine* 11 (1942): 292–303.

Siraisi, Nancy G. *Medieval & Early Renaissance Medicine: An Introduction to Knowledge and Practice*. Chicago: University of Chicago Press, 1990.

Skinner, Mary S. "Lay Sanctity and Church Reform in Early Medieval France." In *Lay Sanctity, Medieval and Modern: A Search for Models*, ed. A. Astell, 27–45. Notre Dame: University of Notre Dame Press, 2000.

Skinner, Patricia. *Health and Medicine in Early Medieval Southern Italy*. Leiden: Brill, 1997.

———. *Living with Disfigurement in Early Medieval Europe*. New York: Palgrave Macmillan, 2017.

Slaveva-Griffin, Svetla. "Byzantine Medical Encyclopedias and Education." In Keyser, *Oxford Handbook*, 965–86.

Smith, Julia M. H. "Einhard: The Sinner and the Saints." *Transactions of the Royal Historical Society* 13 (2003): 55–77.

———. "'Emending Evil Ways and Praising God's Omnipotence': Einhard and the Uses of Roman Martyrs." In *Conversion in Late Antiquity and the Early Middle Ages: Seeing and Believing*, ed. K. Mills and A. Grafton, 189–223. Rochester: University of Rochester Press, 2003.

———. "Gender and Ideology in the Early Middle Ages." *Studies in Church History* 34 (1998): 51–73.
———. "Old Saints, New Cults: Roman Relics in Carolingian Francia." In *Early Medieval Rome and the Christian West*, ed. J. Smith, 317–39. Leiden: Brill, 2000.
———. "Portable Christianity: Relics in the Medieval West (c. 700–1200)." *Proceedings of the British Academy* 181 (2012): 143–67.
———. *Province and Empire: Brittany and the Carolingians*. Cambridge: Cambridge University Press, 1992.
———. "Saints and Their Cults." In Noble and Smith, *Cambridge History of Christianity*, 581–605.
Sot, Michel. "Concordances et discordances entre culture des élites laïques et culture des élites cléricales à l'époque carolingienne: Jonas d'Orléans et Dhuoda." In *La culture du haut Moyen Âge: Une question d'élites?* ed. F. Bougard, R. Le Jan, and R. McKitterick, 341–62. Turnhout: Brepols, 2009.
Souter, Alexander. *A Glossary of Later Latin to 600 A.D.* Oxford: Clarendon Press, 1949.
Squatriti, Paolo. *Landscape and Change in Early Medieval Italy: Chestnuts, Economy, and Culture*. Cambridge: Cambridge University Press, 2013.
Stafford, Pauline. *Queens, Concubines, and Dowagers: The King's Wife in the Early Middle Ages*. Athens: University of Georgia Press, 1983.
Stahl, William H. *Martianus Capella and the Seven Liberal Arts*, vol. 1. New York: Columbia University Press, 1971.
Stannard, Jerry. "Marcellus of Bordeaux and the Beginnings of Medieval Materia Medica." *Pharmacy in History* 15 (1973): 47–53.
Steckel, Sita. *Kulturen des Lehrens im Früh- und Hochmittelalter: Autorität, Wissenskonzepte und Netzwerke von Gelehrten*. Cologne: Böhlau, 2011.
Steele, Robert. "Dies Aegyptiaci." *Proceedings of the Royal Society of Medicine* 12 (1919): 108–21.
Stevens, Wesley M. "Computus-Handschriften Walahfrid Strabos." In Stevens, *Cycles*, 363–81.
———. *Cycles of Time and Scientific Learning in Medieval Europe*. Aldershot: Variorum, 1995.
———. "Walahfrid Strabo–A Student at Fulda." In Stevens, *Cycles*, 13–20.
Stewart, Keith. *Galen's Theory of Black Bile: Hippocratic Tradition, Manipulation, Innovation*. Leiden: Brill, 2018.
Stofferahn, Steven. "The Many Faces in Dhuoda's Mirror: The *Liber manualis* and a Century of Scholarship." *Magistra* 4 (1998): 89–134.
Stoffler, Hans-Dieter. *Der* Hortulus *des Walahfrid Strabo: Aus dem Kräutergarten des Klosters Reichenau*. Sigmaringen: Thorbecke, 1978.
Stok, Fabio. "Fonte e datazione dell'*Epistola* di Vindiciano a Pentadio." *Technai* 3 (2012): 137–43.
———. "Il prologo del *De physiognomonia*." In Santini, *Prefazioni*, 2:499–517.
Stoll, Ulrich. "Das *Lorscher Arzneibuch*: Ein Arbeitsbericht." In Keil and Schnitzer, *Das Lorscher Arzneibuch*, 29–59.
Stone, Rachel. *Morality and Masculinity in the Carolingian Empire*. Cambridge: Cambridge University Press, 2012.
———. "The Rise and Fall of the Lay Moral Elite in Carolingian Francia." In *La culture du haut Moyen Âge: Une question d'élites?* ed. F. Bougard, R. Le Jan, and R. McKitterick, 363–76. Turnhout: Brepols, 2009.

Straw, Carole. *Gregory the Great: Perfection in Imperfection.* Berkeley: University of California Press, 1988.

Sudhoff, Karl. "Die Verse Isidors von Sevilla auf dem Schrank des medizinischen Werke seiner Bibliothek." *Mitteilungen zur Geschichte der Medizin und der Naturwissenschaften* 15 (1916): 200–204.

———. "Eine Verteidigung der Heilkunde aus den Zeiten der 'Mönchsmedizin.'" *AGM* 7 (1913): 223–37.

Sullivan, Richard E. "The Context of Cultural Activity in the Carolingian Age." In *The Gentle Voices of Teachers: Aspects of Learning in the Carolingian Age*, 51–105. Columbus: Ohio State University Press, 1995.

Szarmach, Paul E. "The Latin Tradition of Alcuin's *Liber de virtutibus et vitiis*, cap. xxvii-xxxv, with special reference to Vercelli Homily xx." *Mediaevalia* 12 (1986): 13–41.

———. "A Preface, Mainly Textual, to Alcuin's *De ratione animae*." In *The Man of Many Devices, Who Wandered Full Many Ways*, ed. B. Nagy and M. Sebők, 397–408. Budapest: Central European University Press, 1999.

———. "A Preliminary Handlist of Manuscripts Containing Alcuin's *Liber de virtutibus et vitiis*." *Manuscripta* 25 (1981): 131–40.

Teeuwen, Mariken. "Seduced by Pagan Poets and Philosophers: Suspicious Learning in the Early Middle Ages." In *Limits to Learning: The Transfer of Encyclopaedic Knowledge in the Early Middle Ages*, ed. C. Giliberto and L. Teresi, 63–80. Leuven: Peeters, 2013.

Teeuwen, Mariken, and Sinéad O'Sullivan, eds. *Carolingian Scholarship and Martianus Capella: Ninth-Century Commentary Traditions on* De nuptiis *in Context*. Turnhout: Brepols, 2011.

Temkin, Owsei. *Galenism: Rise and Decline of a Medical Philosophy.* Ithaca: Cornell University Press, 1973.

———. *Hippocrates in a World of Pagans and Christians.* Baltimore: Johns Hopkins University Press, 1991.

Thorndike, Lynn. *A History of Magic and Experimental Science*, vol. 1. New York: Macmillan, 1923.

Timmermann, Josh. "Sharers in the Contemplative Virtue: Julianus Pomerius's Carolingian Audience." *Comitatus* 45 (2014): 1–44.

Tolomio, Ilario, trans. *L'anima dell'uomo: Trattati sull'anima dal V al IX secolo.* Milan: Rusconi, 1979.

Tor, D. G., ed. *The 'Abbasid and Carolingian Empires: Comparative Studies in Civilizational Formation.* Leiden: Brill, 2017.

Tormey, Warren. "Treating the Condition of 'Evil' in the Anglo-Saxon Herbals." In *Bodily and Spiritual Hygiene in Medieval and Early Modern Literature*, ed. A. Classen, 88–113. Berlin: De Gruyter, 2017.

Totelin, Laurence. "Old Recipes, New Practice? The Latin Adaptations of the Hippocratic *Gynaecological Treatises*." *SHM* 24 (2011): 74–91.

Touati, François-Olivier. "Raban Maur et la médecine carolingienne." In *Raban Maur et son temps*, ed. P. Depreux et al., 173–202. Turnhout: Brepols, 2010.

Toubert, Pierre. "La doctrine gélasienne des deux pouvoirs: Propositions en vue d'une révision." In *Studi in onore di Giosuè Musca*, ed. C. Fonseca and V. Sivo, 519–40. Bari: Dedalo, 2000.

———. "La théorie du mariage chez les moralistes carolingiens." In *Il matrimonio nella societá altomedievale*, 233–85. Spoleto: Presso la sede del Centro, 1977.

Touwaide, Alain. "The Legacy of Classical Antiquity in Byzantium and the West." In *Health and Healing from the Medieval Garden*, ed. P. Dendle and A. Touwaide, 15–28. Woodbridge: Boydell, 2008.

Tuten, Belle. "The *Necessitas naturae* and Monastic Hygiene." In *Bodily and Spiritual Hygiene in Medieval and Early Modern Literature*, ed. A. Classen, 129–47. Berlin: De Gruyter, 2017.

Ubl, Karl. "Gab es das Leges-Skriptorium Ludwigs des Frommen?" *Deutsches Archiv für Erforschung des Mittelalters* 70 (2014): 43–65.

van Arsdall, Anne. *Medieval Herbal Remedies: The Old English Herbarium and Anglo-Saxon Medicine*. New York: Routledge, 2002.

Van Dam, Raymond. *Leadership and Community in Late Antique Gaul*. Berkeley: University of California Press, 1985.

———. *Saints and their Miracles in Late Antique Gaul*. Princeton: Princeton University Press, 1993.

van der Eijk, Philip, ed. *Diocles of Carystus: A Collection of the Fragments with Translation and Commentary*, vol. 2. Leiden: Brill, 2001.

———. "The Heart, the Brain, the Blood and the *pneuma*: Hippocrates, Diocles and Aristotle on the Location of Cognitive Processes." In *Medicine and Philosophy in Classical Antiquity: Doctors and Philosophers on Nature, Soul, Health and Disease*, 119–36. Cambridge: Cambridge University Press, 2005.

van Renswoude, Irene. "The Art of Disputation: Dialogue, Dialectic and Debate Around 800." *EME* 25 (2017): 38–53.

———. *The Rhetoric of Free Speech in Late Antiquity and the Early Middle Ages*. Cambridge: Cambridge University Press, 2019.

van Rhijn, Carine. "Introduction." In *Rethinking the Carolingian Reform*, ed. C. van Rhijn, I. Rembold, and A. Westwell. Manchester: Manchester University Press, forthcoming.

———. "The Local Church, Priests' Handbooks and Pastoral Care in the Carolingian Period." In *Chiese locali e chiese regionali nell'alto medioevo*, 689–706. Spoleto: Centro italiano di studi sull'alto Medioevo, 2014.

———. "Pastoral Care and Prognostics in the Carolingian Period: The Case of El Escorial, Real Biblioteca di San Lorenzo, MS L III 8." *Revue Bénédictine* 127 (2017): 272–97.

———. *Shepherds of the Lord: Priests and Episcopal Statutes in the Carolingian Period*. Turnhout: Brepols, 2007.

Vázquez Buján, Manuel E. "Codicologie et histoire des textes médicaux: À propros du codex Paris, Bibliothèque nationale, latin 11219." In *I testi di medicina latini antichi: Problemi filologici e storici*, ed. I. Mazzini and F. Fusco, 75–88. Rome: Bretschneider, 1985.

———. "Problemas generales de las antiguas traducciones médicas latinas." *Studi medievali* 25 (1984): 641–80.

———. "Vindiciano y el tratado *De natura generis humani*." *Dynamis* 2 (1982): 25–56.

Verbaal, Wim. "Eros im Kräutergarten: Eine spirituell-pädagogische Lektüre von Walahfrid Strabos *Hortulus*." *Sacris erudiri* 43 (2004): 131–234.

Vernet, André. "Un nouveau manuscrit du *Manuel* de Dhuoda (Barcelone, Biblioteca central, 569)." *Bibliothèque de l'École des chartes* 114 (1956): 18–44.

Veronese, Francesco. "Contextualizing Marriage: Conjugality and Christian Life in Jonas of Orléans' *De institutione laicali.*" *EME* 23 (2015): 436–56.

Vezin, Jean. "Le point d'interrogation: Un élément de datation et de localisation des manuscrits. L'exemple de Saint-Denis au IXe siècle." *Scriptorium* 34 (1980): 181–96.

Voigts, Linda. "Anglo-Saxon Plant Remedies and the Anglo-Saxons." *Isis* 70 (1979): 250–68.

Voigts, Linda, and Michael McVaugh. *A Latin Technical Phlebotomy and Its Middle English Translation.* Philadelphia: American Philosophical Society, 1984.

von Euw, Anton. *St. Galler Buchkunst vom 8. bis zum Ende des 11. Jahrhunderts*, 2 vols. St. Gall: Verlag am Klosterhof, 2008.

von Staden, Heinrich. "Body, Soul, and Nerves: Epicurus, Herophilus, Erasistratus, the Stoics, and Galen." In *Psyche and Soma: Physicians and Metaphysicians on the Mind-Body Problem from Antiquity to Enlightenment*, ed. J. Wright and P. Potter, 79–116. Oxford: Clarendon Press, 2000.

———. "'In a Pure and Holy Way': Personal and Professional Conduct in the Hippocratic Oath?" *JHMAS* 51 (1996): 404–37.

———. "Liminal Perils: Early Roman Receptions of Greek Medicine." In *Tradition, Transmission, Transformation*, ed. F. Ragep and S. Ragep, 369–418. Leiden: Brill, 1996.

———. "Physis and Technē in Greek Medicine." In *The Artificial and the Natural: An Evolving Polarity*, ed. B. Bensaude-Vincent and W. Newman, 21–49. Cambridge, MA: MIT Press, 2007.

Wagner, David. "The Seven Liberal Arts and Classical Scholarship." In *The Seven Liberal Arts in the Middle Ages*, ed. D. Wagner, 1–31. Bloomington: Indiana University Press, 1983.

Wallach, Luitpold. "Alcuin on Virtues and Vices: A Manual for a Carolingian Soldier." *Harvard Theological Review* 48 (1955): 175–95.

Wallis, Faith. "Bede and Science." In DeGregorio, *Cambridge Companion*, 113–26.

———. "The Experience of the Book: Manuscripts, Texts, and the Role of Epistemology in Early Medieval Medicine." In *Knowledge and the Scholarly Medical Traditions*, ed. D. Bates, 101–26. Cambridge: Cambridge University Press, 1995.

———. "Images of Order in the Medieval Computus." In *Ideas of Order in the Middle Ages*, ed. W. Ginsberg, 45–67. Binghamton: SUNY Press, 1990.

———. "Medicine in Medieval Calendar Manuscripts." In *Manuscript Sources of Medieval Medicine: A Book of Essays*, ed. M. Schleissner, 105–43. New York: Garland, 1995.

———. "Signs and Senses: Diagnosis and Prognosis in Early Medieval Pulse and Urine Texts." *SHM* 13 (2000): 265–78.

Ward, Elizabeth F. "Agobard of Lyons and Paschasius Radbertus as Critics of the Empress Judith." *Studies in Church History* 27 (1990): 15–25.

Wehlau, Ruth. "Literal and Symbolic: The Language of Asceticism in the Two Lives of St. Radegund." *Florilegium* 19 (2002): 75–89.

Weißer, Christoph. *Studien zum mittelalterlichen Krankheitslunar: Ein Beitrag zur Geschichte laienastrologischer Fachprosa.* Pattensen: H. Wellm, 1982.

Wemple, Suzanne. "Claudius of Turin's Organic Metaphor or the Carolingian Doctrine of Corporations." *Speculum* 49 (1974): 222–37.

Westgard, Joshua. "Bede and the Continent in the Carolingian Age and Beyond." In DeGregorio, *Cambridge Companion*, 201–15.

Whitney, Elspeth. *Paradise Restored: The Mechanical Arts from Antiquity Through the Thirteenth Century.* Philadelphia: American Philosophical Society, 1990.

Wickersheimer, Ernest. "Les écrits médicaux attribués à saint Luc." In *Mélanges Alexandre Koyré*, 1:613–18. Paris: Hermann, 1964.

———. "Figures médico-astrologiques des IXe, Xe, et XIe siècles." *Janus* 19 (1914): 157–77.

———. "Un manuscrit médical de l'époque carolingienne ayant appartenu à l'abbaye d'Echternach." *T'Hémecht* 6 (1953): 173–89.

———. *Les manuscrits latins de médecine du haut Moyen Âge dans les bibliothèques de France.* Paris: Éditions du Centre national de la recherche scientifique, 1966.

———. "Une vie des saints Côme et Damien dans un manuscrit médical du IXe siècle, suivie d'une recette de collyre attribuée à la mère des deux saints." *Centaurus* 1 (1950): 38–42.

Wiedemann, Walter. "Untersuchungen zu dem frühmittelalterlichen medizinischen Briefbuch des Codex Bruxellensis 3701–15." Med. Diss., Freie Universität Berlin, 1976.

Williams, James. "Working for Reform: *Acedia*, Benedict of Aniane and the Transformation of Working Culture in Carolingian Monasticism." In *Sin in Medieval and Early Modern Culture*, ed. R. Newhauser and S. Ridyard, 19–42. Rochester: York Medieval Press, 2012.

Winter, Maria. "Corps, maladie et pouvoir dans l'époque carolingienne." Ph.D. Diss., Paris EHESS, 2003.

Wittern, Renate. "Die Wechselfieber bei Galen." *History and Philosophy of the Life Sciences* 11 (1989): 3–22.

Wood, Ian. "Categorising the *cynocephali*." In Corradini, *Ego Trouble*, 125–36.

———. *The Missionary Life: Saints and the Evangelisation of Europe, 400–1050.* New York: Longman, 2001.

Woodruff, Helen. "The Illustrated Manuscripts of Prudentius." *Art Studies* 7 (1929): 33–79.

Wormald, Patrick, and Janet Nelson, eds. *Lay Intellectuals in the Carolingian World.* Cambridge: Cambridge University Press, 2007.

Wright, Jessica. "The Brain as Treasury and as Aqueduct: Metaphors of the Brain in Theodoret of Cyrrhus." *Studies in Late Antiquity* 2, no. 4 (2018): 542–66.

Yearl, Mary K. K. "Bloodletting as Recreation in the Monasteries of Medieval Europe." In Glaze and Nance, *Between Text*, 217–43.

———. "The Time of Bloodletting." Ph.D. Diss., Yale University, 2005.

Zettler, Alfons. "Exkurs I: Zu den Klosterärzten." In *Die Reichenauer Mönchsgemeinschaft und ihr Totengedenken im frühen Mittelalter*, ed. R. Rappman and A. Zettler, 265–78. Sigmaringen: Thorbecke, 1998.

———. "Spaces for Servants and *provendarii* in Early Medieval Monasteries: The Example of the Virtual Monastery on the Plan of St. Gall." *Bulletin du centre d'études médiévales d'Auxerre* 8 (2015): 1–16.

Ziegler, Joseph. "Philosophers and Physicians on the Scientific Validity of Latin Physiognomy, 1200–1500." *Early Science and Medicine* 12 (2007): 285–312.

Zurli, Loriano. "L'epistola a Pentadio (e altre reliquie) di Vindiciano." In Santini, *Prefazioni*, 453–62.

# INDEX

Page numbers in *italics* indicate illustrations. Written works will be found under the name of the author, unless they are anonymous. Manuscripts are listed by city and institution.

# ACKNOWLEDGMENTS

Finishing a first book is (I have heard) never easy. Finishing a first book after having a baby in the midst of a pandemic has made me that much more grateful to all those whose encouragement and assistance have not simply eased the way but crucially underpinned the completion of this project.

The origins of the book reflect a momentous decision to register for a history course on the Carolingians at the University of British Columbia taught by Courtney Booker; he has been an unstinting mentor for nearly twenty years now. To him, Arlene Sindelar, and Joy Dixon I owe deep thanks for nurturing my interest in medieval studies and the history of the body, and to Anne Gorsuch, for enriching my path with her friendship.

This work has benefited immeasurably from the wisdom and guidance of teachers at Princeton, most especially from Helmut Reimitz, whose enthusiasm for intellectual discovery and expertise in conjuring the perfect historical anecdote made the Ph.D. process delightful as well as demanding. Katja Guenther first introduced me to the history of medicine—with great effect—and her thoughtful feedback has done much to structure the current book. It is impossible to encapsulate the breadth of knowledge I have learned from William Chester Jordan, but his honest criticism and finesse for language have consistently sharpened my approach. Others assisted with this project in significant ways: John Haldon, Brooke Holmes, Elaine Pagels, Sally Poor, Jennifer Rampling, Margot Canaday, and Brent Shaw. A seminar with Peter Brown was a highlight of my graduate education, and his generosity in reading my work has been a continual source of inspiration.

At Binghamton University, colleagues in the History Department and Center for Medieval and Renaissance Studies have welcomed me with open hearts and countless favors, none more so than Elizabeth Casteen, whose support and advice have been invaluable. Likewise, Wendy Wall has shared wisdom and warmth as I found my feet as an assistant professor. The greatest challenge of the past few years has been how to maintain an academic position while forging a life with my husband in the same city—that this has just become possible is due to the persistence of innumerable colleagues at Binghamton, especially Heather DeHaan, Marilynn Desmond, Jerry Kutcher, Kent Schull, and Don Nieman.

There are two scholars whose own work initially inspired this research and whose graciousness in providing assistance has been continually uplifting—Faith Wallis and Lynda Coon, the latter of whom also served as a reader for Penn Press. She and James Palmer, the other reader, were the most generous reviewers an author could hope for: their detailed suggestions have improved many aspects of this book. Finally, I give heartfelt thanks to Nate Andrade and Carine van Rhijn, who were both kind enough to read the entire manuscript and offer exceptionally helpful comments.

For conversations that helped shape this project along its winding path, I am grateful to Eliza Glaze, Jinty Nelson, Kate Cooper, Monica Green, David Barnes, Maya Maskarinec, Anna Dorofeeva, Rutger Kramer, Gerda Heydemann, Max Diesenberger, Bonnie Effros, Arsenio Ferraces Rodríguez, Jeff Doolittle, Irene van Renswoude, and Naama Cohen-Hanegbi. John Kuhn, Claire Burridge, Dana Polanichka, Jennifer Davis, Owen Phelan, Delia Wendel, Jacob Doherty, James Bergman, Adam Foley, and Cloudy Fischer have all read pieces in revision and pushed my thought in new directions. Beatrice Kitzinger and Lawrence Nees have kindly shared their knowledge of Carolingian art with me. John Magee was exceptionally generous with his time and expertise in dissecting an obscure Latin text. For the opportunity to participate in invigorating panels, much appreciation goes to Zubin Mistry, Anna Bonnell-Freidin, Aileen Das, Francesco Borri, Deborah Deliyannis, Theresa Holler, and the First Millennium Network in Washington, D.C.

Little could have been accomplished without the help of archivists at the Bibliothèque nationale in Paris, the British Library in London, the Burgerbibliothek in Bern, the University Library in Glasgow, the Badische Landesbibliothek in Karlsruhe, the Bibliothèque royale in Brussels, and the Stiftsbibliothek in St. Gall; special thanks are also due to the late Don Faustino Avagliano at Montecassino, and to Karl Heidecker, Bernhard Zeller, and Philipp Lenz for their assistance with manuscripts from St. Gall. Finally, I am indebted to Kimberly Giambattisto for overseeing the book's production, to Erik Goosmann for crafting maps with wonderful precision, to Kate Mertes for indexing with efficiency, and especially to Jerry Singerman for guiding this project through Penn Press with the greatest patience and geniality.

For a Mellon fellowship that enabled me to write much of this book, I would like to thank the Wolf Humanities Center and the Religious Studies Department at the University of Pennsylvania. Likewise, the Institute for Advanced Studies in the Humanities and a Dean's Research Leave at Binghamton offered crucial time away from teaching, while a book subvention from Harpur College provided funds for images. Research for the dissertation was supported by the Social Sciences and Humanities Research Council of Canada, the Princeton Institute for International and Regional Studies, Princeton's Center for the Study of Religion, and the Institut für Mittelalterforschung in Vienna.

As much as I find the Carolingians endlessly entertaining, it is most certainly friendships in the present that have sustained me in laughter and tears over the last decade. An incredible group of fellow medievalists profoundly shaped my life at Princeton: Rebecca Johnson, Heidi Hausse, Frederic Clark, Jan van Doren, Ian Ward, and Glenn McDorman; Merle Eisenberg, Lee Mordechai, and Molly Lester have continued to animate my work with enlightening discussions. Though not medievalists, Iwa Nawrocki, Margarita Fajardo, and Iain Watts have been dear companions at every stage. And Valerie Garver, Marie Kelleher, Miriam Shadis, Sarah Davis-Secord, and Susan McDonough have smoothed the daily difficulties of writing with exceptional kindness. Finally, to friends who span many cities but have kept me from ever feeling rootless: Yi Wang, Sean Dunwoody, Heather Welland, Frank Chang, Andrew Beaty, Ayşe Baltacıoğlu-Brammer, Ada Kuskowski, Melissa Teixeira, Oscar Aguirre-Mandujano, Arnab Dey, Florian Kuhn, Hilary Geise, Briony Taylor, Kirby Smith, and Ashley Johnson Bavery.

My family is the soul that has carried the body of this book forward (though they may weep at this terrible pun). Lejas and Ainsworths have all lent support, most especially my late grandfather Janek Leja, who pressed me to enjoy a life surrounded by books, and my aunt Andrea Ainsworth, who enlivens dreary days with her wit. Karen and Michael Chase-Levenson have welcomed me into their lives with abiding enthusiasm and sage advice. My parents, Mark and Allison, have unwaveringly bolstered me at every difficulty and continually cultivated a passion for thinking; they are my most devoted readers, and this book is dedicated to them. To my sister, Rebecca, I owe my love for stories, told and retold.

My husband, Alex Chase-Levenson, may keep a millennium of distance from the ninth century, but he has shaped the ideas and perspectives here in a fundamental way. We share a keen love for the study of history, but it is a present and future together that brings the most joy. Although she has caused commotion by consuming (literally) the papers and monographs around me, our daughter Cecily has brightened every break and impelled me to finally finish this book before she grows any older!